Ethical Issues in Pharmacy

Bruce D. Weinstein, Ph.D., Editor
Center for Health Ethics and Law
West Virginia University

Applied Therapeutics, Inc.
Vancouver, Washington

OTHER PUBLICATIONS BY APPLIED THERAPEUTICS, INC.

Applied Therapeutics: The Clinical Use of Drugs, 6th edition
edited by Lloyd Yee Young, Mary Anne Koda-Kimble, Wayne A. Kradjan, and B. Joseph Guglielmo
ISBN 0-915486-23-7

Handbook of Applied Therapeutics, 6th edition
by Lloyd Yee Young, Mary Anne Koda-Kimble, Wayne A. Kradjan, and B. Joseph Guglielmo
ISBN 0-915486-24-5

Applied Pharmacokinetics: Principles of Therapeutic Drug Monitoring, 3rd edition
edited by William E. Evans, Jerome J. Schentag, and William J. Jusko
ISBN 0-915486-15-6

Basic Clinical Pharmacokinetics, 3rd edition
by Michael E. Winter
ISBN 0-915486-22-9

Basic Clinical Pharmacokinetics Handbook
by John R. White, Jr. and Mark W. Garrison
ISBN 0-915486-21-0

A Short Course in Clinical Pharmacokinetics
by Dennis A. Noe
ISBN 0-915486-19-9

Clinical Clerkship Manual
edited by Larry E. Boh
ISBN 0-915486-17-2

Physical Assessment: A Guide For Evaluating Drug Therapy
by R. Leon Longe and Jon C. Calvert
ISBN 0-915486-20-2

Extemporaneous Ophthalmic Preparations
edited by Lois A. Reynolds and Richard G. Closson
ISBN 0-915486-18-0

Drug Interactions & Updates Quarterly
by Philip D. Hansten and John R. Horn
ISSN 0271-8707

Applied Therapeutics, Inc.
P.O. Box 5077
Vancouver, WA 98668-5077
Phone: (360) 253-7123
FAX: (360) 253-8475

Copyright ©1996 by Applied Therapeutics, Inc.
Manufactured in the United States of America

All rights reserved. No part of this book may be reproduced, stored in a retrieval system, or transmitted, in any form or by any means, electronic, mechanical, photocopying, recording, digital, or otherwise now known or by any future method without prior written permission from the publisher.

Library of Congress Card Catalog #95-083225
ISBN 0-915486-25-3

First Printing January 1996

*To David B. Brushwood and Kenneth Mullan with
much appreciation for their support and friendship*

PREFACE

Is a pharmacist's obligation to maintain patient confidentiality absolute? What should a pharmacist do if she or he disagrees with a physician about which medication is best for a patient? Does a pharmacist ever have a right to refuse to fill a prescription? Pharmacists are increasingly facing these kinds of questions, but until now they have not had a resource that comprehensively and systematically addresses them. This book is intended to be such a resource.

Resolving moral problems in pharmacy requires an understanding of both clinical pharmacy as well as philosophical ethics. Each chapter was therefore written and reviewed collaboratively by persons with expertise in one or the other, or both. The topics included are consistent with those identified as the most important by the Ethics Course Content Committee of the American Association of Colleges of Pharmacy,[1] which was charged in 1992 with developing a model ethics curriculum and a list of resources. The book addresses other topics as well, such as the role that the media plays in influencing decisions by pharmacists and physicians. The appendix includes the 1994 revision of the American Pharmaceutical Association's Code of Ethics for Pharmacists and a list of resources in pharmacy ethics.

The book is divided into two sections. The first one, Foundational Issues, maps the terrain of pharmacy ethics. Included here is an examination of whether pharmacy is primarily a business or a profession (Chapter 1), the principles of pharmacy ethics (Chapter 2), the relationship between ethics and the law (Chapter 3), the process of ethical decision making (Chapter 4), and the counterside conversation (Chapter 5). The second

---

[1] Haddad AM et al. Curricular guidelines for pharmacy education: ethics course content committee council of faculties. Am J Pharm Educ. 1993;57:34S–43S.

section, Topical Issues, explores the following subjects: relationships with patients and physicians (Chapter 6) and with the pharmaceutical industry (Chapter 7), the right to medication (Chapter 8), the right to refuse to fill a prescription (Chapter 9), responsibilities toward incompetent or chemically dependent colleagues (Chapter 10), the social context of pharmacy (Chapter 11), the media's role in health care (Chapter 12), and drug research with human subjects (Chapter 13). Ethical issues raised by pharmaceutical care are addressed throughout the text, and in greater depth in forthcoming literature.[2,3]

This text is intended for students and practitioners alike. Students will learn about issues they will soon face in practice, if they have not already done so, and licensed pharmacists will have the opportunity to examine some of the most important matters they confront. Although reflection does not guarantee ethical behavior, the conscientious reader who grapples with the material presented here will be taking an important step toward becoming a better provider of pharmaceutical care.

Pharmacy ethics is a maturing specialty, and continuing interaction among practitioners, ethicists, and students will strengthen the field. Readers are cordially invited to send the editor comments about this book, as well as reports of cases they have encountered that raise challenging ethical issues.

> Bruce D. Weinstein
> Center for Health Ethics and Law
> 1354 HSN, P.O. Box 9022
> Robert C. Byrd Health Sciences Center
> West Virginia University
> Morgantown, WV 26506-9022

---

[2]Weinstein BD et al. Ethical issues in pharmaceutical care. In: Penna R, Knowlton C, eds. Pharmaceutical Care. New York: Chapman and Hall, forthcoming.

[3]Haddad AM, ed. Ethical Issues in Pharmaceutical Care. Haworth Press, forthcoming.

ACKNOWLEDGEMENTS

The author of a handbook for academic authors writes, "Compiling and editing a collection of scholarly articles can be one of the most hair-raising experiences of a lifetime."[4] Fortunately that has not been the case here. I am grateful to each of the contributors to this volume, whose dedication to maintaining the highest standards of scholarship and meeting deadlines I very much appreciate. I wish to express particular gratitude to Dr. Amy Haddad, whose pioneering efforts in the field have made this book possible.

The following individuals also kindly donated their time and energy (in alphabetical order): Marie A. Abate, Pharm.D.; David B. Brushwood, B.S.Pharm., J.D.; Mary Castiglia, Pharm.D.; Arthur L. Jacknowitz, Pharm.D.; Cynthia F. Jamison; Alvin H. Moss, M.D.; Jeanine K. Mount, Ph.D., R.Ph.; Charles F. Ponte, Pharm.D.; Ron Williams; and Susan Winkler. I am especially grateful to George H. Mundorff for his tireless efforts on this book's behalf.

Finally, it has been a distinct pleasure to work with Applied Therapeutics on this project. The publisher and staff provided the kind of support and enthusiasm that an editor wishes for but rarely finds in the publishing industry. My sincerest appreciation goes to Linda McCarley, Nannette Naught, and the publisher Linda L. Young for all that they've done to make this book possible.

---

[4]Luey B. *Handbook for Academic Authors.* Revised ed. Cambridge, England: Cambridge University Press; 1990:96.

CONTENTS

Preface iv

Acknowledgments vii

Contributors x

1. Is Pharmacy a Profession? 1
   William E. Fassett and Andrew C. Wicks

2. The Normative Principles of Pharmacy Ethics 29
   Courtney S. Campbell and George H. Constantine

3. The Relationship Between Ethics and the Law 67
   Kenneth Mullan and James M. Brown

4. Ethical Decision Making 79
   Bruce D. Weinstein

   Applying the Process of Ethical Decision Making 91
   Robert A. Buerki and Louis D. Vottero

5. The Counterside Conversation: Application as Narrative
   in Pharmacy Ethics 97
   Dawson S. Schultz and David S. Ornes

6. Relationships with Patients and Physicians 111
   Stuart G. Finder and David M. DiPersio

7. Relationships with the Pharmaceutical Industry 137
   Carol Bayley and Jeanine K. Mount

8. Is There a Right to Medication? 157
   Robert L. McCarthy and James D. Richardson

9. Do Pharmacists Have a Right to Refuse to Fill Prescriptions
   for Abortifacient Drugs? 175
   Kenneth Mullan and Bruce D. Weinstein

10. Professional Responsibilities Toward Incompetent or
    Chemically Dependent Colleagues 193
    Lisa S. Parker and Michael L. Manolakis

11. Power and Professional Responsibility: The Social
    Context of Pharmacy 221
    Andrew Jameton and Amy M. Haddad

12. Medicating by Media 249
    Pamela L. Redden and Mary Ellen Waithe

13. Drug Research with Human Subjects 281
    Eric D. Kodish and Bruce D. White

Appendices

1. Code of Ethics For Pharmacists 307

2. Resources in Pharmacy Ethics 311

CONTRIBUTORS

Carol Bayley, Ph.D.
Ethics and Justice Education
Catholic Healthcare West
San Francisco, California

James M. Brown, M.A.
Department of Philosophy and Politics
University of Ulster, Coleraine
Northern Ireland

Robert A. Buerki, Ph.D., R.Ph.
Division of Pharmacy Practice and Administration
College of Pharmacy
The Ohio State University
Columbus, Ohio

Courtney S. Campbell, Ph.D.
Department of Philosophy
Program for Ethics, Science, and the Environment
Oregon State University
Corvallis, Oregon

George H. Constantine, Pharm.D.
College of Pharmacy
Oregon State University
Corvallis, Oregon

David M. DiPersio, Pharm.D.
University of Tennessee College of Pharmacy and
Vanderbilt University Hospital
Nashville, Tennessee

William E. Fassett, Ph.D., R.Ph.
Department of Pharmacy Practice
School of Pharmacy
Drake University
Des Moines, Iowa

Stuart G. Finder, Ph.D.
Vanderbilt University Medical Center
Nashville, Tennessee

Amy M. Haddad, Ph.D.
School of Pharmacy and Allied Health Professions
Creighton University
Omaha, Nebraska

Andrew Jameton, Ph.D.
Section on Humanities and Law
Department of Preventive and Societal Medicine
University of Nebraska Medical Center
Omaha, Nebraska

Eric D. Kodish, M.D.
Department of Pediatric Hematology/Oncology
Rainbow Babies and Childrens Hospital
Cleveland, Ohio

Michael L. Manolakis, Pharm.D.
Health Information Designs, Inc.
Fairfax, Virginia

Robert L. McCarthy, Ph.D., R.Ph.
Department of Pharmacy Health Care Systems
Massachusetts College of Pharmacy and Allied Health Sciences
Boston, Massachusetts

Jeanine K. Mount, Ph.D., R.Ph.
Division of Pharmacy Practice
Social and Behavioral Pharmacy Program
University of Wisconsin
Madison, Wisconsin

Kenneth Mullan, M.A.
Department of Public Administration and Legal Studies
University of Ulster
Newtonabbey, Northern Ireland

David S. Ornes, M.B.A., R.Ph.
Department of Pharmacy Practice
College of Pharmacy
University of Colorado Health Sciences Center
Denver, Colorado

Lisa S. Parker, Ph.D.
Department of Human Genetics
University of Pittsburgh, Pennsylvania

Pamela L. Redden, M.D.
Murphy and Redden, M.D.s
Cleveland, Ohio

James D. Richardson, Ph.D.
Division of Arts and Sciences
Massachusetts College of Pharmacy and Allied Health Sciences
Boston, Massachusetts

Dawson S. Schultz, Ph.D.
Department of Philosophy
Colorado State University
Fort Collins, Colorado

Louis D. Vottero, M.S., R.Ph.
College of Pharmacy
Ohio Northern University
Ada, Ohio

Mary Ellen Waithe, Ph.D.
Department of Philosophy
Bioethics Certificate Program
Cleveland State University
Cleveland, Ohio

Bruce D. Weinstein, Ph.D.
Center for Health Ethics and Law
West Virginia University
Morgantown, West Virginia

Bruce D. White, R.Ph., D.O., J.D.
Clinical Ethics Center
St. Thomas Hospital
Nashville, Tennessee

Andrew C. Wicks, Ph.D.
Department of Management and Organization
Graduate School of Business Administration
University of Washington
Seattle, Washington

Ethical Issues in Pharmacy

Chapter 1

Is Pharmacy a Profession?

William E. Fassett
Andrew C. Wicks

When you become a pharmacist, you are expected to behave differently toward people seeking pharmaceutical services than when you were a pharmacy student. Some of these obligations are legal or contractual, but others are ethical or moral in nature. What is it about being a pharmacist that creates these obligations? How does one become adept at fulfilling them? This chapter sets the stage for later discussions of pharmacy ethics by considering whether obligations of pharmacists are best understood by thinking of pharmacy as a profession, akin to medicine and law, or by viewing pharmacy as a business that primarily distributes drug products to customers.

It begins by recognizing that to be a pharmacist sets one apart from other people, and explains how the concept of role is used to explore the special duties owed to others by people in particular occupations. The chapter then considers whether pharmacists have a role similar to other professionals, or more like business persons. The nature of professions is examined, and evidence is presented that supports the inclusion of pharmacy among those occupations regarded as professions.

Next, we consider arguments for and against the proposition that professional ethics and business ethics are quite distinct. If they are distinct, then pharmacists face a quandary: how can they operate pharmacy businesses and still fulfill their professional obligations? Ultimately, the chapter concludes that strong distinctions between professional and business ethics are less realistic today than they once were, and that the long tradition of pharmacists combining both a business and a professional role orientation demonstrates the two perspectives are compatible. It is possible that pharmacists are, therefore, better prepared for the realities of practice after health care reform than other health professionals.

Finally, the chapter examines how knowledge of what is right and a desire to do the right thing are combined to produce a pharmacist who actually does the right thing most of the time. It concludes that the development of professional virtue is the process that enables the pharmacist to become the type of practitioner who fulfills professional ideals in practice. After suggesting particular virtues that are desirable for the practice of pharmacy, it recommends some specific ways in which you can apply the lessons of this textbook to become and remain ethical in today's complex practice environment.

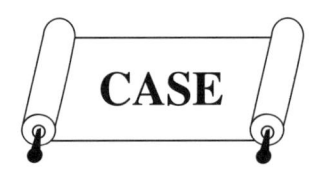

CASE

Anstar Pharmaceuticals recently has introduced Anstrol-DR, a delayed-release dosage form. Although it contains the same ingredient as Miratrol-DT (the originator's product), it is not considered a generic equivalent because the release characteristics of the two products are not equivalent. However, Anstrol-DR is a therapeutic equivalent for the originator's product. Its major advantage is that its average wholesale price is about 10% lower and its introductory price is approximately 30% lower than Miratrol-DT. Anstar recognizes that pharmacists might be instrumental in converting existing Miratrol-DT patients to Anstrol-DR, but that it will require more effort to substitute the latter because it is not generically equivalent. Therefore, Anstar is offering pharmacists a "cognitive service" fee of $25 during the next six months for each patient converted to Anstrol-DR. To receive this payment, the pharmacist must submit a voucher to Anstar indicating the date of service, the prescriber, the prescription number, and the quantity of Anstrol-DR dispensed.

J.T., president of Bay City Pharmacy, is enthusiastic about this opportunity. The typical patient taking one Miratrol-DT tablet daily pays $65 for 30 tablets, and J.T.'s cost for these tablets is $48. He can purchase 30 Anstrol-DR for $34, and he can sell these to patients for $59. He also can get the $25 fee from Anstar for each of the 40 or so patients currently on

Miratrol (for up to $1000 additional income). J.T. makes a better profit for his effort and the patients save money. It seems like a good thing to do.

As a business owner, J.T. needs to do those things that allow his business to be profitable and to grow. Opportunities such as the one presented by Anstar's promotion of its new product appear to help accomplish these goals. Yet, as a pharmacist, J.T. realizes he must temper his judgment regarding business opportunities by considering the effect of his actions on his patients' welfare and interests. This opportunity appears to be good for business; is it also right for his patients?

Duties, Expectations, and Professional Roles

When J.T. considers this question, he is asking a moral or ethical question: "What is the right thing to do?" J.T. may recognize that, from a moral point of view, some of the options open to him are better than others. In reflecting on J.T.'s situation, we will be concerned with those options that concern the webs of relationships among people, especially those in which persons can be characterized according to the roles they play within the relationship. For example, women and men who assume the professional roles of pharmacist, priest, teacher, or lawyer are involved with others who assume the client role, and societies have expectations about how professionals and clients should behave.

Each role functions within a constellation of relations, known as its role-set. For example, a pharmacist's web of relationships includes patients, employers, fellow pharmacists, other health practitioners, and past and present teachers. The obligations to each of these others and their duties to him or her differ, but are consistent across many pharmacists.

Finally, each person simultaneously performs in multiple roles. Every pharmacist also may be husband or wife, father or mother, and each is son or daughter, student or teacher, and citizen. Many pharmacists are also attorneys, and airplane pilots, and soldiers, and parishioners. Most are also investors in corporations and many are small business owners.

Sociologists suggest that we share notions of correct action within these common relations because of our expectations about the roles we assume.[1] In this chapter, we discuss how the expectations for right actions of pharmacists might differ if we assume that the pharmacist's role is that of a business person as compared to that of a health professional.

The Nature of Professions

Most Americans participate in society as private economic agents, selling skills and labor in return for the goods and services they desire: we work for a living. Certain understood responsibilities and rights are associated with various economic roles such as wage earner, employer, entrepreneur, client, and consumer. Occupations have been classified further in a variety of ways, such as agricultural, "blue collar," skilled trades, technical and managerial, entrepreneurial, mercantile, and professional.

Expectations vary somewhat for persons acting in different occupational roles, but they differ most markedly for those occupations known as professions. Professionals are expected to exercise special skill and care, to place the interests of their clients above their own immediate interests, and they often provide services in spite of the client's inability to pay. On the other hand, merchants, tradespeople, and technicians are expected to exercise the "ordinary care" demanded from all competent adults, and may honorably refuse service to indigent customers.

Professionals obtain several benefits in return for these more demanding societal expectations. They have greater control over the organization and conduct of their work than other workers, and members of the professions predominate in agencies that regulate them. Managers of professionals are nearly always members of the profession as well. The training and nurturing of professions occurs primarily within universities by faculties largely drawn from professional ranks. Finally, the social position and financial security of employed professionals in the United States is substantially better than employees in most other occupations, and professionals in solo, entrepreneurial practices consistently inhabit the highest economic echelons of American society.

One of many models that explain this reciprocity between professional perquisites and societal demands is the "functionalist" model outlined by Kultgen: professionals are privileged by society because they master essential tasks we cannot fully discharge for ourselves.[2] Therefore, they "function" in society in a special way that sets them apart from lay persons. In return, professionals are expected to provide their skills and knowledge to society and to individuals irrespective of the client's social status, and relatively unmindful of the professional's immediate interests. Because the terms of this "implied contract" are widely understood by those who enter the professions, they are bound thereby.

Medieval professions (medicine, the clergy, law), demanded entering practitioners to publicly affirm their willingness to adhere to the moral standards of the profession by the swearing of an oath or a "profession."

The most famous physician's oath was modeled after one attributed to Hippocrates. Members of clerical orders frequently swore vows of "poverty, chastity, stability, and obedience."[3] This public proclamation of adherence to particular values of conduct separated professionals from other occupational groups by virtue of what has been called an "atypical moral commitment."[4] Thus, professions are best understood as "moral communities" which share certain values and commitments.[4]

Entry to modern practice is marked less often by public oath-taking than in the past, but the delineation of professional claims is made in other ways. Major professional associations have codes of ethics, and have promoted mandatory state licensure as a requirement for professional practice. Licensing and examining boards in turn often include explicit or implicit moral requirements in regulations. Also important is the vast body of common law that allows clients to sue for damages when professionals fail to exercise the skill and care expected of them.

If pharmacy, too, is a profession, the pharmacist will be seen to have made commitments by which he or she can be judged morally praiseworthy or morally wrong. Thus, it may matter very much whether a pharmacist is a member of a profession, or whether his or her commitments are of the more ordinary type expected of citizens generally. An examination of the characteristics of professions will help us make this determination.

The Attributes of Professions

One method to decide whether a particular occupational group is, in fact, a profession relies on the "attribute theory of professions," formulated by writers such as Parsons[5] and Greenwood.[6] One identifies important functional or structural[a] characteristics of professions and then examines occupational groups to see if they possess these attributes.

Greenwood, for example, began by examining the list of occupations included in the U.S. Census Bureau's "professional" category:

> ... accountant, architect, artist, attorney, clergyman, college professor, dentist, engineer, journalist, judge, librarian, natural scientist, optometrist, pharmacist, physician, social scientist, social worker, surgeon, and teacher [citation omitted]. What common attributes do these professional occupations possess which distinguish them from the nonprofessional ones? After a careful canvas of the sociological literature on occupations, this writer has been able to distill five elements, upon which there appears to be consensus among the students of the subject, as constituting the distinguishing attributes of a profession.[7]

---

[a] *Functional refers to those activities that are unique to a given profession, whereas structural refers to the way in which a profession is organized.*

He extracted five attributes: 1) a systematic body of theory; 2) professional authority; 3) sanction of the community; 4) a code of ethics; and 5) a professional culture. Examining each attribute as it relates to pharmacy helps illustrate what it is about pharmacy that helps define it as a profession.

Systematic Body of Theory

Professionals exercise skill in the performance of their work that seldom is possessed by their clients. However, other nonprofessional occupations (e.g., hair styling, air conditioning repair, computer programming) also require superior skill. The skills of the professional, however, "flow from and are supported by a fund of knowledge that has been organized into an internally consistent system, called a *body of theory*."[7] Thus, a professional must learn the body of theory, as well as master basic skills needed to apply that theory. For this reason, as much as any other, the university is the essential training ground for professionals.

Professionals once jealously guarded their theory and kept knowledge of it away from the public; the Hippocratic Oath-taker promised never to reveal the secrets of the profession to the laity.[8] In the 20th century, however, professions have relied extensively on systematic scientific research to expand the knowledge base applied to their daily work. As professional knowledge has become more systematic and less arcane, it has become more public. Some economic entities outside the professions, therefore, are prominent users of professional knowledge. For example, the compounding and manufacturing of drug products, once the exclusive province of pharmacy, has become the economic and technical forte of the pharmaceutical industry, and for several decades pharmacy has struggled to find a new basis for professional standing.

In response to industry usurpation of its original reason for being, pharmacy has identified two new bodies of theory. The Millis Commission recognized pharmacy as a "system concerning itself with knowledge about drugs and their effects upon men and animals."[9] This emphasized understanding a theory of drug action, interaction and reaction, heavily dependent on the interaction of drugs with the biological system, by which pharmacists would be able to predict and prevent drug misadventures and assure desired therapeutic results. More recently, the concept of *pharmaceutical care*, defined as the "responsible provision of drug therapy by a pharmacist for the purpose of achieving specific outcomes that improve a patient's quality of life,"[10] has encompassed additional theory arising from the social, behavioral, and administrative sciences to inform the practice decisions of pharmacists. Pharmacists now acknowledge an independent responsibility to individual patients to exercise the unique perspective of pharmacy on their behalf to achieve results of treatment that are "good" for the patient and desired by the patient. The theory underlying this commitment focuses on drugs, how they work, how they interact, and on the interaction of patients and their body systems with drugs. Pharmacy will be seen as more fully an independent profession to the extent that pharmacists understand this body of theory more perfectly, and can apply it more effectively, than other professions.

Professional Authority

The authority of the professional arises (according to attribute models) when the client acknowledges the superior competence of the professional. As a result, the client surrenders a portion of his or her autonomy to the professional, and trusts the professional's judgment about which course of action will meet the client's needs. Not only is the client ill-prepared to judge independently what is best for him or her to do, he or she has difficulty judging the quality of service provided by the professional.

However, the professional's authority is limited to his sphere of expertise. Outside the professional domain, the professional is akin to all other citizens, and has no particular competence to prescribe what her client should choose to do. This is a key concept in emerging theories regarding patient autonomy. For example, the pharmacist can better predict than the patient the effectiveness of alternative therapies for palliating the pain of terminal cancer; she cannot, however, determine for the patient the wisdom of seeking treatment in the first place.

Community Sanction

The policy making power of a professional community often reinforces the profession's control over its organization and practice and greatly enhances its authority. Important community sanctions include restrictions on use of a professional title, license requirements for the practice of the profession, accreditation of professional training centers, and granting of professional privileges such as the duty (or right) to respect client confidentiality.

Pharmacy enjoys all these forms of community support. No person may advertise traditional pharmacy services to the public unless they are both professionally trained in an accredited school of pharmacy and have been licensed by the state. These sanctions have, for example, prohibited the use of the word "Drugs" on signs above the nonprescription medication section of grocery stores. In addition, the regulation of the profession normally is vested in a state Board of Pharmacy, all or the majority of the members of which must be pharmacists. Virtually all states protect prescription records from public scrutiny without the patient's permission, except in accordance with appropriate law enforcement.

Code of Ethics

Pharmacy and the paradigm professions of law and medicine have adopted formal codes of ethics within national professional organizations. Although professions no longer are dominated by monolithic national organizations, professionals at one time could not practice unless they held membership in these associations. For example, membership in the American Medical Association (AMA) was once a prerequisite to physicians being allowed to admit patients to hospitals.[11] Violation of the code of ethics brought not only the opprobrium of one's colleagues, but could result in expulsion from the professional association and exclusion from hospital-based practice.

Whether codes of ethics are useful or even desirable is now subject to debate among ethicists.[12] Their inclusion as an attribute of a profession is perhaps the weakest part of attribute theory. Not only do some professions lack an enforceable code of ethics, it is not clear that a nonprofession can become a profession by adopting a code. However, the American Pharmaceutical Association (APhA) has a long tradition of adopting and periodically revising its code of ethics,[13] and writers on pharmacy ethics have benefited from observing the changes in the code over time, and from relying on the current code as a point of departure for ethical discussion.

Even without a formal code of ethics, there is generally an informal understanding within a profession of appropriate behavior, and professional forces act to compel adherence to this informal code. For example, no part of the 1994 APhA code expressly forbids pharmacists from exchanging professional services for sexual favors; yet one scarcely can imagine that such an action, at any point in pharmacy's history, would not have been repugnant to the professional conscience and considered destructive to pharmacy's image.

Professional Culture

The inculcation and enforcement of informal professional standards is but one function of the professional culture, which Greenwood set forth as his fifth professional attribute. Three essential elements of professional culture are its *values, norms,* and *symbols.*[14]

Professional values must include a belief in the importance and merit to society of the profession's unique professional expertise. The profession must understand that it offers a service that cannot be better provided by another occupation. This service also must be essential, in that society would suffer if the service was withdrawn. A corollary to these two beliefs is the assumption that society is improved when the profession maintains a monopoly on the provision of this service.

Pharmacy has experienced a period of shaken confidence in its professional status. The old monopoly on compounding was usurped by industry and, seen particularly from the perspective of independent community pharmacists, the resulting monopoly on distribution of pharmaceuticals has been under constant attack. Pharmacists have responded to encroachments such as mail-order distribution by emphasizing the professional role in encouraging compliance and preventing therapeutic misadventures. Other pharmacists have sought to provide new services anchored in therapeutic knowledge. Many pharmacists believe the profession must espouse a new role centered in pharmaceutical care and less reliant on drug distribution to secure the profession's future. Current research concerning reimbursement for pharmacists' cognitive services may be as useful for convincing pharmacists of the value of these services as for convincing society.

Values are the central beliefs of a profession; its norms are accepted ways of social behavior within the professional culture. Pharmacists differ from other professions, such as medicine and law, in that professional specialization has been slow to develop, and until recently the profession has been relatively undifferentiated. Observers now can recognize distinct subgroups within pharmacy in which individual pharmacists gain status in subtly different ways.

Most professions use symbols to identify their calling. These include insignias (an ongoing debate within pharmacy over the adoption of a single symbol finds the mortar and pestle, the bowl of Hygeia, and the "Rx" as principal contenders), vocabulary, and dress. A recent egalitarian etiquette has reduced health professionals' former adherence to standards of professional dress, but vestiges of the "white coat" tradition persist in settings that feel the need to reinforce a "professional image." One example of health professions' efforts to preserve the symbolic value of professional dress is AMA and APhA success in obtaining agreement by advertisers not to costume drug product spokespersons (i.e., actors or actresses) in white coats for television or magazine ads.

The Importance of Client Trust

Recent writers have emphasized professional authority as somewhat more important than the four other attributes listed above. Professional authority originates when clients place trust in the professional to make decisions about matters the clients are not competent to handle. In return for this trust, the professional implicitly promises the client that he will act in the client's best interests. This type of relationship is said to be fiduciary in nature.

Professional power in this relationship is made possible by some fundamental human need which the professional has become particularly adept at meeting. Such fundamental needs include the need to restore health when one is ill, the need to learn new things, and the need for access to justice. The professions of medicine, teaching, and law, respectively, have developed to meet these needs. Were there no such professionals as teachers, society would have to invent them, and if the need to learn suddenly disappeared, teachers would become unnecessary. Thus, each profession exists to meet a fundamental need, and even though our reasons for becoming professionals might spring from personal desires for recognition or fortune, that does not change the underlying nature of our professions.[15]

Seen in this light, pharmacy is a distinct profession when it facilitates the use of drugs—a behavior whose long history suggests it must be a uniquely human activity[16]—rationally and effectively. This notion is compatible with the concept of pharmaceutical care, and suggests that the scope of the profession ranges beyond merely carrying out the orders of physicians.

Emmet argued that "social action depends on there being mutual reciprocal expectations as to how people are likely to act, and on these expectations not being too often disappointed."[17] Pharmacy's high level of generalized public esteem may have developed because pharmacists are particularly consistent in refraining from disappointing their clients' expectations.

What reasonable expectations might patients hold for their pharmacists? Certainly accuracy in drug distribution is the essential foundation for patient trust. Barker's studies of drug distribution in hospitals confirm that the reputation of the pharmacy department is based first on timeliness and dependability in drug distribution, and then on clinical prowess.[18]

Second, patients must be confident in the advice and counsel rendered by pharmacists. DeSimone and his colleagues examined the types of information and advice requested of pharmacists by patients, and discovered in community pharmacies that the most common request was for the pharmacist to recommend a specific nonprescription therapy for a patient's condition. However, the majority of all requests for advice and information concerned prescription drugs, including what the drug was intended to do, whether it should be refilled, and what the correct dosage should be. A very common request was for "triage": asking the pharmacist to recommend a course of action and to estimate how urgent it would be for the patient to seek a physician's care. They concluded that pharmacists

> ... must be skilled in certain types of diagnoses. Such diagnostic skills would allow the pharmacist, when appropriate, to advise the patient that: 1) no drug therapy is needed; 2) a specific nonprescription product can be used to treat the problem; 3) the patient should see a physician; or 4) any combination of the above.[19]

Patients seeking pharmacists' counsel must place two types of trust in the pharmacist: trust in affirmative statements made by pharmacists, and trust that the pharmacist will not withhold information important to them. Of the first type, the patient expects that the pharmacist knows what he or she is talking about, and also that recommendations made take cognizance first and foremost of the patient's interest, not the self-interest of the pharmacist.

J.T. legitimately might ponder whether his recommendation of Anstrol-DR over similar drugs meets the requirements of the trust placed in him by his patients, and whether making such recommendations in return for drug company "cognitive service" payments would in any way diminish his patients' future trust. For example, he might worry that if patients learned of the $25 fee it would lead them to suspect his motives and would diminish their reliance on his advice. Also, J.T.'s consideration of the Anstar offer was predicated on keeping the introductory savings and not passing them on to his patients (otherwise, he will just have to raise the price in the future when the introductory price expires). It seems that J.T.'s acceptance of this offer involves some deception on his part. Finally, does J.T.'s acceptance of this fee make him more likely to accept similar offers in the future? If so, can his patients ever rightly trust that his recommendations are motivated primarily by their best interests?

On the other hand, J.T. may argue that patients do not have such high expectations of pharmacists, but rather that pharmacists are just business persons. Patients can shop around to get the best prices, and if he offers them a savings on Anstrol-DR compared to Miratrol-DT, they are free to check with their physician regarding its suitability for their condition and can compare his offered price with that of other pharmacies. Therefore, he has no obligation to disclose either the fee from Anstar or the introductory discounts he obtains from the manufacturer.

Professional versus Business Ethics

This reasoning suggests that whether a pharmacist is primarily a professional or a business person matters because the expectations patients hold are different for the former in some critical way. Put differently, it matters because patients dealing with a pharmacist on a professional level likely would be disappointed if the pharmacist's presumption regarding their relationship is that it is purely business. We, therefore, turn to the suppositions concerning commerce that are thought to be held by business clients, and see how they compare to those discussed above for professionals.

We will offer general descriptions of both business and a profession that suggest inherent differences, but these comparisons can be exaggerated. Indeed, there are many reasons for us to soften many distinctions made between businesses and professions, particularly as they pertain to health care. We first will present arguments favoring the proposition that the ethics of professions are quite different from those of business, then we will consider arguments that business and professional ethics are more similar in many ways than previously thought.

The Argument For a Business and a Profession as Sharply Differentiated

Writers emphasizing differences between business and professional ethics argue that the purpose of entering a profession differs from that of opening a business: the professional person defines success in practice in terms of how well clients' needs are served; the business person is considered successful when a large profit is made.[20] Status in business often is reflected in one's personal income or net worth, but status in the profession is recognized more frequently by awards, offices in professional societies, and certifications of special competence.[21]

Accordingly, the professions and commerce are concerned with proper allocation of societal resources in two different domains: the professions provide their expertise and services under circumstances where the client is in an unequal position either to judge quality or to bargain concerning price, whereas commercial interests deal in goods and services where we believe the consumer has significant power through the price mechanism and open competition among providers.

Consider the consumer of two different products often available in community pharmacies: film and prescription drugs. The customer-as-photographer can judge the worth of different types of film for his or her photographic needs, and also may comparison shop among various dealers in photographic supplies. Thus, film is readily available in self-service retail outlets, stores compete on price for most common types of film, and often advertise heavily. If the customer selects slide film when he or she wants prints, few film dealers will refund the purchase price. *Caveat emptor* ("let the buyer beware") characterizes the relationship between film dealer and customer.

On the other hand, the customer-as-patient (particularly for drugs to treat acute illness) is hard pressed to shop on the basis of price and almost never can select the product themselves. Furthermore, advertising of prescription products is much more restricted than is film, and much less commonly done. The pharmacist and/or prescriber selects the product and source of supply, and is liable for errors in product selection.

Many commentators have suggested such a fundamental distinction between the health professions and business, as exemplified by physician-editor Arnold Relman:

> ... [M]edical care ... is in many ways uniquely unsuited to private enterprise. ... [I]t cannot meet its responsibilities to society if it is dominated by business interests.[22]

Relman saw business in the image of a used car salesman (greedy, purely self-serving, untrustworthy) while the health professional is envisioned as a benevolent public servant (altruistic, putting others before the self, trustworthy). There are several reasons to reject these polar opposites.

Rejecting the Distinction Between Health Professions and Business

First, clear incentives in the present system of fee-for-service remuneration of health professionals encourage excessive treatment for patients. This seems more benevolent than alternative arrangements where professional and patient interests are at odds, but it does cause problems.

Overtreatment is expensive, inherently risky, and where there are limited resources to provide health care, overtreatment of some individuals denies needed care to others.

Second, the stance of professional associations such as the AMA on such issues as HMOs, Medicare and Medicaid, and health care reform has led some observers to question the fundamental altruism of health care professionals. Similarly, segments of organized pharmacy often oppose or favor changes in health care on the basis of the impact of the proposed changes on the financial health of the pharmacy profession.

Finally, the relatively high salaries of health professionals, the growth of medical specialties, the decline in indigent care, and the geographic maldistribution of health professionals toward affluent areas provide further evidence that health professionals act in their own interests much of the time.[23] In short, the structure of professional responsibilities tends to place patient and professional interests in the same general direction, such that activity may appear benevolent when in fact, on closer inspection, it is self-serving, often dangerous, and sometimes abusive. The noble ideals of the professions may mask the considerable room left for personal gain and may not, as such, prevent patient abuse.

The Superior Knowledge of Professionals and Client Vulnerability

The bargaining power of the consumer relative to the "seller" often is thought to be different in business relationships than in professional-client encounters. In health care, it is argued, consumers need a professional to serve as their advocate because it is extremely difficult for them to obtain sufficient information to make informed choices and to bargain effectively. "Bargaining power" seems an almost absurd concept: whether or not to undergo emergency surgery for a bleeding ulcer has far different consequences than the decision to buy a BMW.

This notion can be taken too far. First, not all health care decisions are made in extreme circumstances and patients have many more sources of health information than in the past. Second, as business technology advances and consumer products become more complex, customers are also increasingly dependent on the individuals and firms that make and sell them. Purchasing a VCR, a computer, or a car also is a daunting task for most consumers. Each of these activities has taken on a level of complexity which makes it very difficult for the average consumer to be "informed." Other business-related choices such as insurance coverage, home financing, investment opportunities, and planning for college expenses all put important personal projects at risk. The easy distinction between professionals and business persons on the basis of relative levels of consumer knowledge is less appropriate than it once was, largely because the obligations of business persons are becoming more like those of professionals.

This discussion raises an additional issue concerning our view of health professions. The idea of the uninformed and vulnerable patient tends to reinforce a paternalistic model wherein health care professionals are the primary decision makers while patients passively assent, and the "good patient" is one who complies with his or her prescribed therapy. We should challenge this characterization for several reasons, particularly for the implications it has for the economic health of the health care system. Suspicious of the ability of centralized health planning to reduce waste in our current system, many critics urgently advocate the creation of better educated, more selective, fiscally aware patients (i.e., they need to become "better customers"). If patients remain uninformed and vulnerable, then health professionals bear the burden of examining alternatives, weighing costs, and making choices. Clearly, fiscal limits will become a more explicit part of the health care encounter, if not as detailed restrictions on the physician-patient experience, then as a set of external limitations on the forms it can take. Even assuming this change, patients must become more assertive, more informed, more like customers in the business sense if the crisis in health care is to be resolved.

Changing Images of Business

Not all businesses operate in the model of the used car salesman.[b] Legal rights, government regulations, and other enforceable protections for a wide array of stakeholder groups[c]—including customers, employees, local communities, and the general public—forbid management to focus strictly on profit and the interests of stockholders. These modern intervenients in the operation of businesses have made *caveat emptor* an untenable management perspective.

---

[b] Indeed, there are several "business"-related groups that also constitute professions. One such group is accountancy. Accountants have adopted a set of professional standards, known as "Generally Accepted Accounting Principles (GAAP)," that govern their activities, and they stand in important fiduciary relationships to their clients.

[c] Stakeholders are individuals or groups who can affect or who are affected by the operation of the firm. Primary stakeholders, those who are directly involved in the firm's operations, include employees, suppliers, stockholders, customers, and the local community. Secondary stakeholders, who are affected indirectly by the business, may include government, the public, the media, and others. For further discussion of the stakeholder concept and the idea of stakeholder management (i.e., managing a firm for all primary stakeholders), see Freeman RE. Strategic Management: A Stakeholder Approach. Englewood Cliffs: Prentice-Hall; 1984. Also see Freeman RE, Gilbert DR. Corporate Strategy and the Search for Ethics. Englewood Cliffs: Prentice-Hall; 1988.

Many firms now prosper by adopting a proactive and principled approach to management. Companies like Johnson & Johnson, Merck, Corning, and Xerox base their business strategy on a wide mandate; they exhibit explicit concern for stakeholder groups, as well as stockholders, in formulating managerial policy. Johnson & Johnson's successful handling of the Tylenol product tampering crisis, and Merck's decision to develop a drug for treatment of river blindness, and then to give it to patients at no charge, provide two examples drawn from the pharmaceutical industry. Both firms went to extraordinary lengths and risked millions to act in the interest of stakeholders other than corporate owners. These actions alter the traditional understanding of "business" and take moral values like trust, respect for others, and fairness to develop a formula for doing business that does not put profits at odds with enriching the entire community. These firms recognize that, as do professionals, they require the trust and respect of customers, suppliers, employees, and the general public if they are to enjoy long-term success.[d]

Of course, although this value-driven approach has taken root and become more influential in our society, it is not yet dominant. Many firms still see profit maximization as their central goal. However, even these firms have had to show respect for various stakeholder groups in order to survive in the emerging business environment. These changes indicate that any sort of strict dichotomy between health care professions and business is misleading. General distinctions between the two still exist, but three themes are cogent: 1) these differences are not between an approach that is "moral" (a profession) and one that is "amoral" (a business); 2) differences that are present are of degree more than kind; and 3) numerous variations of for-profit businesses make any "model" of business extremely limited in application. This reasoning suggests as well that, just as businesses no longer can hide behind a profit motive to escape responsibility to stakeholder groups, neither may a health practitioner avoid duties to patients by disingenuously claiming that his or her practice is a business and not a profession.

---

[d] See the writings of management guru Tom Peters, including *In Search of Excellence. New York: Warner Books; 1984*, and *A Passion for Excellence. New York: Warner Books; 1985*, for a flavor of this kind of approach to management and a range of examples that demonstrate his ideas. One particularly notable passage maintains, "[s]ome colleagues who have heard us expound on the importance of values and distinctive cultures have said in effect, 'That's swell, but isn't it a luxury? Doesn't the business have to make money first?' The answer is that, of course, a business has to be fiscally sound. And the excellent companies are among the most fiscally sound of all. But their value set integrates the notions of economic health, serving customers, and making meanings down the line. As one executive said to us, 'profit is like health. You need it, and the more the better. But it's not why you exist.'" [Peters T, Waterman RH Jr. In Search of Excellence: Lessons from America's Best Run Companies. New York: Warner Books; 1984:103.] Similar expressions are found in the works of Freeman and Gilbert.

Is Pharmacy a Profession? 17

J.T. must recognize that Bay City Pharmacy will flourish as its community prospers and as its customers are able to trust it in all of their dealings. As a practical consideration, if the substitution of Anstrol-DR for Miratrol-DT is, in fact, in his patients' interest, disclosing information to them about the Anstar promotion would be an excellent demonstration of his commitment to a value-driven business philosophy. As patients and customers learn that he will be open about items he easily could conceal, this is a powerful way to build their trust and admiration. Armed with knowledge that both they and Bay City Pharmacy could benefit from the offer, and also understanding more fully its application to their own situation, potential Anstrol-DR users are likely to agree with the substitution of Anstrol-DR for Miratrol-DT, and J.T. can obtain the additional income as well as patient loyalty and respect.

Professions and Businesses: Serving the Public Interest

Neither the professional model nor the business model alone best serves both patients and the general community. The problem of paternalism and pressure to provide greater access to cost-efficient health care creates a need to infuse health care practice with forms of thinking commonly associated with a business orientation. While this is a very different proposition than suggesting that health professionals come to see themselves as business people, it does indicate that the two perspectives can combine in a complementary way. In addition, examples from value-driven companies suggest clear affinities between these successful business philosophies and the ideals of the professions.

Imagine structuring the interaction between a health professional and patient in a business context. Concerns about profit and efficiency will become highly significant, to both parties. However, the professional also will understand the importance of maintaining trust and high standards of care, not just because it is rooted in the profession's traditions, but because it is good business. In our current social context, where patients and the public generally expect much from the health care system, health care businesses likely will opt to retain most, if not all, of the ethical constraints and moral charges that have resulted from the professional tradition. These standards will be seen as making for satisfied customers who will maintain long-term relationships, and as helping to avoid lawsuits, while at the same time providing for a reasonable income. While other plausible scenarios allow that approaching health care as a business could erode these traditions, increase health care consumption, and facilitate the trend toward high-technology specialization, there are legitimate constraints on these potential abuses within a business framework.[e]

Such a thought experiment may well have already occurred in the development of modern entrepreneurial pharmacy practice. Chappell and Barnes examined the professional and business role orientations among practicing pharmacists in Canada. Pharmacists were evaluated on their orientation toward professional and business roles, and could be counted in one of four groups: high professional, high business; high professional, low business; low professional, high business; or low professional, low business. More pharmacists expressed the importance of the professional role than the business role, but the largest number of pharmacists practicing in community retail settings scored high on both professional and business role orientations. The authors concluded that although a high business orientation might be detrimental to provision of patient care, such an effect was not observed.[24] The high public esteem for pharmacists reported in the Gallup polls, even given the highly entrepreneurial setting in which the majority of patient-pharmacist encounters occur, suggests that for pharmacy, such a fusion of professional ideals with business practices has occurred, and is successful in providing highly regarded patient care.

Sorting Out Similarities and Differences

Amid our attempts to soften many of the traditional assumptions about business and the professions, it is nonetheless apparent that there are certain basic differences. The two occupational domains are distinct, although the difficulties of defining one specific account of "business" makes distinguishing these domains an arduous task. If we work from functionalist theory, business seems to have many of the characteristics associated with professions. Business generally fails to meet the first two conditions (systematic body of theory, professional authority), but possesses aspects of the next three (sanction of the community, a code of ethics, and a professional culture). Of particular importance are the moral dimensions of business. Business need not concern itself solely with profit. There is room for other moral considerations and priorities serving a broad range of interests within the context of for-profit operations. Indeed,

---

[e] *This could include the continuance of fiduciary duties to the patient and high standards of care where failure to provide them would lead to legal sanctions and loss of privilege; continuance of Hippocratic and other professional traditions and ethical standards imposed by health care providers; other forms of legal and ethical directives mandated by the public which then would shape how the business enterprise operated. Such limitations would not undermine our ability to call what resulted a "business"—indeed, given the legal and regulatory restrictions facing most businesses today, and the ethical directives adopted by many of the firms we have discussed, the differences are only of degree.*

though most businesses are not fully value-driven firms, most American businesses have codes of ethics and many others have mission statements, stakeholder representatives on Boards of Directors, policy committees, review boards, and a variety of other mechanisms that make ethics a part of modern U.S. business.

Our moral expectations for health professionals generally are greater than those for people in business (and our wariness is correspondingly greater in business relationships), but this is seen best as a difference of degree rather than kind. If health professionals generally are obliged to put their patients' interests first, this rarely is seen as incompatible with making a good living. And while businesses must make profits over the long run to survive, this is not incompatible with including important moral values in decision making. These insights project the possibility of constructively combining professional ideals and business principles to provide value-driven yet cost-effective health care. The long tradition in pharmacy of combining business and professional roles may have prepared pharmacists well for a special place in a reformed health care system that attempts to balance therapeutic possibilities with economic realities.

Professional Virtues

The above approach to defining professions and professionals is grounded in the relationship between professional and client, or between business person and customer. It is an analysis, essentially, of dyads. Such an analysis may miss important considerations. It fails to place the profession or the corporation in a larger social context. It further ignores competing obligations among multiple clients, to non-clients, and to causes.[25] Dyadic analysis also may lead us to think of ourselves as split into roles, the "wearers of many hats," and we may allow ourselves to act in one role in a way we would regard as reprehensible when we occupy a different role.[26] The chilling cinema image of the mob boss casually ordering the murder of a competitor while indulgently bouncing his baby daughter on his knee captures what is troubling about such a result.

Our analysis also ignores issues of professional character and virtue. William May underscored the importance of these by noting that

> a person's character and virtue often determines which "cases" he [or she] chooses to notice, the level on which he [or she] tackles them, the personal presence he [or she] brings to them, and the resources which enable him [or her] to survive a given crisis and function another day.[27]

We understand May's use of terms as follows: *character* refers to the person's basic nature, and includes traits such as honesty, aggressiveness, reticence, introspection, and thoroughness; *virtue* describes a person's moral excellence, and his or her tendency to behave in accordance with moral values. A virtuous person is one who wants to have virtue, who wants to act in morally acceptable ways.

Professional virtue has an additional meaning. Not only must the professional possess the tendency to act in morally acceptable ways, but also the propensity to behave in ways which further professional competency, or to be able to carry out professional work.[28] These additional "professional virtues" may differ somewhat across professions. For example, all professionals must exhibit industriousness and intelligence, but success as a clinical pharmacist may not require the "combative traits of cunning"[29] needed to excel as a trial lawyer. With these notions in mind, we may examine the professional virtues of pharmacists, and how the profession selects or produces individuals with these traits.

Desirable Characteristics of Pharmacy Practitioners

Gorovitz has outlined characteristics of the "good physician":

- has and maintains a high level of technical competence, including both the knowledge and the skills appropriate to his [or her] specialty;
- is unfailingly thorough and meticulous in his [or her] approach to his [or her] specialty;
- is aware of the dependence of clinical medicine on medical research and equally aware of the experimental nature of clinical medicine;
- sees patients as persons with life stories, not merely as bodies with ailments;
- sees beyond simplistic slogans about health, nature, and life to the complexity involved in selecting goals for treatment;
- has a breadth of understanding that enables transcending the parochialism of his [or her] own specialty;
- understands his [or her] own values and motivation well enough to recognize that they can be in conflict with the patient's interests;

Is Pharmacy a Profession?

- is sensitive to the diversity of cultural, interpersonal, and moral considerations that can influence a patient's view of what is best, in process or outcome, in the context of medical care, and has the judgment to respect that diversity without undermining the integrity of his [or her] own moral commitments;

- has a respect for persons that shapes his [or her] interactions with patients, staff, and colleagues alike;

- has the humility to respect patient autonomy, the dedication to promote it through patient education, and the courage to override it when doing so seems justified;

- has the honesty to be truthful both with him- or herself and with his [or her] patients about his [or her] own fallibility and that of his [or her] art; and

- has the sensitivity to recognize moral conflict where it exists, the motivation to face it where it is recognized, the understanding to consider it with intelligent reflection where it is faced, and the judgment to decide wisely following such consideration.[30]

Technically competent, thorough and meticulous, sensitive, introspective, respectful of persons, humble, courageous, honest, intelligent, and judicious: "It is a tall order," Gorovitz admitted. "But many physicians meet it, and more approximate to it reasonably well."[30] Substitute "pharmacy," "pharmacist," and "pharmaceutical" for "medicine," "physician," and "medical" in Gorovitz's list and few who are knowledgeable about the practice of pharmacy would disagree that these traits are desirable for pharmacists as well as for physicians.

Other writers include professional virtues such as honesty, candor, competence, diligence, loyalty, discretion, tenacity, and self-discipline. These lists are as interesting for what they omit as for what they contain. Terms such as aggressive, decisive, passionate, innovative, venturesome, enterprising, and fierce infrequently comprise descriptions of professional persons. One writer noted, in addition, that "While altruism is not a necessary condition for expert work, we are able to trust the occasional selfish professional because he works within a social network of ethical persons."[31]

If professional practice requires certain characteristics, and if the professional culture encourages and rewards individuals who possess these virtues and discourages those who do not, then long-term job satisfaction will likely accrue to practitioners who either possess these innately or develop them over time. Students oriented by nature to professional service will be attracted to the professions and will not seek training in other fields. Entrants to the profession lacking most of these characteristics are likely to move on to other occupational pursuits. However, many potential practitioners possess professional virtues only latently, and develop these characteristics more fully as they are socialized into the profession during college and early practice. In the last section of this chapter, we consider how professionals turn a desire to become professional into the fact of being professional in their behavior.

Development of Professional Character

For most aspiring pharmacists, mere knowledge that certain virtues and positive characteristics are essential to a successful career in pharmacy leaves them well short of their goal: embodying those qualities in their daily activities. As Aristotle maintained, knowing the good and desiring to do the good are important components of virtue; but they are incomplete unless one can connect right thoughts with right actions.[32] Becoming virtuous involves modeling virtuous behavior in our own actions: having role models who we believe are virtuous that we can imitate, finding ways to "practice" virtuous activity, and cultivating habits which embody these positive qualities. To become good, one must do the good. This sounds simple, but Aristotle described it as a difficult and lengthy process which requires commitment and training not unlike that of a craftsperson learning a trade or an athlete preparing for competition. Indeed, it is a pursuit to which one must dedicate an entire lifetime. Thus, if what this textbook imparts can be described as "knowledge of the good" or a model of virtue for pharmacists, we are still a long way from putting that knowledge to use.

Virtue focuses on habituation because our character defines much of who and what we are. The character traits we possess shape how we act most of the time. Especially important is how we act in situations of moral complexity or when we lack time to reflect carefully on our options. Absent certain traits and virtues ingrained in our character and conduct, we may fail to act virtuously just when virtue is most necessary. To fully learn from this textbook demands a continual effort to reflect its wisdom in our daily professional conduct. The following suggestions are made directly to the reader in aid of this goal.

One important step along the path to a virtuous professional life is to find a mentor or role model whom you believe embodies the traits desirable in a pharmacist. (We who have practiced for years continue to seek mentors, even as we serve as mentors for others.) Endeavor to recognize your mentors' particular features that make you believe they are virtuous: how do they behave, what do they say, how do they think that embodies honesty, integrity, fortitude, or compassion more completely than others? Try to learn from them and model your behavior after their own. You should not, however, literally mimic all that they do. The apprentice imitates the craftsperson, but along the way introduces a distinctive flair. Similarly, your own modeling of the behavior of others should let your own character shape and influence how you express particular values. Also know that you will honor your mentor most by growing beyond his or her perspective, adding your own to the profession's recognition of its obligations and opportunities. Isaac Newton recognized this when he alluded to the principle that dwarfs standing on the shoulders of giants may see further than giants themselves.f

Professional norms and traditions established by pharmacists also may guide you. They provide important indicators of virtue and vice in a context that is more concrete and action oriented (e.g., do not accept kickbacks from drug companies) than the more general notion of virtue (e.g., you should have integrity). A careful study of the history, norms, and traditions of pharmacy is extremely useful for reflecting on how certain behaviors might or might not express virtue.

One great challenge to virtue lies in the dynamics of individual behavior within organizations. The Milgram studies on obedience to authority suggest a disturbing ability in people to distance themselves from their actions when commanded to do so by an authority figure. People may perform acts with only minimal discomfort which, in other contexts, they would see as highly unethical and abhorrent.g This distancing provides the

---

f "If I have seen further than you and Descartes, it is by standing upon the shoulders of Giants." Newton, Isaac [1642–1727]. Letter to Robert Hooke, February 5, 1676. Cited in Beck EM, ed. Bartlett's Familiar Quotations. 15th ed. Boston: Little, Brown & Co.; 1980:313.

g In Milgram's famous study, research subjects were told that they were part of a study on learning under conditions of stress. In fact, the study was an attempt to see to what lengths individuals would go when ordered by an authority figure. The experiment called for the subject to ask questions of the "learner," and whenever they got a question wrong, to administer an electric shock. With each incorrect answer, the shock level increased 15 volts. (The "learner" actually did not receive a shock, but the subject was led to believe that the shock was real.) The majority of subjects agreed to continue asking questions and giving shocks of levels exceeding 400 volts, even though the "learner" began to express increasing pain, complained of a heart condition and demanded to be let out of the experiment, and then ceased to respond at all by the time the 250-volt "shock" was given. Research subjects expressed concern for the learner and asked to stop, but when told by the scientist that the study was necessary and that the scientist would take full responsibility, the subjects returned to the protocol and continued to increase shock levels. The experiments are described in Milgram S. Obedience to Authority: an Experimental View. New York: Harper & Row; 1974. Interestingly, Milgram's work later was criticized by ethicists because of the deceit involved and because some of the student subjects suffered emotional trauma from their participation.

means through which much unethical and illegal activity is permitted within organizations. Practitioners of virtue must "own" their actions and the consequences which derive from them. As individuals assert their right to consider the morality of their actions as a basis for deciding whether to proceed, regardless of whether they are "ordered" to, organizational misconduct is less likely.

Virtuous organizations promote individual virtue. Cultivation of virtue is a difficult and delicate process made easier by organizational support and positive reinforcement. Several preconditions to ethical and virtuous organizations include: 1) clear codes or standards of conduct that embody worthy and relevant moral ideals; 2) overt managerial commitment to these values and to the importance of moral and professional standards more generally; 3) rewards, incentives, and discipline reinforcing these standards; and 4) support for open discussion of ethical problems, including protection for internal "whistle blowers."

A corollary is that corrupt organizations tend to corrupt their members. A pharmacist wishing to remain virtuous must prepare to depart when the organizational culture is inimical to professional virtue. Leaving an undesirable position is easiest for the pharmacist who has continued to perfect his or her technical and professional skills and is therefore desirable to some other firm. For this reason, assiduous study and continuing education are aids to achieving professional virtue.

Finally, you must value debate with colleagues about matters of the profession, its ideals and standards, and how one's activities may or may not constitute virtue. Aristotle thought friendship profound for those dedicated to the pursuit of virtue. Friends sharing one's values provide a kind of mirror to the self, to help appraise one's behavior, and to reinforce one's commitment to moral ideals.[33] Colleagues in your profession can serve in an analogous role: sharing the identity of "pharmacist," they allegedly are committed to mutual aims.

These suggestions only initiate the task of doing and embodying the good. To see it through and become a pharmacist who routinely lives up to professional ideals is more arduous, and demands practice, patience, commitment, and creativity. Ultimately, however, you will be rewarded with satisfaction in your chosen career and, we believe, in yourself.

Discussion Questions

Review the case at the beginning of the chapter, and consider the following questions.

1. As J.T. considers whether to begin promoting Anstrol-DR to his patients, what might be some important issues he should consider: a) what duties does he owe to patients and to others that might help him decide whether to do this (this is called the deontological approach); b) what are the possible good and bad effects of promoting Anstrol-DR to his patients (this is the utilitarian approach); and c) how would a decision to promote Anstrol-DR to his patients represent acting according to professional virtues (e.g., integrity, honesty, fairness), and which virtues would be promoted or diminished?

2. How would a professional approach this sort of decision? How might the business viewpoint lead to a different kind of analysis? Are there ways to bring both of these approaches together to offer a defensible resolution to the case?

3. Is it any more or less acceptable for a physician to receive the $25 fee from Anstar to convert patients to Anstrol-DR than it is for the pharmacist to receive the fee? If you conclude that there is a difference, how do you explain it in terms of the professional-client relationships involved?

4. Patients invest a certain amount of trust in pharmacists. Does accepting this kind of arrangement and increasing one's own "payoff" violate that trust? Is it a conflict of interest? Are there ways of maintaining trust and accepting these financial incentives?

5. If it is permissible for J.T. to accept the payment from Anstar in these particular circumstances, are there circumstances in which similar payments from other manufacturers would not be acceptable?

6. Would the widespread acceptance of this type of fee from manufacturers have any effect on the image or reputation of the profession in general?

7. What sorts of rules and directives ought to exist for the relationships between pharmacists and their "business" counterparts to preserve the integrity and virtue of the profession?

REFERENCES

1. Emmet D. Rules, Roles and Relations. New York: St Martin's Press; 1966.
2. Kultgen J. Ethics and Professionalism. Philadelphia: University of Pennsylvania Press; 1988:72–98.
3. Schurr GM. Toward a code of ethics for academics. Journal of Higher Education. 1982;53(3):318–34.
4. Camenisch P. Grounding Professional Ethics in a Pluralistic Society. New York: Haven; 1983:33.
5. Parsons T. The professions and social structure. Social Forces. 1939;17:457–67.
6. Greenwood E. Attributes of a profession. In: Baumrin B, Freedman B, eds. Moral Responsibility and the Professions. New York: Haven; 1983:20–32.
7. Greenwood E. Attributes of a profession. In: Baumrin B, Freedman B, eds. Moral Responsibility and the Professions. New York: Haven; 1983:21.
8. Veatch RM. Medical ethics: an introduction. In: Veatch RM, ed. Medical Ethics. Boston: Jones and Bartlett; 1989:8.
9. Anon. Pharmacists for the Future: The Report of the Study Commission on Pharmacy. Ann Arbor, MI: Health Administration Press; 1975:14.
10. Hepler CD, Strand LM. Opportunities and responsibilities in pharmaceutical care. Am J Hosp Pharm. 1990;47:533.
11. Starr P. The Social Transformation of American Medicine. New York: Basic Books; 1982:168.
12. Manolakis ML. Why APhA should reject its code of ethics. Am Pharm. 1991;NS31(11):46–8.
13. Buerki RA, ed. The Challenge of Ethical Professional Practice, Publication No. 8, New Series. Madison, WI: American Institute of the History of Pharmacy, 1985. (Note: The APhA Executive Board approved another revision of the Code of Ethics at the March 1994 annual meeting.)
14. Greenwood E. Attributes of a profession. In: Baumrin B, Freedman B, eds. Moral Responsibility and the Professions. New York: Haven; 1983:29.

15. Sokolowski R. The fiduciary relationship and the nature of professions. In: Pellegrino ED et al., eds. Ethics, Trust, and the Professions. Washington, DC: Georgetown University Press; 1991:35–6.
16. Brecher EM. Licit and Illicit Drugs. Boston: Little, Brown; 1972.
17. Emmet D. Rules, Roles and Relations. New York: St. Martin's Press; 1966:7.
18. Barker K et al. Consultant evaluation of a hospital medication system: analysis of the existing system. Am J Hosp Pharm. 1984;40:2009.
19. DeSimone EM et al. Pharmacist-patient interaction and patient expectations. Am J Pharm Educ. 1977;41:167–71.
20. Kultgen J. Ethics and Professionalism. Philadelphia: University of Pennsylvania Press; 1988:77.
21. Barber B. Some problems in the sociology of the professions. In: Lynn K, ed. The Professions in America. Boston: Houghton Mifflin; 1965:19.
22. Relman A. What market values are doing to medicine. Atlantic Monthly. 1992;March:106.
23. Brock D, Buchanan A. Ethical issues in for-profit health care. In: Bradford G, cd. For Profit Enterprise in Health Care. Washington, DC: National Academy Press; 1986:241–42.
24. Chappell NL, Barnes GE. Professional and business role orientations among practicing pharmacists. Soc Sci Med. 1984;18(2):103–10.
25. Gorovitz S. Professions, professors, and competing obligations. In: Pellegrino ED et al., eds. Ethics, Trust, and the Professions. Washington, DC: Georgetown University Press; 1991.
26. MacIntyre A. Why are the problems of business ethics insoluble? In: Baumrin B, Freedman B, eds. Moral Responsibility and the Professions. New York: Haven; 1983:357.
27. May WF. Notes on the ethics of doctors and lawyers. In: Baumrin B, Freedman B, eds. Moral Responsibility and the Professions. New York: Haven; 1983:94.
28. Callahan JC, ed. Ethical Issues in Professional Life. New York: Oxford University Press; 1988:388.
29. Eshete A. Does a lawyer's character matter? In: Callahan JC, ed. Ethical Issues in Professional Life. New York: Oxford University Press; 1988:394.

30. Gorovitz S. Good doctors. In: Callahan JC, ed. Ethical Issues in Professional Life. New York: Oxford University Press; 1988:425.
31. Kultgen J. Ethics and Professionalism. Philadelphia: University of Pennsylvania Press; 1988:95. Citing Michael Bayles. Professional Ethics. Belmont, CA: Wadsworth; 1981.
32. Aristotle. Nichomachean Ethics. Ostwald M, translator. New York: Macmillan; 1986:book 2.
33. Aristotle. Nichomachean Ethics. Ostwald M, translator. New York: Macmillan; 1986:books 8 and 9.

Chapter 2

The Normative Principles of Pharmacy Ethics

Courtney S. Campbell
George H. Constantine

Pharmacists have undertaken a professional commitment to the care and interests of patients. A tradition of ethics is thus integral to the self-understanding of pharmacy as a profession. This chapter identifies five normative principles in the ethical tradition of pharmacy—nonmaleficence, beneficence, respect for persons, loyalty, and distributive justice—and displays their relevance for pharmacy practice through illustrative clinical cases. Normative principles establish moral duties, obligations, and rights, and provide an evaluative standard for justification of moral choices.

Pharmacists may confront three forms of moral conflict in their practice. Moral weakness refers to a conflict between a person's ethical responsibility, as established by a normative principle, and self-interested inclinations. Apparent moral dilemmas arise when two or more normative principles appear to be in conflict and may be resolved through closer factual scrutiny of the situation or discernment of alternative courses of action. A genuine moral dilemma occurs when two principles conflict and signals that a moral agent will be unable to act fully on his or her responsibilities and duties.

A central task of pharmacy ethics is to probe the meaning of the normative principles through these different forms of moral conflict, examine the implications of the principles for professional identity and integrity, and discern priorities when principles conflict. Nonmaleficence, which requires avoiding harm, also provides a context for trust in the pharmacist-patient relationship. The ethical tradition of pharmacy historically has been expressed in an ethic of beneficence and patient-benefit. However, especially in cases of paternalism, a commitment to beneficence may conflict with patient autonomy and dignity, including a patient's right to respect for his or her informed and voluntary decisions. Loyalty and fidelity engage the conscientious pharmacist in an ongoing process of negotiation and a thoughtful deliberation about personal and professional roles. Justice demands of pharmacy professionals that they seek a fair allocation of benefits and burdens in pharmacy practice.

Depending on interpretations of the meaning and priority of these normative principles, a pharmacist may affirm a professional self-understanding of technician, parent, advocate, or partner. Such models also have ramifications for the conception of the "patient" in pharmacy practice.

The principles of pharmacy practice are most appropriately understood as presumptions or *prima facie* obligations rather than moral absolutes or moral maxims. This method permits flexibility to the particularities of a clinical situation without compromising the obligatory force of ethical principles. Deliberation and discernment among conflicting principles can enable better patient care and a pharmacy practice that embodies professional ideals.

THE NORMATIVE PRINCIPLES OF PHARMACY ETHICS
The Moral Reality of Pharmacy

The fundamental reality that pharmacy is a moral practice and profession can be difficult to discern. Pharmacy often has been characterized as a "product" rather than a "service" oriented profession, which suggests professional identity is bound up more with commodities than with persons. Two contemporary pharmacists have described the traditional "technical model" of pharmacy, for example, in which pharmacists function as "mechanical prescription processors, typing labels and counting pills. ... The pharmacist's primary activity is oriented more toward the product rather than the patient."[1]

Moreover, an individual pharmacist might find that many decisions central to the health of a patient are largely out of his hands. The pharmacist sometimes is perceived as an "extension" of the physician,[1] and his exercise of moral agency can be severely circumscribed not only by the directives of physicians, but also by the regulations of government and the marketing methods of the pharmaceutical industry. The ethical choices a pharmacist might make about patient care have, in short, often already been made by someone else, and the role of pharmacist may thereby seem largely restricted to the activities of "filling and following orders."

The technical model of pharmacy practice renders it an amoral profession and it is the basic premise of this chapter that this amoral model is mistaken. Pharmacists are much more than technicians of transfer for health-related products. They instead have undertaken a professional commitment to the care and interests of persons who present themselves as patients. A moral choice about providing benefits to fellow human beings is integral to the self-understanding of pharmacy. As articulated in the 1994 revision of the American Pharmaceutical Association's (APhA) Code of Ethics, "a pharmacist promises to help individuals achieve optimum benefit from their medications, to be committed to their welfare, and to maintain their trust."[2] The ethical tradition embedded in pharmacy has been formalized since the 1850s through various codes of ethics,[3] which express a collective "profession" of moral self-identity.

It also is not the case that pharmacists are mere passive puppets of physicians, regulators, or entrepreneurs. The discrete encounters and ongoing relationships between pharmacists and patients continually confront practitioners with perplexing moral choices that require the exercise of personal and professional autonomy. Consider the following case.

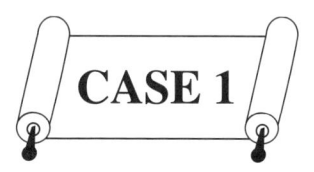

CASE 1

R.P. is a pharmacist in a small community pharmacy. In the morning paper, he reads that one of his regular customers, C.E., had a car accident the evening of her granddaughter's recent wedding. Concerned, R.P. checks C.E.'s medication profile and notes her regular use of the antihypertensive enalapril (Vasotec) for moderate hypertension, sporadic use of diflunisal (Dolobid) for mild intermittent arthritis, and significantly increased refills for the hypnotic flurazepam (Dalmane) over the past two years since the death of her husband. According to the records, all refills were approved by C.E.'s physician, but R.P. calculates her present level of consumption of Dalmane to be 60 mg per day. Two weeks following the accident, C.E. returns for an approved refill of her prescription. In the wake of her accident, R.P. believes a modification of C.E.'s medication patterns may be called for, and considers whether he should discuss this with her before refilling the prescription.

Case Discussion

If R.P. is a product technician, then C.E.'s situation presents little more than technical questions about altering dosages or medications. If, however, R.P.'s professional commitment to patient health and safety constitute his paramount responsibility, then he is confronted with several layers of ethical questions and choices. A first set centers on the best interests of his patient, C.E. The tranquilizing and depressant effects of Dalmane produce drowsiness, an effect that is intensified with alcohol use (which might have been consumed at the wedding). This may have been a contributing factor in the accident. R.P. has good reason to determine whether C.E. was given necessary information about the side effects of her medication, whether she paid adequate attention to these warnings, or whether she might be displaying a pattern of noncompliant behavior. In short, is C.E.'s current (and increasing) medication use serving her interests in health and safety?

Yet, R.P.'s commitment to his patient's health and safety also is embedded in intertwining professional relationships. The increased use of Dalmane has been approved and prescribed by her primary physician. Is there a medically indicated reason for this pattern or does it suggest an emerging problem of drug dependency? If so, the medication is working to C.E.'s harm rather than benefit. The request for another renewal could give R.P. an opportunity to inform the physician of C.E.'s increasing dependency on Dalmane, and to suggest that the current prescription practice appears to have placed her in some danger. Indeed, the information provided in the profile might indicate R.P. is in the best position of anyone to offer this assessment. Yet, this may be perceived as intrusive by the physician, who might feel his competence and care are being questioned. R.P. thereby is faced also with a moral issue of whether a pharmacist may have a moral responsibility to intervene in the physician-patient relationship.

R.P. also needs to engage in some self-scrutiny. His pharmacy practice, after all, followed the physician's prescribing patterns thus far; it need not take an automobile accident to suggest something might be amiss in C.E.'s increased use of an addictive medication. In that respect, R.P. has acted primarily as the dispensing arm of the physician in his dealings with C.E. Moreover, R.P.'s privileged access to the information in the medication history does not permit him to overstep boundaries of privacy and confidentiality; under the 1994 APhA Code of Ethics, "a pharmacist focuses on serving the patient in a private and confidential manner."[2] The patient has rights of control regarding the information contained in the profile and to whom this may be disclosed, a moral dimension downplayed by the codified language of "professional" records. A professional commitment to patient health and safety, which may have prompted an earlier review and intervention before the accident, here seems to conflict with a patient claim to respect for privacy, which can limit access to the records. C.E. can reasonably request an explanation for how her medication patterns have come under scrutiny in the first place.

R.P. has a set of issues to confront and choices to consider about patient welfare, collegial collaboration, and personal and professional integrity. He is on moral terrain because the decisions he makes (and those he does not) will affect other persons. He has several options available before him, including 1) assume that C.E.'s physician knows best and fill the renewal without questions; 2) use the trust established in his previous dealings with C.E. to discuss with her the necessity of the medication increases and provide counsel on appropriate use; 3) refuse to fill the prescription before a detailed conversation with the physician; and 4) arrange a consultation between C.E., the physician, and himself to discuss her medication practices.

Whatever course of action R.P. adopts, he will need to give reasons for his choices, not only to himself, but to his patient(s) and other professionals. This process of deliberating about alternative courses of action and then offering reasons for the course chosen is what philosophers refer to as *moral justification*. Moral justification affirms that as responsible persons, we are to be held accountable and answerable for our actions. The Preamble of the 1994 APhA Code of Ethics suggests several audiences of justification towards whom a pharmacist may be responsible and accountable, including "patients, health professionals, and society."[2]

A character in a film by Jean Renoir observes, "You see in this world there is one awful thing, and that is that everyone has his reasons."[4] Yet, not all reasons are equally valid and justifiable, and a central task of ethics in pharmacy practice is to offer normative principles that set out general guidelines of moral and immoral conduct and provide an evaluative standard for moral justification. Normative principles give us direction when we confront complex ethical decisions such as those encountered by R.P. and help us differentiate justifiable from unjustifiable reasons. This essay will identify and discuss the importance of five normative principles for pharmacy ethics—nonmaleficence, beneficence, respect for persons, loyalty, and distributive justice—and display their relevance in illustrative clinical cases. These principles establish duties and give action-guides regarding, respectively, refraining from harm, providing benefits, respecting rights and autonomy, giving others their due, and distributing benefits and burdens. In addition, the normative principles of pharmacy ethics validate important rules such as informed consent, fidelity (promise-keeping), veracity (truthfulness), confidentiality, and privacy. These principles and rules constitute an embedded common morality for social and professional conduct. Thus, they provide a common ground for ethical discussion and justification not only for pharmacists but also between other participants in the moral world of pharmacy, including colleagues, other health care professionals, and the persons who present themselves as patients.

Moral Perplexity and Ethical Justification

The process of moral justification can be conceived in terms of an ascending and descending relation of judgments regarding particular choices or actions, moral rules, and normative principles.[5]

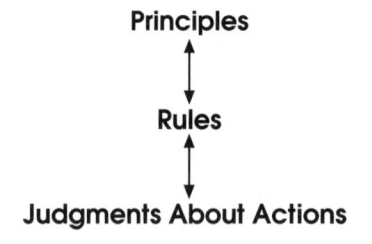

Principles
↑↓
Rules
↑↓
Judgments About Actions

For example, in a standard clinical encounter with a patient, a pharmacist might make a judgment to fill a prescription based upon a professional rule to promote patient health, which in turn is rooted in the principle of beneficence (patient benefit). The pharmacist might make a second judgment to inform the patient of the nature of the medication, its prescribed dosage, any side effects, etc., based upon a rule of informed consent to medical treatment, which in turn is derived from a principle of respect for persons. (A beneficence-based commitment to patient safety also would support such disclosures.) The process is dialectical and corrective, moving back and forth between particular judgments in specific situations and the general guidance offered by the principles and rules, with judgments and choices being modified or changed by different and competing principles in more complex circumstances. Let us illustrate this method of justification and moral decision making by reference to some cases.

The nature of ethical justification in pharmacy practice will reflect different kinds of moral situations. Not all moral problems are as complex as that experienced by R.P.; in many instances, as in the standard encounter portrayed above, a person's ethical responsibility is clearly evident, and his performance of it is justified by appeal to one (or more) normative principles. Alternatively, we may know what our responsibility is and fail to do it. As philosopher John Lemmon observes, the experience of moral weakness (acrasia) is a "dilemma," because we experience conflict between moral principle and personal desires, but it does not constitute a moral dilemma because "our moral situation (responsibility) is perfectly clear."[6] Imagine that you are eagerly anticipating an arranged discussion with your professor of a case in pharmacy ethics, but the professor fails to attend. It turns out that the professor found a day of blue sky and snow-covered mountains irresistible and headed for the local ski resort. We can correctly conclude the person failed to meet moral and professional responsibilities set by rules of fidelity or promise-keeping and principles of justice and respect for persons. In a conflict of moral weakness, a person may offer excuses or explanations for action that fails to meet a moral requirement, but such reasons (e.g., "It was such a nice day"; "You could read the book"; "I forgot") cannot be justified with reference to a moral principle. There is very little experience of perplexity about what one should do in a dilemma of moral weakness; the problem is doing what one knows to be right or good.

We face some situations in the moral life generally and in pharmacy practice in particular, however, where the experience of perplexity expresses a genuine moral dilemma because it is unclear what the right or good thing might be, all things considered. As two medical ethicists have written, "In a moral dilemma, an agent morally ought to do X and morally ought to do Y, but the agent is precluded by circumstances from doing both."[7] It may turn out, for example, that your professor did not meet with you for a quite different reason: While preparing for the discussion, her daughter took ill and required attention at the local clinic. The professor has a moral responsibility to meet with you because of her antecedent promise, but she also has a moral responsibility to obtain necessary care for her daughter. To be sure, there may be alternatives to avoid the dilemma, such as contacting you in advance to explain and reschedule the meeting, or seeking another family member to take her daughter to the clinic, but these options might be foreclosed (e.g., you can't be reached, no other family member is available, the daughter's need is immediate).

The language of "moral dilemma" signals that the person will be unable to act fully on her responsibilities because of a conflict of principles and duties. Our professor, for example, cannot both render necessary aid to her daughter and fulfill her promised teaching commitment. Thus, in a moral dilemma, moral considerations could be offered for alternative and seemingly incompatible courses of action, and careful deliberation is necessary to determine which principle or rule, that of familial beneficence or that of fidelity, should have moral priority. The nature of moral justification in a dilemma involves discerning which of the conflicting actions has greater moral weight or strength and offering persuasive reasons to various audiences of justification (e.g., conscience, a student, a child, and others) for the decision. Moreover, while some moral dilemmas are only apparent because acceptable reconciling alternatives can be explored, a genuine dilemma cannot be resolved solely by more extensive investigation of the facts, needs, and capabilities demanded by the situation. It requires a value choice that expresses the moral character of the person.

It is important in pharmacy ethics to determine whether a situation calling for moral choice is a result of weakness of will, an apparent dilemma that can be resolved through alternatives, or a genuine conflict between principles. The relationship between the kind of perplexity experienced and the process of ethical justification can be displayed concretely by recollecting the choices confronting pharmacist R.P. If his decision to review his patient's records was rooted in a desire to determine whether dosage or frequency level could be altered to increase his financial remuneration, we would not consider that a justifiable reason for the action. Patient privacy would be infringed, and the patient perhaps placed at greater risk, without any correlative concern for C.E.'s health and safety. An act of exploitation of a vulnerable person would exemplify unprofessional conduct and moral weakness for which no justification could be offered.

The moral perplexity displayed in the actual choices facing R.P. seem more suggestive of an apparent or genuine dilemma. His actions cannot be construed as exclusively self-interested; C.E. is a regular customer and the moral choice required by the record review and refill request stems not from concern for his bank balance but an interest in her present and ongoing welfare. His uncertainty about which course of action is morally justified can perhaps be alleviated by some "fact-finding" about C.E.'s knowledge level regarding proper prescription drug use and patterns of compliance, and the physician's awareness of her use and general health condition. Good ethical reasoning requires a sound factual basis and obtaining this information is necessary for R.P. to make a justifiable ethical decision. In this respect, R.P.'s dilemma may be only apparent because alternatives could exist to resolve the problem short of moral compromise.

Yet, even if he receives satisfactory answers to his inquiries, R.P.'s perplexity also might reflect the experience of a genuine moral dilemma. His commitment to patient health and safety, as expressed in the principle of beneficence, might require active intervention to modify her medication or arrange a consultation, but his interest in preserving professional loyalty and collegiality might stipulate a hands-off approach. The physician could acknowledge R.P.'s concerns but adamantly insist his prescribing pattern is in the best interests of patient C.E., her recent accident notwithstanding. In short, R.P. might find himself with conflicting interests and divided loyalties, such that any decision he makes will require justification to some others who may feel he has compromised their trust and breached his responsibilities.

Assume, for example, that R.P. chooses to initiate a conversation with C.E. about her medication in response to her presentation of the refill order, and on the basis of her response, seeks to arrange a caregiving consultation with C.E. If challenged by others, such as the physician, to defend or justify this approach, he might cite a rule that patients have rights to be informed about and consent to their medication program. R.P. might then have justified such a rule by appealing to a more general principle of respect for persons (self-determination). In this scenario, his justification could be structured as follows:

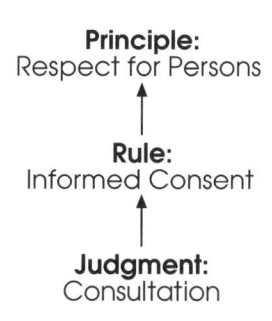

Principle:
Respect for Persons
↑
Rule:
Informed Consent
↑
Judgment:
Consultation

Others might seek to persuade R.P. that other rules or principles, such as respect for the integrity of relationships of other professionals with their patients, or loyalty to professional colleagues, are more compelling. The moral reasoning in this instance might begin at the level of the normative principles and "work down" to a specific choice.

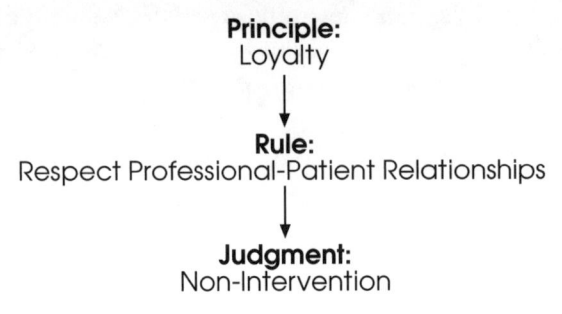

Principle:
Loyalty
↓
Rule:
Respect Professional-Patient Relationships
↓
Judgment:
Non-Intervention

R.P. could contend in response that a principle of beneficence (patient benefit) generates for pharmacists the primary consideration of promoting patient health and safety, including that they not be subjected to undue risk of harm from their medication. This in turn supports an obligation to engage in a consultation with the patient. The reasoning behind this conclusion might be structured as follows:

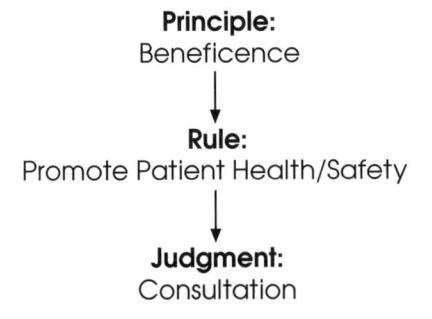

Principle:
Beneficence
↓
Rule:
Promote Patient Health/Safety
↓
Judgment:
Consultation

This discussion illustrates that clarification and resolution of moral problems in pharmacy ethics is influenced by the meaning of the normative principles, a determination of their priorities when they conflict, and professional moral identity. We want to probe these issues in greater depth through a series of cases organized around the basic principles.

The Principle of Nonmaleficence

A fundamental duty in patient care and in social life generally consists in the noninfliction of harm, injury, or death to other persons. This duty is expressed in the normative principle of nonmaleficence. This principle is implicit in the Hippocratic maxim of *primum non nocere*, "first of all, or at least, do no harm." We also acknowledge this moral duty in our legal and philosophical traditions that allow a broad scope to personal freedom but permit the imposition of moral and legal restrictions when individual actions pose risks of harm or injury to others. The principle of nonmaleficence is a bedrock of social life and it is difficult to conceive of a society or a profession functioning without a commitment to it. Indeed, philosophers who have imagined the human condition without a duty of nonharm have referred to it as a "state of nature."

A commitment to nonmaleficence by contrast provides a context for the expression of trust in human relationships, and this capacity for trust is especially significant in health care because of the vulnerability of patients. Patients give over to professional caregivers privileged access to their bodies and selves in the trusting expectation that they will not be harmed unnecessarily; that is, that any harm inflicted (e.g., drawing blood) is done only for the purpose of the interests and welfare of the patient. Trust is so vital to the encounters of caregivers and patients that we commonly perceive their relationships as embodying a "fiduciary" character. The cultivation of reliance and confidence is especially relevant to pharmacist-patient relationships; in marked contrast with the levels of trust expressed in other health care professions, pharmacists are "considered to possess high levels of integrity; they are afforded a social trust generally given to friends, neighbors, and relatives."[1]

While the principle of nonmaleficence is clearly essential to ethical research and testing for safe and effective drugs, it plays no less a significant role in the activities of the practicing pharmacist. To avoid harming patients, even if unintentionally, the pharmacist must be technically competent and knowledgeable about new product developments, the interactive qualities of various medications, and the characteristics of the particular patient, who may suffer an allergic reaction to a medication that will be entirely safe for most others. The principle of nonmaleficence thereby provides justification for specific professional duties delineated in the 1994 APhA Code of Ethics, including the duty "to maintain knowledge and abilities as new medications, devices, and technologies become available and as health information advances."[2] The principle of nonmaleficence, as well as respect for persons, also supports professional duties of honesty and integrity:

> A pharmacist has a duty to tell the truth and to act with conviction of conscience. A pharmacist avoids discriminatory practices, behavior or work conditions that impair professional judgment, and actions that compromise dedication to the best interests of patients.[2]

If pharmacists fail to observe these duties, patients may be harmed due to dated knowledge or technical skills and can rightly claim that their trust in the fiduciary relationship has been violated.

Of course, such a relationship entails that the expression of trust is mutual, and the pharmacist can be placed in a difficult situation if patients or their proxies seek to exploit the trust. Consider the following case.

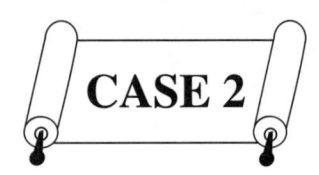

CASE 2

During a social gathering, V.R., a pharmacist at the local chain-store pharmacy, is approached by a neighbor he has not met before, who is introduced as A.G. After social pleasantries are exchanged, the conversation is directed toward the beneficial effects the hematopoietic agent epoetin (Epogen) may have for athletes. A.G. is particularly involved in the discussion because his son J.G. is a long-distance runner in high school. As the conversation winds down, A.G. turns to V.R. and informs her: "If my son qualifies for the state finals, he will undoubtedly receive a large scholarship for college. I would be very grateful if you could investigate epoetin for me so that J.G. can obtain some." V.R. is not comfortable with this request, but she informs A.G. that she will look into the properties and use of epoetin and get back to him about the situation.

Case Discussion

There are several avenues by which V.R. might obtain more extensive information about epoetin (e.g., a Drug Information Center, the manufacturer). In the course of her search, she most likely will discover that epoetin is banned for use by athletes by both the U.S. Olympic Committee and the National Collegiate Athletic Association as a form of blood doping.

Having engaged in this necessary "fact-finding," there would appear to be little in A.G.'s request to create moral perplexity for V.R. To agree to encourage the use of an agent for a nonapproved use would constitute a violation of nonmaleficence (and perhaps legality) for several reasons. First, no fiduciary relationship exists. Not only is A.G. a relative stranger, but the prospective "patient" isn't even present in the discussion to give his opinion or consent about the proposal. V.R. knows virtually nothing about J.G., other than that he excels at track and may have a promising career. Dispensing or encouraging the prescribing of epoetin for a person she doesn't even know, except through the idealized image of his father, would violate the trust and confidence society has invested in pharmacists to act in the best interests of patients.

Even if a therapeutic relationship previously had been created, however, V.R. has solid reasons based upon nonmaleficence for saying "no" to A.G.'s request. There are several medical indications for epoetin as a medication for anemia; enhanced athletic performance, by contrast, is quite clearly a nonmedical indication that falls outside the realm of V.R.'s professional interests and concern. It is not V.R.'s place to question the priorities A.G. apparently has assigned to J.G.'s athletic and academic potential, but it is even more misguided for A.G. to expect or V.R. to agree to use her professional expertise for engineering rather than therapeutic purposes. In short, the request is not only for a blood product but that V.R. compromise her moral integrity.

Perhaps A.G.'s interest in the college scholarship stems not principally from a desire that his son's athletic prowess receive public display, but rather that athletic excellence is the only way J.G. will be able to attend college, due to underlying financial hardship. V.R. may wish to do some fact-finding to determine the authentic reason for A.G.'s request, but economic deprivation is nonetheless not a medical indication. An issue of educational equality may be embedded in the need for a scholarship, but that is a question of social ethics and justice that is beyond V.R.'s capacity and expertise to resolve. The inequity may evoke her sympathy but not her therapy.

It also is possible that making arrangements for J.G. to obtain the agent could harm J.G. While it is unlikely J.G.'s use would be detected in high school meets, were he to obtain a prestigious scholarship on the basis of epoetin-enhanced performance, it would be offered under false and deceptive circumstances. His subsequent participation in a program where he would not have access to epoetin could mean diminished performance and recriminations about being "cheated" by athletic officials, who might well have offered the scholarship to another person. The end result could be that the scholarship offered to J.G. is withdrawn. The use of epoetin may pose risks of harm to J.G.'s identity and integrity. The principle of nonmaleficence and the prospects of harm to many persons from providing epoetin should give clear direction to V.R. in her response to A.G.

The Principle of Beneficence

Only a very minimalistic morality would claim that our moral responsibilities are exhausted by duties to refrain from harming or injuring others. Our common life requires affirmative efforts to benefit others by promoting their welfare, although disagreement often ensues about who is obligated to assist or provide the benefits. Few persons dispute, for example, that receiving health care is of substantial benefit; there is, however, controversy over whether a person's access to health care should be based upon need, personal responsibility, or ability to pay, as well as who should be obligated to provide access.

The principle of beneficence expresses this sense that morality requires more than just "staying out" of another's way but rather that on occasions we may be obligated to "step in" and aid others, or that we may already be in relationships, such as families, whose very viability requires mutual assistance. In most instances, duties of positive benefit are accepted as part of the various roles and relationships we assume, such as husband-wife, parent-child, teacher-student, pastor-parishioner, and health care professional-patient. Indeed, what makes the health care professions morally distinctive is the prominence of duties of positive benefit as part of the profession's self-identity. We have already seen, for example, how patient health and safety are deemed the "first consideration" of the ethical pharmacist, and fulfilling that duty requires both acts of nonmaleficence and the positive concern for patient benefit expressed by beneficence. It is arguable whether a society can survive without beneficence; our society, for example, has largely repudiated legally compelled beneficence expressed in so-called "Good Samaritan" laws, preferring to leave acts of charity and love to personal ideals and discretion. It is clear, however, that a health care profession cannot survive morally without beneficence: the act of "professing" is just that a person voluntarily assumes certain affirmative responsibilities towards a patient's or client's welfare.

Philosophers often have specified a three-fold content to beneficence, holding that it encompasses duties to 1) prevent harm, 2) remove harm, and 3) provide benefits.[8] The professional responsibilities of pharmacists can reflect each of these dimensions of beneficence. One rationale for disclosing the potential effects of a medication to a patient or in monitoring patient compliance is clearly to prevent harm to the patient. Pharmacists do not perform the kinds of invasive procedures that remove harm as a surgeon or dentist might, but as was suggested in our discussion of Case 1, a pharmacist might take steps to intervene in medication patterns to alleviate or minimize causes of harm. Finally, the intention and expectation of dispensing drugs and medications is that they will bring benefit to the patient by improving his health condition.

While beneficence is integral to the profession's sense of moral identity and integrity, its priority is a source of controversy in pharmacy ethics (and in health care ethics generally). Ethicist Robert Veatch, for example, has characterized the historical ethical orientation of pharmacy as a "tradition of faithful commitment to patient benefit." Veatch observes the ethic of beneficence recently has been subject to increasing criticism from an ethic of autonomy and patient rights.[9] The dispute is not over whether pharmacists should express commitment to patient health and safety, but rather who defines "health and safety": the pharmacist (or physician) or the patient. The patient's understanding of health or safety is set in relation to his or her particular way of life and set of values, and on that basis he or she might, for example, be willing to accept certain levels of risks or side effects that are different from the standard professional recommendation. Or, some patients with protracted terminal illness (e.g., cancer, AIDS) may be willing to trade safety for a chance at health by seeking to use nonvalidated drugs.

The conflict between the professional's and the patient's perspective over health and safety constitutes the moral conflict of paternalism. The paternalistic medical model depicts the relation of professional and patient in terms of parent and child. The parent/professional makes decisions and provides directive information, based upon his experience and specialized knowledge, to enhance the child/patient's best interests as perceived by the parent/professional. The beneficence-based rationale of paternalism is that the professional, like one's parents, "knows best." The child/patient thereby is excluded from the decision-making process because of lack of education and minimal understanding about the consequences of his choices. It becomes clear that because of significant disparities in power, information, and experience the potential for paternalistic practice is embedded in all interactions between health care professionals and patients. As an important participant in these relationships, pharmacists can find themselves involved in paternalistic conflicts regarding refusals of patient requests for a particular medication or disclosure and nondisclosure of information. Veatch, for example, describes a situation in which a pharmacist is asked by a physician to make a placebo compound in an effort to wean a patient off a dependency on sleeping medication.[10] The physician's approach reflects an attitude of "what you don't know won't hurt you" and the pharmacist is invited to participate in a conspiracy of beneficent paternalism to assist the patient without her knowledge or consent.

In other instances, a pharmacist may experience the conflict of paternalism directly, as illustrated in the following case.

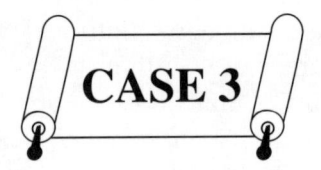

CASE 3

J.E. is a 50-year-old pharmacist working for a relief pharmacist agency that places him in a relatively isolated rural farming community with only one pharmacy. The owner-pharmacist, who is out of town for a convention, is heavily relied upon by his clientele since the nearest medical services require a round trip of over 100 miles. Just before closing on a weekend night, a young couple, apparently in their early teens, enters and wishes to talk with the owner-pharmacist. After J.E. convinces them that he can be of assistance, they ask for his advice about the most effective over-the-counter contraceptive.

Case Discussion

J.E. could render the requested "advice," but should he? He might simply refuse because of the age of the couple, his unfamiliarity with their situation and relationship, his own personal convictions about sexual relationships, or because the "most effective" method of preventing pregnancy is abstinence. Alternatively, he might consider that "it's their lives," and simply recommend "Product X" out of deference to their apparently mutual decision. Neither of these approaches, however, seems morally preferable, and J.E. should instead seek to balance his commitments to beneficence and respect for privacy.

The significant moral feature for J.E. should be the expression of trust in him by the couple. The couple most likely had anticipated being able to raise their query with their regular pharmacist, trust that has been transferred to him, a relative stranger. That expression of trust is reinforced by the couple's willingness to raise with him a potentially embarrassing, but nonetheless vital, concern about their relationship and health. That trust needs to be reciprocated, and the first moral imperative for J.E. should be to commend the couple for giving such careful consideration to this important aspect of their relationship and for their courage in seeking out some professional advice rather than taking the risks of either ignorance or unprotected sex.

That approach should help establish mutuality and a fiduciary relationship, which is necessary if J.E.'s advice, whatever its content, is going to be effective. Once mutual trust is present, the couple may be willing to consider several forms of advice about effective contraception, including alternatives and risks of each different method. J.E. must avoid the role of parent towards the couple, or expressing personal convictions about sexuality in the guise of a professional recommendation, but at the same time, responding to their request for advice by directing them to "Product X" expresses indifference rather than the sensitive advice the situation calls for.

The presence of a paternalistic ideology and practice in pharmacy recently has come under sharp criticism from pharmacist-ethicists. Michael C. Shannon[11] and Michael Manolakis[12] drew attention to the paternalism embedded in the 1981 APhA Code of Ethics and argued that this document failed to consider the patient as a participant in decision making. Manolakis held that the 1981 Code should have been rejected even before the development of the 1994 revision, in part because it "affirm[ed] an outdated paternalistic style of practice that other health care professions have long since replaced in their codes."[12] The paternalistic attitude of "doctor knows best" needs to be discarded in principle and in practice by values of "cooperation" and "participation" and by "the concept of shared decision making between pharmacists and patients." Indeed, the 1994 revision of the Code of Ethics speaks directly to the "covenantal relationship" between pharmacist and patient which requires that "a pharmacist respect the autonomy and dignity of each patient."[2] Such arguments invoke a third normative principle for the moral terrain of pharmacy, that of respect for personal autonomy.

The Principle of Respect for Autonomy

The philosopher Immanuel Kant held that a fundamental requirement of morality consisted in treating other persons "always as an end and never as a means only." This moral vision of the intrinsic dignity of human beings lies behind the normative ethical principle of respect for autonomy (self-determination). This dignity is expressed in our capacities for free action and rational choice, and in our political culture generally and in health care specifically, the possibility of exercising these capacities without interference from others commonly gives rise to the language of "rights." For example, a claim of a patient "right" to information (i.e., informed consent) about a proposed medication allows the patient to make a rational choice about whether to use the medication and accept its risks, or seek other alternatives. We treat others as ends and respect their autonomy by allowing them a zone of personal liberty in which to enact their ways of life and world views and by requiring that they offer reasons for their choices and decisions regarding their interests. That is, the necessity of moral justification is itself a part of what it means to express respect for another person as an end.

Conversely, the principle of respect for autonomy prohibits us from treating a person merely as an instrument or means to achieve our own ends and purposes, or to achieve ends and purposes they do not share with us, even if we think they should. This is what makes paternalistic pharmacy practice morally problematic. A patient who unknowingly receives a placebo in place of his or her standard medication, as in the previous illustration, is being treated as a means to the end of health as defined by the physician or pharmacist. It neither respects the patient's liberty of action nor provides the information the patient requires to make an autonomous and voluntary choice.

Current trends in pharmacy ethics and practice clearly signal an ascendancy of respect for personal autonomy. A shift in language from "patient" to "client" or "consumer" to describe the recipient of the pharmacist's services reflects this trend: a "patient" embodies the passivity of "the sick role," in contrast to the more informed and participatory role required of a client or consumer. This emerging moral vision of the person who requests medication requires a corresponding modification in the understanding of the moral role of the pharmacist. Thus, Schulz and Brushwood have articulated a model of pharmacist as an "advocate" for the patient in relations with physicians as well as in providing information. The pharmacist as advocate seeks to rectify some of the disparities in power and knowledge that support a paternalistic medicine, and instead permits patients to "develop their *own* medication practice."[13] (Our emphasis.)

The ascension of autonomy does not mean it is the only or supreme principle in pharmacy ethics. We can consider two kinds of limitations on autonomy, internal and external limits, as portrayed below.

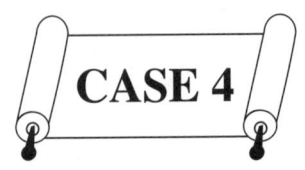

CASE 4

K.M. is a pharmacist-consultant at Golden Years Retirement and Convalescent Center. While evaluating patient charts and refill orders, he notes that D.K. has not been taking her daily dose of 10 mg of the antihypertensive nifedipine (Procardia), but has maintained her use of the laxative, docusate and the miotic, pilocarpine (Pilo-20), and the nonsteroidal anti-inflammatory agent naproxen (Naprosyn). During the last month, her blood pressure has increased from 165/110 to 210/155 mm Hg. K.M. questions the nursing supervisor, who informs him that D.K. told the medication nurse, "I don't plan to live forever, so why should I prolong my lonely, miserable life with medicine that sometimes makes me feel worse?" K.M. inquires why D.K. is continuing to take her other medications but not the one that affects her blood pressure, and learns that D.K. commented, "I want to die but I don't want to be uncomfortable until then."

Case Discussion

The meanings of personal autonomy in this case create significant moral perplexity for K.M. In one perspective, D.K.'s refusal to take prescribed nifedipine displays noncompliance, and in the "sick role" model of the patient, that is in itself a sufficient indication of nonautonomous behavior. Sickness or illness already compromises not only bodily functions but the capacities of the patient for effective deliberation and rational choices. On this understanding, K.M.'s obligation lies in the direction of having D.K. resume taking her blood pressure medication.

Yet, this perspective on noncompliance may convey paternalistic attitudes. Peter Conrad, for example, argued that noncompliance is an expression of patient autonomy, rather than a sign of its absence, that is particularly focused on obtaining or maintaining control over one's health condition.[14] D.K., for example, is seeking to achieve comfort and freedom from pain and distress. Her refusal of medication may then be interpreted as a quest for control as she anticipates her dying and death.[a]

This interpretation of noncompliance does not mean K.M. should simply proceed to the next patient's chart. Acquiescing in a patient's choices, uncoupled from care for the patient's welfare, can express indifference and apathy rather than respect. K.M. instead needs to do some fact-finding to determine whether D.K.'s refusal is an authentic expression of autono-

---

[a] The enhancement of quality care for patients by assuring appropriate drug therapy is one goal of drug use review programs. In an ambulatory care setting, an assumption was traditionally made that patients complied with prescription directives. It is now known that $1/3$ to $1/2$ of all patients fail to take their medications as prescribed. This pattern has significant health care implications (e.g., increased hospitalizations, lost work days). Many pharmacy groups have engaged in efforts to stimulate practitioners to become more assertive in changing patient behaviors through a variety of patient education activities. To date, however, there are few published studies documenting the effectiveness of these activities in an ambulatory care setting. The emphasis on stimulating proper drug use must be to improve the quality of life of the patient and not to increase consumption.

my. It surely is not an unreasonable request or choice to seek comfort (and all that request symbolizes, including the preservation of dignity, self-identity, and control) in the face of one's mortality. However, D.K.'s refusal of nifedipine may have precisely the counter-effect of her expectations, increasing her discomfort and perhaps hastening her death.

An autonomous choice presupposes background conditions of decision-making capacity, adequate knowledge and understanding, and a freedom to act without compulsion. These conditions refer to the capacities of the person making the choice. Conditions of incompetence, insufficient disclosure of information or lack of comprehension of the information, or insufficient free will to choose without undue influence identify internal limits on the autonomous nature of a person's choice. The presence of these latter conditions indicates a situation of compromised capacity for autonomy.

While D.K. has demonstrated decision-making capacity in that she can offer reasons for her refusal, K.M. needs to determine that she understands or comprehends the nature of her refusal. Respecting and promoting her autonomy requires K.M. to consult with D.K. about her refusal, its effects on her blood pressure, and the relation of both to her stated objective of comfort. The outcome of this conversation may be a resumption of nifedipine, or an alteration in the medication to assuage her concerns about physiological discomfort, or perhaps some other approach. At the least, however, a concern for a patient's autonomy requires communication and conversation about the medications, their risks and benefits, and alternatives, including the alternative of no medication through refusal. In this respect, ensuring autonomous decisions requires a convergence of the science, the art, and the ethics of pharmacy practice.

In the course of the conversation, for example, D.K. may disclose that she wishes to discontinue the medication due to side effects of dizziness, nausea, and frequent headaches. K.M. then will be in a position to assure her that these may decrease with time and perhaps to suggest that she may wish to talk with her physician about an alternative calcium channel blocker which may have fewer side effects.

K.M. also may question whether D.K.'s refusal of medication reflects involuntary limits on her autonomy. Her comments about a "lonely, miserable life" may indicate a cry for help rather than a desire for death. She may not be objecting to continued life as such, but rather to the quality of her anticipated life as deprived and diminished. There may be no pharmaceutical cure for loneliness and the psychic misery present in the experience of feeling isolated or abandoned, but clearly there are social and interactive programs of care available at a retirement center that can assist D.K. What appears to be a medical problem of refusal based upon discomfort may be resolved through social and relational alternatives. K.M. may intervene on behalf of D.K. by informing the resident social worker of her expressed loneliness or by reporting his concern at the monthly patient care conference. An assessment of the autonomous nature of D.K.'s decisions, then, also needs to explore whether a background condition of insufficient freedom to choose without undue influence may be present.

There are clearly instances where a patient who "wants to die" is making a capable, informed, and voluntary choice. Ethics, medicine, and the law have gradually moved during the last two decades in the direction of respecting patient autonomy by permitting competent patients (or authorized proxies for incompetent patients) to request the termination of life-prolonging medical treatment. The question of whether autonomy should be respected when the patient requests assistance in dying continues to create substantial ethical and professional controversy that can encompass the pharmacist through cases of "stockpiling." Consider the following case.

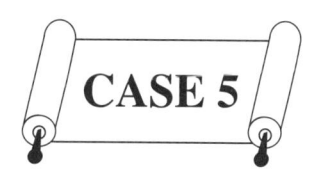

CASE 5

P.N.'s pharmacy is located adjacent to a large retirement community, whose members recently have engaged in several vigorous discussions about end-of-life decisions. The discussion groups have listened to speakers and reviewed reading material regarding living wills and literature from death-with-dignity advocacy groups that provide information on how persons who so choose may use certain medications to ensure their own death.

Several weeks later, as part of a routine inventory, P.N. observes a 20% increase in the volume of prescriptions of certain medications, including the sedative-hypnotic, secobarbital, described in the advocacy literature. She is concerned that some patients appear to be refilling these prescriptions more frequently than needed, and that in the wake of their recent discussions, may be engaged in "stockpiling" for a suicide attempt. P.N. has just been presented with a prescription for an additional refill of secobarbital and considers whether she has a professional responsibility to refuse such a request.

Case Discussion

P.N. is confronted with a dilemma whose moral contours are quite distinct from that faced by K.M. Patients who are stockpiling medications based upon literature that is, after all, publicly accessible, are likely to be well-informed about the nature of their decision, its potential consequences, and alternatives. There may be, in short, little basis upon which to challenge the autonomous character of such a choice, as was possible for K.M. in his relation with D.K.

Assuming a background of personal autonomy for the stockpiling of medications: does P.N. have any moral ground upon which to defend a stance of refusal or nonparticipation? She would rightly be concerned with the legal and professional appraisals of her dilemma. Some pharmacists have had legal proceedings initiated against them in situations where patients have committed suicide after using prescribed and stockpiled medication, but the pharmacists have been exonerated in such cases because they were not aware of the patient's intentions.[15] This seems an accurate portrayal of P.N.'s situation at this stage, in that she has no definite knowledge of any intentions by patients to use the medication for purposes of suicide. She cannot be held legally or morally accountable for performing her professional responsibilities in good faith and trust that the medication would be used as prescribed.

P.N. nonetheless is involved in a professional predicament that is likely to become more prominent in the years ahead. The medical literature in the last five years has witnessed a proliferation of proposals from philosophers and physicians advocating physician-assisted suicide,[16] and some studies have indicated a sizable proportion of physicians treating seriously ill patients either have or would help the patient stockpile sufficient medication for suicide.[17] That end can be accomplished only by making the pharmacist a knowing or unknowing participant in the stockpiling or by engaging in a conspiracy of silence that excludes the pharmacist from the relationship altogether.

In this respect, P.N. could well be caught in a dilemma not of her own making. There is a sense in which she appears to have been excluded rather than accepted as a partner in the decision-making process. The fiduciary relationship appears not to have been respected but compromised by dissembling or deceit, though it is not yet clear whether this is attributable to the patient, the prescribing physicians, or both. Respect for personal autonomy is not a one-way street; neither the patient nor the physician should perceive the pharmacist as a mere technocratic tool to the achievement of mutually agreed upon ends. P.N.'s autonomy as a person and as a professional also demands respect and it would be entirely appropriate for her to seek ways to insert herself into the relationship as a participating partner.

The dilemma may well dissolve once her presence in the relationship is acknowledged by the other parties. Some fact-finding with the prescribing physician is a necessary initial step, because the physician may be unaware of the timing and frequency of the refill requests, or may present additional information about the medical status of the certain patients that validates the frequent refills. This conversation may confirm or invalidate her suspicions about stockpiling and patient intentions, but it would be premature for her to refuse a refill request in the absence of this information. The pharmacist's role and responsibility in patient care can also be acknowledged through conversations with patients. Our general claim here is that P.N. cannot act responsibly on her suspicions while remaining in the dark.

It also is possible, of course, that the dilemma could intensify rather than dissolve as a consequence of these inquiries. Some physicians with whom we are acquainted, for example, have commented that while they also have had suspicions of patient stockpiling on occasion, they would find it intrusive or disrespectful of the patient's privacy to probe his intentions regarding use of medication. Other physicians act on their moral sympathy for a patient suffering from a terminal illness or a debilitating chronic ailment and have knowingly assisted patient stockpiling. In other situations, some patients may be open and candid about their intentions. These responses would clearly intensify the dilemma for P.N.

P.N.'s moral justification in the presence of some confirming evidence of stockpiling for a subsequent suicide may assume several different forms. She may refuse to be a participant in the relationship on grounds that it would violate her conscience, personal autonomy, and moral integrity to use her professional skills in the knowledge that they could contribute to a person's death. This claim of conscientious refusal would be applicable only to her particular moral framework and values. She could, on this view, refuse a refill request, but if asked, recommend other pharmacists.

At a second level, P.N.'s response might be shaped by her sense of professional moral integrity. She might claim that it is incompatible with the paramount professional commitment of pharmacy to patient health and safety to provide some form of assistance, such as distributing medication, that can bring about a patient's death. This claim from the standpoint of professional integrity would entail not only a refusal of the refill request but also a refusal to recommend alternative pharmacists. This is not to say every pharmacist would embrace this moral ideal of the profession; indeed, the advocacy model might direct a quite different approach. Our point here is that P.N.'s refusal could be grounded not only in a claim of personal conscience, but also of professional conscience, of an understanding of the moral vocation of pharmacy.

At a third level, P.N.'s refusal could express moral convictions about suicide, rooted in the principle of nonmaleficence, as distinct from concerns about her profession's assistance in suicide. Suicide might be considered to contravene the sanctity of human life or prohibitions against killing, even if the choice reflects rational and autonomous deliberation. Although society has decriminalized suicide, morally it is both possible and necessary to distinguish between a (legal) right to choose and (morally) right choices. P.N. might well claim that the moral integrity of society is at stake in her dilemma, in addition to personal and professional integrity, and that literature describing methods of suicide should not be publicly accessible.

The question of assistance or participation in a patient's suicide will likely become even more contested for the health care professions over the next several years, and it is not our purpose here to propose a normative stance for the pharmacy profession. We have used the case of P.N. to illustrate three major points relevant to the principle of respect for autonomy. First, in addition to internal limits on autonomy that reflect issues of patient decision-making capacity, comprehension, or free will, there may be external limits on patient autonomy that derive from convictions about moral integrity at a personal, professional, or social level. These limits can permit pharmacists to refuse to acquiesce in some patient requests even if those requests are autonomous; that is, when there are no unresolved questions regarding internal limits or patient capacities.

Secondly, the moral source of a refusal by a pharmacist to acquiesce in a patient request reflects different forms of paternalism that may be more or less justifiable.[18] A refusal rooted in issues of internal limits of patient autonomy displays weak paternalism. It is typically justifiable inasmuch as the patient lacks the capacities for autonomous choice and only so long as he lacks them. A refusal based upon concerns that cooperation will compromise the pharmacist's personal moral ideals displays passive paternalism and should be considered justifiable because of the threat such participation poses to one's sense of personal moral integrity. Moreover, a patient typically will have recourse to other alternatives (another pharmacist) to pursue his own ends.

In contrast to this justification, a refusal based upon prospects of harm to the patient exemplifies strong paternalism. Strong paternalism can be very difficult to justify because the patient's autonomy is compromised for his welfare, with the professional rather than patient view of what constitutes "welfare" predominating. A refusal that appeals, by contrast, to harm to others or to third parties may be justifiable based upon the principle of nonmaleficence. However, we would first need to consider whether the act contemplated would in fact injure or harm others or society. It may be hard to argue, for example, that suicide from stockpiled medication injures society or damages societal regard for the value of life. It may well harm identified others, and we would then need to ask whether the harm experienced by these specific persons or groups (a family) is greater than the harm to the person whose self-determination is denied or violated.

Finally, moral resolution of these and other issues in pharmacy ethics will be influenced by a pharmacist's perception and enactment of professional self-understanding and moral integrity. The course of action P.N. chooses may well be different according to whether she embraces a moral vision of a pharmacist as a product technician, or a parent, a partner, or a patient advocate. The differing role expectations of other parties—patients, physicians, professional colleagues, society—may themselves create conflicts of interest and loyalties for the pharmacist. Thus, part of professional autonomy and responsibility involves an ongoing reassessment of the moral vocation and identity of pharmacy. The conflicting ideals of professionalism in pharmacy likewise create moral tensions for the normative principle of loyalty.

The Principle of Loyalty

Philosopher John Ladd describes loyalty as "an essential ingredient in any civilized and humane system of morals."[19] The moral necessity of loyalty in a humane system of pharmacy morals has already been anticipated somewhat in our previous case discussions. In one of its aspects, loyalty is concerned with the fulfillment of the moral self. It therefore overlaps with issues of personal autonomy and integrity, although it entails more than self-determination in decision making. Loyalty in addition requires commitment and deep devotion to the kind of person (or professionally, the kind of pharmacist) one aspires to be.

Loyalty also presumes a social and institutional context to our moral choices. It reveals a relational dimension to the moral life that an exclusive focus on personal autonomy, for example, can conceal. We do not find ourselves to be free-floating, unencumbered atoms in a moral universe; instead, our moral responsibilities are interwoven with and mediated by our interrelationships with others, which in the context of pharmacy may include family, patients, physicians, professional colleagues, administrators, employers, and others. We express concern about devotion, fidelity and "betrayal," the antithesis of loyalty, in these relationships that are core to our sense of self-identity. Loyalty answers to our need for a unification of the personal and relational dimensions of our lives, a harmony of the private and public moral worlds.[20]

It would be incorrect, then, to associate the principle of loyalty with the model of pharmacy as a technical, amoral practice. Loyalty instead engages a conscientious moral agent in an ongoing process of negotiation and accommodation through which commitment and faithfulness are displayed to sometimes converging, sometimes diverging, claims. It requires thoughtful, discriminating deliberation about priorities and the relative importance of responsibilities, be they personal, professional, or institutional. The principle of loyalty is thus morally richer than a professional model of following and filling orders, and within which to question an order is itself a form of disloyalty, rather than an autonomous expression of devotion and fidelity.

As a normative principle, loyalty requires that we give the persons to whom we are loyal what is their moral due. It often is expressed in interpersonal or interprofessional relationships in the rule of fidelity, including the keeping of promises, while in broader social settings, loyalty overlaps with the normative principle of justice (which we discuss below in Case 6). That is, the answer to the question of what is "due" another on the principle of loyalty is conditioned by the nature of the roles and relationships of the persons. That requires, in turn, that we give meaningful content to professionalism in pharmacy.

The participation in many relationships can, on occasion, make conflicts of loyalty an unavoidable part of the moral life of the pharmacist. Resolving the conflict could involve extricating oneself from the relationship, but this obviously does not occur without moral loss. We have already discussed conflicting loyalties in professional and patient relationships (see Cases 1, 4), so in Case 6 we wish to focus on the institutional contexts of such dilemmas.

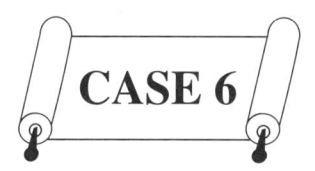

CASE 6

L.J. is a consultant pharmacist and one of three buyers for XYZ, a large (1100-bed) for-profit nursing home chain. In renewing contracts with providers of generic amitriptyline (an antidepressant), he notes that bids from three different providers vary by as much as 35%. L.J. seeks information from each provider individually, and the high bidder, S.W., indicates that if her company is given the contract, not only will XYZ show a better profit margin but that she will help XYZ to become the pharmacy provider for two other large nursing homes. XYZ previously has made unsuccessful attempts to make these homes part of their chain, and L.J. is skeptical that S.W. can make good on her proposal. Still, he is aware that if he were to be instrumental in securing the new homes, there would be benefits not only to XYZ but also to himself in the way of a needed promotion.

Case Discussion

The conflict of loyalties confronted by L.J. is created by the various roles he assumes. He is, first, a pharmacist and his patients can rightly make a claim to his loyalty. In particular, he has an obligation to provide safe and effective medications, such as amitriptyline, and other professional services, according to a standard of "fair and reasonable" remuneration.[21,22] L.J.'s inclination to engage in business with a particular company could, however, increase patient costs significantly without offering any medical benefit. The patients might then make claims about "unfair" pricing and express a sentiment of betrayal, recriminations that over the long term could be harmful to the objectives of XYZ.

L.J. is not only a pharmacist but also embodies the entrepreneurial or market model of medicine. As a buyer or employee for a very substantial "chain" of nursing homes, he has accepted certain obligations towards his employer. These most likely include seeking to enhance the competitive position of XYZ in the health care industry and to improve its profitability, both of which may be aided by securing the deal with S.W. This approach also may not compromise L.J.'s loyalty to the patients as radically as may appear; while an increased profit margin could be used by XYZ for several different purposes, one alternative might be to lower costs of some drugs, including amitriptyline, to patients in the XYZ chain. Patients might not have to absorb the 35% differential in price all by themselves while the company could better pursue its entrepreneurial objectives.

Finally, it appears that L.J. could well advance his own career as a professional through this arrangement. We previously have described acts performed purely out of self-interest in the face of a competing moral obligation as exemplifying moral weakness, but L.J.'s situation is more complicated than that framework. While it is true he may benefit from the transaction, this would be an indirect or side effect of the benefits realized by XYZ. He cannot achieve his needed promotion entirely on his own efforts. Moreover, it may well be that the promotion is "needed" so that he can bring benefits to immediate others, such as providing a college education for his daughter or ensuring financial stability for his family. In such a setting, his role in a family offers a quite different motive than an aspiration to climb a rung on the corporate ladder.

In contemplating these alternatives, it is important to distinguish possibilities from high probabilities and to identify those stakeholders who will benefit and those who might be burdened. The virtual certainty of a completed transaction with S.W. is substantially increased costs to patients of XYZ when lower alternatives are available; the possibility, and therefore, uncertainty, is whether XYZ will acquire its desired nursing homes through the transaction. That uncertainty also means the prospects of securing the promotion also fall within the realm of possibility, not probability. Thus, the transaction risks the certainty of burdens to patients, without any correlative guarantee of anticipated benefits (except perhaps those accruing to stockholders). Moreover, however the transaction turns out, it does seem certain that the burdens and benefits will not fall on the same groups of persons. The agreement thereby risks inequitable distribution, and as suggested above, could actually have a negative impact on the company if clientele discontent over high prices becomes extensive.

This analysis suggests a compelling moral direction for resolving L.J.'s conflict of loyalties. There are occasions where advancement of patient, employer, and professional career interests can converge, or where advancing one set of interests does not directly jeopardize another set. The proposed transaction with S.W., by contrast, appears to treat patient welfare merely as an instrument to the achievement of certain business and career ends. While that may be compatible with L.J.'s role either as employee or as professional, it seems to contravene his fundamental commitment of loyalty to patients. Indeed, in this situation, it may be very important for L.J. to assume a patient advocacy role, for while patients clearly have a stake in the decision, they are (apparently) being denied a voice. The principles of respect and loyalty are violated when we impose burdens on a class of persons without their having a say in the matter and without expectation of comparable benefits.

S.W. has not made an offer that is too good to refuse. Other alternatives will likely present themselves in the future for XYZ to obtain its desired nursing homes or for L.J. to secure a deserved promotion, ones that can be consistent with his professional commitment to patient loyalty. This commitment explains why society has conferred upon pharmacy the special status of "profession," with its accompanying privileges and responsibilities, rather than subsuming it to a market model in which the ethic of the "bottom line" predominates.

The Principle of Distributive Justice

We have seen that it is not always ethically possible in pharmacy practice to avoid harms (nonmaleficence) and provide benefits (beneficence). In such situations, we need to be concerned with who receives the benefits and who bears the burdens or harm. The question of the allocation of benefits and burdens is the focus of the principle of distributive justice. It is a central principle for pharmacy ethics because of the broader social context in which pharmacists practice, one aspect of which is that some persons may be restricted in terms of their ability to have access to the services of a pharmacist. The principle of distributive justice requires the pharmacist to consider whether the resources he provides to patients are distributed fairly and equitably.[23] Consider the following case.

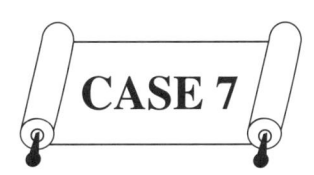

CASE 7

M.Z., a patient with hypertension, visits his pharmacist, H.B., to obtain a previously authorized refill for his antihypertensive medication, a slow-release calcium channel blocker. The medication is expensive, but in the past M.Z.'s insurance plan paid for the medication with a $5 co-payment. However, M.Z.'s employment recently has been terminated as part of a company restructuring plan, and M.Z. admits he is experiencing even higher levels of stress as a result of being unemployed. In addition, he no longer has medical insurance coverage, and when informed by H.B. of the cost of the refill, remarks: "That's outrageous. I can't possibly afford to pay that."

H.B. is aware that there are many alternative antihypertensive medications that cost significantly less than what was originally prescribed for M.Z. and may well be within M.Z.'s income range. However, these alternative agents perhaps may not be as optimal as the slow-release calcium channel blocker, and the diminished efficacy may be compounded by the additional stress M.Z. is now experiencing. Given M.Z.'s comment, H.B. considers whether he should propose to M.Z. and his physician a less expensive and possibly less optimal medication.

Case Discussion

It can be tempting to see the issue for H.B. as a "social" problem that is really beyond his professional purview. There are obviously background conditions of social inequity and economic dislocation that enter into M.Z.'s situation that neither H.B. by himself nor the pharmacy profession as a whole can remedy. Yet, it would simply be callous to add professional abandonment to the vocational and social abandonment M.Z. has already experienced. The foundational ethical (and increasingly, political) question is whether the basis for distributing health care services, including pharmaceuticals, is need or ability to pay. M.Z. unquestionably has need but is unable to pay: are there moral alternatives to abandonment for H.B.?

H.B. is confronting several features of the "stratification" of care characteristic of the American health care system, which frequently results in inefficient and unfair patterns of distribution. The first form of stratification occurs within the pharmaceutical industry, which inevitably influences professional practice. There are, for example, different "tiers" of antihypertensive medication in which greater efficacy and selectivity is correlated with substantially higher cost. Safe, but perhaps less effective medications may be available to virtually all persons at some minimal level of cost, while access to the most efficacious may be limited to persons with generous insurance coverage.

For example, there are some 30 different antihypertensive medications, 24 NSAIDs, 40 oral contraceptives, 35 antianxiety agents, and 20 antihistamines. The choice from among these agents in independent medical practice is typically up to the discretion of the physician in an informed consultation with a patient. In more restricted settings, such as hospitals or HMOs, the choice of the most appropriate agent is commonly determined by a formulary committee that evaluates the cost/benefit ratio for one agent of choice from among all the others. Are there, or should there be, mechanisms whereby independent physicians and pharmacists can assist patients in determining which level of therapy they wish to receive, based upon all relevant factors, including ability to pay? Such a procedure may require alterations from patterns of the current model of practice in which all persons should be able to receive the newest and most effective medications, a model that does not conform to reality in all cases.

The stratification of pharmaceuticals through ability to pay is of course just the tip of an iceberg that this country is now desperately trying to correct. M.Z. represents more and more the changing face of persons who are denied access to necessary medical services. Some 37 million citizens do not have insurance coverage for basic health care; many of these persons are unemployed, while others are part-time employees whose income is higher than eligibility levels for government assistance, but simply insufficient to purchase an adequate private insurance plan. Such persons, and their dependents, are not adequately protected by any type of social "safety net" for health care. The general distribution of health care is stratified according to income levels, and for some persons, that may mean receiving no medical care until they enter an emergency room with an acute condition.

H.B.'s ethical response to his dilemma thus will be influenced by these constraints of stratification within pharmacy and within health care generally. Nonetheless, there are constructive steps he can take, both in his role as professional and in his role as citizen, to ensure a sphere of relatively equitable allocation of those health care resources distributed through his practice. H.B. first needs to be clear about the alternatives that might be open to M.Z. He needs to determine that the increased stress of M.Z. under the prior medication is not, for example, attributable to noncompliance. If M.Z. has not been faithfully adhering to a prescribed regimen, it will be that much more difficult to gauge the impact of a shift to a different medication that is taken regularly. H.B. also needs to involve the prescribing physician in a consultation about alternative medications that could be equally as effective as the prior medication, but also be less expensive. Since the refill had been authorized in advance, the prescribing physician may be aware only of M.Z.'s symptoms and not of the recent change in his insurance status.

If the loss of his insurance coverage has rendered M.Z. medically indigent for all prescription medicines, a couple of alternatives may still be open. It is possible that the manufacturer of the previously-prescribed medication has established an indigent patient program in which M.Z. could be enrolled. Such programs typically allow free access to the medication for qualified patients, and H.B. could in this instance be an advocate on behalf of M.Z. Finally, H.B. could fill the authorized prescription without charge or at reduced charge to M.Z., thus adding to the expanding pool of "uncompensated care" in medicine. This approach, however, could itself face objections from the standpoint of distributive justice: M.Z. would be receiving a benefit that other patients are not, and moreover their willingness to pay the requisite price provides a kind of subsidy or "free ride" for M.Z. Clearly, if every patient of H.B.'s asked for treatment similar to that offered to M.Z., H.B.'s pharmacy practice would cease quickly.

In a broader perspective, the social status of "profession" entails that reciprocal and correlative responsibilities exist in the relationship between society and pharmacy. The health care professions, including pharmacists, cannot be expected to fulfill the trust society has invested in them to care for patients unless the society is itself willing to commit the necessary financial resources. The stratification of health care, including inadequate coverage of prescription medicines, treats what are necessary medical services as discretionary commodities, which is clearly mistaken in the case of most patients. A person can choose to forgo purchasing a television set or choose amongst different varieties of food at a grocery store. This consumer model of choice, however, is simply inappropriate for the situation of a patient who needs a particular medication for hypertension, and for whom forgoing medication may mean not merely a change in lifestyle (though that is clearly one method of lowering blood pressure) but may also present a risk to life. Thus, part of the answer to the problem confronting H.B. is not to require him to universalize his altruism, but to require society to universalize access to basic health services, including prescribed medications, so that ability to pay is not a barrier to receiving necessary medical care.

It is only a partial answer, however, because it is equally mistaken for any health care profession to claim moral independence from the society of which it is a part. William F. May has rightly identified the "indebtedness" of a profession to the society, which confers upon the profession its special status, commits resources for the training and education of practitioners, and presents patients in their vulnerability for "practice" as part of professional education.[24] The reciprocal responsibilities of pharmacists in the context of distributive justice include critical scrutiny of the emerging entrepreneurial ethos of medicine, which has an immense impact on the distribution of health care resources and also can create an insular professional community. The responsibility of reciprocity also encompasses an informed professional critique of the pricing patterns of drug companies, which have clearly limited the access to very basic health services for thousands of persons. Such patterns can be criticized from the standpoint of distributive justice because persons like M.Z. suffer the burdens of illness without sharing in the benefits of the health care system.

These "macro" considerations will not resolve the microcosm of the social dilemma standing immediately before H.B. in the presence of M.Z. M.Z. has not asked for a "free ride" but to be treated fairly and respectfully. The principle of distributive justice does not permit M.Z. to receive benefits at the expense of H.B.'s other patients, but it supports H.B.'s efforts to pursue creative alternatives that make both medical, ethical, and economic sense. It no less requires sustained efforts for reform within the profession and in society as a whole to ensure that the future M.Z.s are the rare exception rather than the rule of pharmacy practice.

The Moral Status of Principles

We have identified five normative principles of pharmacy practice and displayed their relevance through illustrative cases. It has been our contention that the meaning and priority of these principles is in part conditioned by prior conceptions of professionalism in pharmacy. It will be useful in conclusion to address the question of priorities among conflicting principles.

One possible interpretation of the moral status of principles is to understand them as expressions of moral absolutes (i.e., prescribing moral norms and obligations which have no exceptions). This interpretation can be difficult to sustain when, as in our view of pharmacy ethics, an ethical framework offers a plurality of principles. It simply is not always possible to avoid harming and provide benefits and respect rights without moral conflict arising. One method of resolving this sense of incompleteness associated with moral absolutism is to prioritize one principle, and consider others to reflect important but subordinate responsibilities. The 1981

APhA Code of Ethics was suggestive of this method in its designation of patient health and safety as the "first" consideration of the pharmacist. Yet, as we have noted in describing the embedded paternalism of this version of the Code, prioritizing one principle can neglect some moral matters such as patient and professional autonomy, which should be more prominent.

A third alternative is to treat moral principles as maxims that may illuminate a situation of moral conflict but do not themselves give moral direction or prescribe moral obligations. On this account, the principle of loyalty, for example, would have a moral status analogous to the medical maxim, "Take two aspirin, get plenty of rest, and call me in the morning." A moral maxim expresses the generalized experience and wisdom of the past, but can be set aside or ignored in the exigencies of any situation.

While the flexibility of this approach is appealing, we believe it is possible to accommodate flexibility and sensitivity to the distinctive setting of a moral problem without abandoning (as the maxim method does) the normative or obligatory force of a principle. Following the suggestions of philosopher W.D. Ross,[25] our proposal is that the principles of pharmacy ethics be understood as establishing presumptive or *prima facie* duties or obligations. All other things being equal, a pharmacist is obliged to avoid harming, promote welfare, respect autonomy, express loyalty and fidelity, or distribute benefits equitably. However, as displayed in our cases, often (as with moral dilemmas) things are not equal, and the ethical pharmacist is required to choose one principle that provides definitive moral direction in the dilemma.

An instructive analogy for presumptive or *prima facie* principles can be drawn from the law. A basic principle of our legal system is that a person is "presumed innocent until proven guilty." The legal presumption of innocence imposes a burden of proof on those who seek to establish guilt. Similarly, the moral decision to infringe one principle, such as beneficence, for the sake of another, such as loyalty, imposes a moral burden of proof on the pharmacist, which can be met through the reason-giving process we described earlier as moral justification. Thus, unlike the absolutist approach, this account accommodates both moral conflict and flexibility, but unlike the maxim account, it demands conscientious deliberation and public accountability rather than allowing for laxity.

Under what circumstances might it be morally permissible to infringe one principle (and thus an obligation) in order to meet an obligation deemed weightier in that situation? Consider a scenario in which a pharmacist is confronted with a choice about disclosing confidential information about a patient to a third party to benefit the patient. The moral burden of proof for disclosure here consists in meeting five "justificatory conditions:"[26]

1. Effectiveness—The disclosure will benefit the patient.
2. Proportionality—The benefits of the disclosure will outweigh the harms of infringing confidentiality.
3. Necessity—The disclosure is a last resort; the need of the patient is significant and there is no alternative to meet the patient's need short of disclosure.
4. Least Infringement—The circle of disclosure is narrow, involving only the person(s) who can directly bring about the patient benefit.
5. Explanation and Justification—The patient should be informed of the infringement of his or her confidentiality and the disclosure defended by the overriding principles and rules.

In actual practice, very few disclosures of confidential information would be able to meet the burden of proof demanded by these justificatory conditions. Our general claim, however, is that this process of balancing conflicting obligations and determining whether an infringement of one principle is justifiable is a necessary part of moral justification for the responsible pharmacist. This process can ensure better patient care and a pharmacy practice that embodies professional ideals.

Discussion Questions

1. Which form of moral conflict arises most frequently in pharmacy practice? Give illustrations of each and discuss how the conflicts were resolved.

2. The authors offer a hierarchical method of moral reasoning and justification, moving from the particular and concrete to the general and abstract, and back again. Does this method of moral justification account for personal or professional experience of moral issues, and if so, how?

3. Does the medical maxim, *first of all do no harm*, imply that avoiding harm (nonmaleficence) would be a more rigorous or prior duty for pharmacists relative to other normative principles? Why or why not?

4. What models of pharmacy practice seem most persuasive to you? Will different models be appropriate for different patients? Is a paternalistic model of pharmacy practice ever morally justified?

5. How can conflicts between moral principles be resolved? Are the normative principles of pharmacy ethics best understood as absolutes, maxims, or presumptive obligations?

REFERENCES

1. Schulz RM, Brushwood DB. The pharmacist's role in patient care. Hastings Cent Rep. 1991;21:13.
2. American Pharmaceutical Association: Code of Ethics for Pharmacists; 1994.
3. Lawall CH. Pharmaceutical ethics. In: Smith M et al., eds. Pharmacy Ethics. New York: Pharmaceutical Products Press; 1991:5–19.
4. Renoir J. The Rules of the Game: A Film. 1970.
5. Beauchamp TL, Childress JF. Principles of Biomedical Ethics. 3rd ed. New York: Oxford University Press; 1989:6.
6. Lemmon J. Moral dilemmas. In: Ramsey IT, ed. Christian Ethics and Contemporary Philosophy. New York: The Macmillan Company; 1966:266.
7. Beauchamp TL, Childress JF. Principles of Biomedical Ethics. 3rd ed. New York: Oxford University Press; 1989:4.
8. Beauchamp TL, Childress JF. Principles of Biomedical Ethics. 3rd ed. New York: Oxford University Press; 1989:121.
9. Veatch RM. The pharmacist and the patient's rights movement. In: Smith M et al., eds. Pharmacy Ethics. New York: Pharmaceutical Products Press; 1991:254–56.
10. Veatch RM. Case analysis in ethics instruction. In: Haddad AM, ed. Teaching and Learning Strategies in Pharmacy Ethics. Omaha: Creighton University Biomedical Communications; 1992:85.
11. Shannon MC. Ethical decision making in practice: current problems and future concerns. In: Haddad AM, ed. Teaching and Learning Strategies in Pharmacy Ethics. Omaha: Creighton University Biomedical Communications; 1992:75–82.
12. Manolakis ML. Why APhA should reject its code of ethics. Am Pharm. 1991;31:46.
13. Schulz RB, Brushwood DB. The pharmacist's role in patient care. Hastings Cent Rep. 1991;21:16.
14. Conrad P. The noncompliant patient in search of autonomy. Hastings Cent Rep. 1987;17:15–17.
15. LeBlang TR. What if prescription medication is used for suicide? Am Druggist. 1989;199:64.

16. Quill TE et al. Care of the hopelessly ill: proposed clinical criteria for physician-assisted suicide. N Engl J Med. 1992;327:1380–384.
17. Smith M et al., eds. Pharmacy Ethics. New York: Pharmaceutical Products Press; 1991:477-84.
18. Childress JF. Who Should Decide?: Paternalism in Health Care. New York: Oxford University Press; 1984:16–21.
19. Ladd J. Loyalty. In: Edwards P, ed. Encyclopedia of Philosophy. New York: Macmillan Publishing Co. Inc. & The Free Press; 1972:97.
20. Royce J. The Philosophy of Loyalty. New York: The Macmillan Company; 1908.
21. American Pharmaceutical Association: Code of Ethics. In: Smith M et al., eds. Pharmacy Ethics. New York: Pharmaceutical Products Press; 1991:74.
22. American Society of Consultant Pharmacists: Code of Ethics. In: Smith M et al., eds. New York: Pharmaceutical Products Press; 1991:76–8.
23. American Pharmaceutical Association. Proposed Code of Ethics for Pharmacists. Personal Communication with Marsha S. Holloman. 1993.
24. May WF. The Physician's Covenant. Philadelphia: The Westminster Press; 1983.
25. Ross WD. The Right and the Good. Oxford: The Clarendon Press; 1930.
26. Childress JF. Mandatory HIV screening and testing. In: Reamer FG, ed. AIDS and Ethics. New York: Columbia University Press; 1991:53–5.

Chapter 3

The Relationship Between Ethics and the Law

Kenneth Mullan
James M. Brown

Pharmacists are often faced with situations that raise both ethical and legal questions. We will tease out the knotted relationship between ethics and the law so that you may use each field constructively and knowledgeably in the professional setting. In many cases, what is required of you legally is also what is required ethically. This is not always so, however; sometimes what is permissible legally is unethical, and sometimes what is required ethically is illegal. After unpacking the concepts of law and ethics, we will use two case studies that demonstrate how the question, "What should I do?" may be answered differently depending upon whether one takes ethics or the law to establish the ultimate standards for deciding how one should act.

The pharmacist's primary role in patient care is to use his or her technical expertise to interpret the details of a physician's prescription; to ensure that the prescription is valid; to dispense the drug product which has been prescribed or, in certain circumstances, an equivalent drug; and to give instructions to the patient on the use of the drug, including possible side-effects, through appropriate verbal or written directions. Without this technical expertise, the patient is not in a position to complete treatment. The pharmacist is, therefore, a crucial member of the health care team.

In addition to the fundamental technical decisions a pharmacist has to make, she often is faced with other difficult decisions requiring immediate resolution where technical expertise cannot provide the answer. Certain important factors may arise and even conflict with each other so that the pharmacist is faced with a dilemma of whether to provide the treatment in question. A dilemma occurs when a person must choose between two courses of action and both have valid reasons for being selected. It is a moral dilemma if the reasons on both sides are moral reasons and it is a legal dilemma if the reasons on both sides are legal reasons. The practice of pharmacy often raises both legal and moral dilemmas for pharmacists. Let us briefly examine the nature and sources of law.

What Is Law and Where Does It Come From?

Law concerns the regulation of human affairs and human relationships. Every modern society has a legal system which includes a set of general rules regulating the conduct of the society's members. The regulation is not perfectly effective, and the system includes provisions for cases where the rules have been breached or appear to have been breached and for cases where there is dispute among members of the society as to how the rules apply to matters affecting their interests.

In a modern state many of the rules in the legal system are based on actions undertaken by parliaments, regional assemblies, and the like, and written down as a matter of public record. This is known as *legislation*. Courts and judges also play a part in formulating laws and perhaps in making them. This is called *case law* or *common law*.

The difference between legislation and case law is that the former consists of a body of rules that have been formally enacted by the legislative or executive branches of government, and the latter is a legal position in a particular case based on the decisions of previous courts in similar cases. Both case law and legislation are classified into the divisions of criminal and civil law. Criminal law concerns the relationship between an individual and the state, and civil law is concerned with the relationships between individuals. Criminal law is usually enforced by punishing offenders with imprisonment, fines, and the like. Civil law is usually enforced when the offended party files a lawsuit against the offender.

Both case law and legislation are relevant to the practice of pharmacy. For example, the Federal Controlled Substances Act (21 USC 801) regulates the production and distribution of chemical substances with the potential for abuse or dependence. Failure to adhere to the requirements of the Act may render a noncompliant pharmacist liable to criminal sanction. Similarly, in the case of *French Drug Company vs. Jones* [367 So 2d 431 (Miss 1978)], the court confirmed that a pharmacist has breached the duty of care owed to the patient where he or she fills a prescription in a manner other than that called for by the physician. Such a breach might render the pharmacist liable to pay damages in a civil action.

What Is Ethics in General and Pharmacy Ethics in Particular?

Ethics is the attempt to answer the question, "What should I do?," when that question has a direct reference to the rights and welfare of other people. The question, "Should I make an effort to return this $20 bill I found, or keep it for myself?" is an ethical question, because the person who lost the money is entitled to its return, all things being equal. The question, "Should I wear the red outfit or the blue one?," is not an ethical question, because it has nothing to do with anyone else's rights or welfare; this kind of question is a matter of aesthetics.

Pharmacy ethics is the attempt to answer the question, "What should I do as a pharmacist?" For example, when you ask yourself whether you should dispense pills that have accidentally dropped on the floor of the pharmacy, you are asking an ethical question, because the rights and perhaps the welfare of patients is at stake. Most of the time, when you ask yourself "What should I do?" in the context of practicing pharmacy, you are asking an ethical question, because your conduct almost always has a direct reference to the rights and welfare of patients.

We will follow the convention in the literature by using the terms "ethical" and "moral" synonymously.

What Is the Relationship Between Law and Morality?

There are many laws that attempt to codify morality; the laws concerning abortion and euthanasia are two examples. Not all acts that are immoral are illegal, however. Generally speaking, it is unethical for parents habitually to lie to their children, but it is not illegal. Because laws are an attempt to regulate large numbers of people, it is sometimes the case that a practice is illegal, even though there are instances where no harm is likely to occur from engaging in it (e.g., driving through a red traffic light late at night when no one else is around).

Pharmacy law might, at first blush, not appear to have anything to do with ethics. For example, regulations concerning the maintenance of pharmacy records have no appeal to morals. Let us consider a case, however, that raises both legal and ethical considerations for a pharmacist.

CASE 1

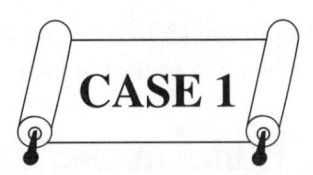

A.K. is a pharmacist-owner of a community pharmacy. One of her patients, G.M., is a bookkeeper with a local lumber firm. A.K. knows G.M. well because they live in the same apartment complex. G.M. has had some emotional problems and has been treated with temazepam, amitriptyline, and fluoxetine.

A.K. learns that G.M. has been fired from his job as bookkeeper. There are allegations that G.M. has embezzled money from the lumber firm. In fact, the firm has filed a lawsuit against him to recover the lost money. A.K. was told that the owner of the lumber firm said that he does not want "nutcases working for me and stealing my money." People in town believe, however, that although there is evidence that money is missing, G.M. is one of a number of people who might have taken it.

A.K. received a subpoena commanding her to appear in court and bring her records of medications dispensed to G.M. The lawyers for the lumber firm intend to use this information to show that G.M. had emotional problems. A.K. contacted G.M. and learned that his physicians have refused to testify regarding his medical condition, citing physician-patient confidentiality. The court has agreed not to require the physicians to testify.

A.K. told G.M. that if she is made to testify, the substance of her testimony would be that nothing in the medication record indicates any predisposition to embezzle money. She would tell the court that it is preposterous to think that the medications a person takes could cause them to steal. Although her testimony would support G.M., he told A.K. that he wanted her to refuse to testify. G.M. feels that his medication record simply is nobody else's business, and also that it would be a bad precedent for a patient's medication use to be discussed in open court.

Case Discussion
What Should Pharmacist A.K. Do and Why?

In all lawsuits, each party to the action may seek to obtain documentary or other evidence to try the case and may ask a court, in certain circumstances, to order the other side, or indeed, a third party, to produce this evidence. Such an order is legally enforceable and is an example of the rules and regulations pertaining to civil and criminal law. The threat of such enforcement is often hidden in the language used to describe the order (e.g., "subpoena" literally means "under pain"). A.K. has been served with such an order, and if she chooses to ignore it or appears in court but refuses to testify, the judge may require her to be brought before the bench to explain her actions. If that happened, A.K. might argue that, just as physicians have a duty to protect confidential patient information, so should pharmacists be obliged.

Would a court extend the physician-patient privilege to a pharmacist in these circumstances? According to Brushwood,[1] the law does recognize that the forced disclosure of a pharmacist's documents such as prescriptions or adverse drug reaction reports that are covered by the physician-patient privilege may amount to a breach of that privilege, even when the documents are no longer in the possession of the physician. In addition, there may be public policy arguments against forced disclosure of pharmacist records. The constitutionally protected right to privacy may uphold a pharmacist-patient privilege.

To convince the court that the privilege already granted to the physicians in this case ought to be extended to her as G.M.'s pharmacist, A.K., will need to argue one of the three legal positions outlined above. She may point out that the records contain documents that were originally covered by the physician-patient privilege and communicating them to her does not mean that the privilege has been waived. Because the court already has been convinced of the validity of the physician-patient privilege, she may be in a strong position to persuade them that the documents in her possession also ought to be covered by that privilege.

Second, A.K. may indicate that public policy dictates that the records ought not to be disclosed. In this regard she will have to note that a previous court, in the case of *State vs. Mark* [23 Wash App 398, 597 P2d 406 (1979)], has found that the interest that an individual has in the nondisclosure of pharmacy records may be overridden by the public interest served by the investigation of fraud in pharmacy practice. The facts of this case are similar. G.M.'s employers are anxious to recover lost moneys which they believe have been embezzled from their firm. However, in *State vs. Mark* the fraud against the pharmacist had already been proved and the records were being sought to determine the amount of compensation payable as a result. It may be possible to argue in the present case that the claims against G.M. amount to unproven allegations.

Finally, A.K. may argue that forcing her to testify and reveal the contents of the medication record might amount to an interference with

G.M.'s right to privacy as guaranteed by the constitution. Previous judgments of the U.S. Supreme Court may be against her in this proposition. However, Brushwood[1] has argued that the rulings in the reported cases on this point are narrow and as such, A.K., or more probably her legal representatives, may seek to persuade a judge to distinguish them. If A.K. is unable to persuade the court to extend the patient-physician privilege to her and continues to refuse to abide by the terms of the subpoena and testify, a judge then may find her in contempt of court and impose whatever penalty he sees fit. This penalty may include fines, imprisonment, or both.

The language of these orders and the nature of the action enforcing them sums up the law's attitude toward them. A citizen ignores such orders of a court at his or her peril. Continued disregard leaves them in contempt of the authority of the law manifested through the court.

Nevertheless, A.K. may feel that she cannot in good conscience comply with the court order, even if this holds significant legal consequences for her. A.K. may believe she has a moral obligation to assist a person who is part of the same community (the apartment block) as herself. She also might note that the 1994 version of the American Pharmaceutical Association's Code of Ethics for Pharmacists requires the pharmacist to serve the patient "in a private and confidential manner," and "to act with conviction of conscience." She also might hold that, although citizens generally have a moral duty to obey the law, this duty is not absolute, particularly when the rights or welfare of a patient are at stake. Thus, A.K. could reason, she is ethically obligated to engage in an act of civil disobedience and not comply with the court order, because her first duty is to her patient. This case suggests that what is illegal may be not only ethically *permissible* but ethically *required*.

To continue exploring the relationship between ethics and the law, let us consider a second case.

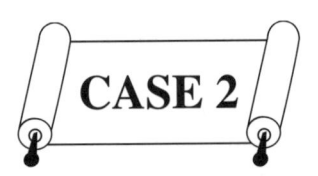

CASE 2

J.W. recently passed the state board of pharmacy licensure examination, and was granted a license to practice pharmacy. She accepted a job with a large chain store, working in a pharmacy in her home town.

On her first day at work, a young woman presented to J.W. a prescription for four tablets of Ovral, with directions to take two tablets immediately and two in 12 hours. J.W. told K.O., Pharm.D., the pharmacy manager, that she could not fill the prescription because of her religious beliefs. These beliefs preclude her from dispensing medications that interrupt a pregnancy after fertilization.

Dr. K.O. tells J.W. that before accepting the position she should have realized that all sorts of drugs have to be dispensed as part of the job. Dr. K.O. states that there is no room in pharmacy for individual pharmacists to assert their personal beliefs about medications. J.W. is ordered to dispense the medication, and not to talk with this patient or any other patient about her personal beliefs or other factors unrelated to the therapeutic aspects of the patient's drug therapy.

Case Discussion

At least three parties have an interest in this case. The patient has an interest in having her prescription filled. J.W. has an interest in exercising her right to practice her religion freely, even if this conflicts at times with her duty to practice pharmacy in accordance with the standards of the profession. Her employer has an interest in seeing that patients receive their prescriptions without undue interference. Whose interests ought to take precedence if there is an unresolvable conflict among them?

Federal legislation prohibits an employer from using religion as a basis for the terms, conditions, or privileges of employment. Regulations made under the legislation indicate that employers, in seeking to comply with the duty not to discriminate, are obliged to accommodate the reasonable religious needs of employees where such an accommodation can be made without undue hardship to the conduct of the business. As will be explained in greater detail in Chapter 9: Do Pharmacists Have a Right to Refuse to Fill Prescriptions for Abortifacient Drugs?, this legislation is a part of the civil law, and when an employer violates this law, an employee is entitled to compensation.

Because of the law that prohibits religious discrimination in the employer-employee relationship, J.W. may believe that she has a legal right to not fill certain prescriptions. She might also hold that, whether or not a law allows for her refusal, she has a moral right to practice her religion freely, even if this means that, on occasion, she will not be able to perform the duties of a pharmacist. The pharmacist could reason that she would like to fulfill her obligations both to her profession and to her faith, but if there is a conflict, the latter takes precedence for her. In other words, J.W. could claim that ethics, and not the law, ultimately establishes the standards of conduct.

Suppose J.W. explained this in private to Dr. K.O. and she replied that, although she appreciates J.W.'s situation, a pharmacist's first responsibility is to serving the health care needs of the public. When a patient presents with a valid prescription of any kind, the pharmacist has a moral duty to fill the prescription, Dr. K.O. continues. "Frankly, I think you have your priorities in the wrong order," she tells her employee. "You should have known when you were in pharmacy school that you might have to subordinate your religious beliefs to meet the needs of patients."

"Yes, I did know what I was getting into," J.W. replies, "but I figured that health care professionals would make some allowances for people like me who have strong moral convictions. As you know, I worked very hard in pharmacy school and did very well, and I just assumed that someone with my knowledge and skills still would able to make a significant contribution to the welfare of patients, even if I wouldn't be able, in good conscience, to do everything that was asked of me. After all, a Catholic physician isn't legally or morally obligated to perform abortions. Why should I be obligated to dispense birth control pills?"

"You know, in most workplaces, people put aside their personal convictions for the sake of getting along with others. The workplace is called that because it's where we *work*. If you are troubled by the work that pharmacy entails, then I suggest that you look for another profession," Dr. K.O. tells her directly.

"That's such an inflexible position," J.W. says with some hesitancy. "Can't you just excuse me from having to fill prescriptions for contraceptives? I mean, I'm not asking that you not stock these drugs, or that I be free to counsel patients about my views. I'm just requesting that my right to practice my religion be respected, that's all."

If Dr. K.O. chooses to fire J.W. on the grounds that the employee is unwilling to perform the duties expected of her, J.W. could choose to file a wrongful discharge suit. Ironically, it is often only through such a suit that an employee will be able to enforce specific employment rights. Would J.W. win such a suit? If the court determines that the law does apply to her case, and the employer did not make a reasonable attempt to accommodate her religious beliefs (for example, by reallocating her duties when patients present with prescriptions for contraceptive medications), then she very well may be entitled to compensation.

CONCLUSION

The good pharmacist takes the law seriously, because she is legally required to do so, and because we all are morally obligated to be law-abiding citizens. Nevertheless, sometimes laws are outdated, incomplete, or even unjust. Laws prohibiting women from voting, or requiring African-Americans to sit at the back of the bus were simply wrong. Conversely, even if it is legally permissible to do X, it might be inappropriate or unethical to do X. We hope that in this chapter we have suggested when the pharmacist is faced with a quandary, the good pharmacist looks to the relevant law, but also thinks carefully about their moral obligations. In many cases, there will not be a conflict between the two. Sometimes, however, he or she may need to rely upon the skills of ethical decision making to provide a satisfactory answer to the question, "What should I do?" Chapter 4: Ethical Decision Making, will help you develop this skill.

Discussion Questions

1. Can you think of a situation where you might be ethically *required* to do something that is *illegal*? How might you respond to this challenge?

2. Write a scenario in which a pharmacist is asked to do something that is legally *permissible*, but is either ethically *inappropriate* or even blatantly *unethical*. What should the pharmacist do, and why?

3. Discuss a present or historic law that you believe is unethical. Why is or was such a law on the books? What does this suggest for the ways in which laws are developed and passed?

4. Why does it make sense to say that there is a moral obligation to take the law seriously? Why does it also make sense to say that this obligation is not absolute?

REFERENCES

1. Brushwood D. Pharmacy Law. Colorado Springs: McGraw-Hill; 1986.

Chapter 4

Ethical Decision Making

Bruce D. Weinstein

When you are faced with a moral problem, how should you proceed? There are many ways of answering this question, but a particularly useful way is to approach the problem *systematically*. This chapter proposes a four-step approach: 1) gather the relevant *facts*, 2) identify the *values* that play a role, 3) generate *options* open to you, and 4) *select* an option and *justify* it. I apply this approach to two clinical cases involving pharmacists faced with common ethical dilemmas. After identifying the ethical questions the case raises, and showing why these questions are ethical ones, I ask us to consider what facts we need to answer the ethical questions responsibly. These facts include, but are not limited to, medical, social, and psychological information.

Facts are necessary, but by themselves they are inadequate for answering ethical questions. In addition to facts, values play an important role, for they give rise to *moral rules*. I show which values are imbedded in the cases before us, and which moral rules correspond to those values. The next step is to consider options open to the pharmacist, or in other words, to answer the question, "What *could* be done?" It is in picking an option and supporting it with reasons that put us in the position of stating what *should* be done.

Each step in the protocol builds logically on the preceding steps. Still, some steps may be easier than others; you may find it easier, for example, to gather facts than to identify values, and to generate options than to justify one. This may be because pharmacy education focuses on the technical aspects of pharmacy, and on developing problem-solving skills. One of the themes that emerges from this book, however, is that pharmacy is not merely a technical enterprise. As a profession, values, especially moral values, determine what pharmacists ought to do in their care of patients, as well as shape what pharmacists actually do. The purpose of this chapter is to help you to identify some of these values, to see how they sometimes come into conflict, and to use them (along with the relevant facts) to support the choices you make. In developing such skills you will be taking important steps toward improving patient care and doing for patients what they want to have done for themselves. (Please see an additional commentary by two noted pharmacists follows this chapter.)

Consider the following scenario.

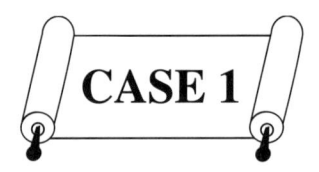

CASE 1

M.M. is a 76-year-old patient of Dr. T.D. and is being treated for hypertension. She had previously been treated with diuretics and β-blockers separately, but the drugs had been stopped because of side effects (orthostatic hypotension in the case of the diuretics). Dr. T.D. decides to try Ismelin (guanethidine) and prescribes 20 mg daily. Patient M.M. presents the prescription to her pharmacist, P.L., but pharmacist P.L. knows that there are potentially severe side effects, especially orthostatic hypotension, with this drug, and that it is no longer commonly used. Pharmacist P.L. believes that alternative antihypertensive medications would be more appropriate. When she calls Dr. T.D. and suggests this, the physician becomes irate and tells her angrily, "This is not your area of expertise. You don't even know this patient. Leave prescribing drugs to me, and just fill the prescription." P.L. hangs up the phone and is troubled by the situation.[a]

Case Discussion

There are many different kinds of questions suggested by this case. They include, but are not limited to, the following:

---

[a] *Portions of this chapter appeared in Weinstein BD. Teaching Pharmacy Ethics: The Case Study Approach. In: Haddad AM, ed.* Teaching & Learning Strategies in Pharmacy Ethics*. Omaha: Creighton University; 1992:9–20. Weinstein BD. Ethical Issues in Pharmacy. In: Abood RR, Brushwood DB.* Pharmacy Practice and the Law*. Gaithersburg, MD: Aspen Publishers; 1994:310–23. Weinstein BD, Brushwood DB. Counseling: The Courts' Decisions.* U.S. Pharmacist*. 1992 March:76–7,81.*

1. What is the best drug treatment for patient M.M.'s hypertension?
2. What might happen to M.M. and to others if she takes the Ismelin?
3. Does M.M. have a right to know of the disagreement between the pharmacist and the physician?
4. Should the physician consider the pharmacist's suggestion?
5. Does the pharmacist have a right to refuse to fill the prescription for guanethidine?
6. Does the pharmacist have a responsibility to attempt to persuade the physician that guanethidine is potentially harmful to the patient?
7. Ought the pharmacist fill the prescription but counsel the patient about the potentially harmful side effects?
8. What are the pharmacist's duties to the profession and to society?

The first question is really one of efficacy, assuming that the physician, pharmacist, and the patient all are trying to achieve the same goal (i.e., the use of an antihypertensive medication that lowers blood pressure without significant side effects). The second question addresses the personal, medical, and social consequences of taking guanethidine. Although it is important to know these consequences when answering the relevant ethical questions, as we will see momentarily, question number two is not itself an ethical question. The remainder *are* genuine ethical inquiries, as certain key terms suggest: "right" (in the sense of entitlement) in number three and number five, "should" in number four, "responsibility" and "harmful" in number six, "ought" in number seven, and "duties" in number eight. Questions from three to eight, and only those questions, raise concerns about the appropriate *conduct* of someone, and/or have a direct reference to the welfare or rights of others. Whenever a question has such elements, it may be considered an ethical one.[b]

The purpose of this chapter is to present a method for approaching these and other ethical problems that arise in the clinical setting. Let us begin with a brief description of the field of ethics and the role it plays in the pharmacy profession.

---
[b] *Some might take question number one to be an ethical one because it appears to meet these criteria, but if one reasonably assumes that there is no dispute among the three parties about the goals of therapy, then the question may be translated, "Which drug is most likely to achieve the stated aims of the patient?" Seen this way, question number one is clearly not an ethical question.*

WHAT IS ETHICS AND WHAT DOES IT HAVE TO DO WITH PHARMACY?

Ethics is the systematic study of what is right and good with respect to conduct and character. As a branch of both philosophy and theology, ethics seeks to answer two fundamental questions: 1) *What* should we do?, and 2) *Why* should we do it? As an intellectual discipline, ethics is concerned not only with making appropriate decisions but with *justifying* them. Unlike other forums for the discussion of moral issues (e.g., television talk shows, barroom debates), ethics seeks to provide good reasons for our moral choices. In fact, it is the attempt to justify our actions that gives ethics its distinctive character.

Pharmacy ethics is an application of ethical rules and principles to the practice of pharmacy. To ask what a pharmacist should do in a particular case is to ask an ethical question, and to justify our answer we appeal to the same rules and principles that apply to persons in society generally.[1] For example, the pharmacist's obligation to protect patient confidentiality is merely an application of the rule that all of us have to guard carefully information that is entrusted to us. Sometimes, however, health care professionals are ethically required to assume risks not shared by laypersons, such as caring for persons with AIDS.[2] To be a professional thus involves having certain obligations not shared by nonprofessionals. To understand why this is, it is helpful to examine what it means to be a pharmacist, and how pharmacy differs from other occupations.

Pharmacy as a Moral Practice

Pharmacy is a moral practice, because pharmacists are concerned primarily with using their knowledge and skills to advance the interests of patients, and to do for patients what patients wish to have done for themselves. Unlike members of other occupations (e.g., business), the pharmacist places the interests of others above his or her own interests. Indeed, this feature of pharmacy is one of the defining characteristics of the health care professions in general. Every encounter between a pharmacist and a patient implicitly raises ethical issues, because a pharmacist may—and indeed must—ask questions about how the welfare of the patient should be promoted.

Although every encounter between pharmacist and patient raises ethical issues, these issues are not necessarily ethical *problems* or *dilemmas*. A situation in which two or more choices are morally justifiable, but only one is capable of being acted upon at a particular time, represents a moral dilemma.[3] A pharmacist who has to decide between protecting a patient from harm and filling a prescription, as is the case with pharmacist P.L., is caught in an ethical dilemma, since there are moral reasons for justifying each of two mutually exclusive options. No moral dilemma exists for a pharmacist when a patient provides a legitimate prescription to be filled and is able to pay for the medication, but the situation raises a moral *issue*, namely whether the pharmacist ought to act in the best interests of the patient and fill the prescription. Moral issues are unavoidable in pharmacy because of the nature of professions in general and pharmacy in particular.

To ask what one should do as a pharmacist is often to ask a legal question as well, but it is incorrect to *reduce* the question to a matter for the legislature or the courts to resolve. Indeed, for any legislative or judicial resolution to a problem concerning appropriate conduct, we may—and indeed should—ask, "Is the law a *good* one?," or "Was the court *right*?" It will be the assumption of this chapter that ethics, and not the law, establishes the ultimate standard for evaluating conduct.[4] Still, there is a moral obligation to obey the law, and thus ethical analyses need to take into account the relevant statutes and court decisions.

A difficult problem in ethics concerns the *source* of ethical standards. People have appealed to many sources of authority in ethics: religious texts (e.g., the Bible, the Koran), natural law, philosophical argument (reason), intuition, personal experience, governmental decree, and the free negotiations of persons within a community. Traditionally in pharmacy, it has been the members of the profession who have selected its ethical norms and established codes of ethics. Because laypersons have a significant stake in the way that professionals conduct themselves, however, it is appropriate to include them in the selection of these norms.[5] Our discussion thus will be based not only on what the profession of pharmacy has held to be right and good, but more broadly upon what a reasonable person with knowledge of the relevant facts might hold to be appropriate.

All moral problems have both a technical and an evaluative component. That is, the answer to the question, "What should we do?," requires technical information as well as information about values. Suppose, for example, that a 63-year-old patient states that, although she cannot pay for a medication she claims she needs, she has a right to it. The expertise that pharmacists have by virtue of their scientific education and technical experience may allow them to decide to what degree her *clinical* claim is justified (i.e., whether the medication would promote her physical health). This technical expertise does not, however, confer an ability to assess the *moral* claim that the patient has a right to the treatment.[6,c] How, then, are such claims to be evaluated, if not through technical expertise? Let us turn next to a protocol that may help one to systematically consider ethical problems that arise in the clinical setting, or anywhere else for that matter.

ETHICAL DECISION MAKING IN PATIENT CARE

After identifying an ethical question facing you in patient care:

1. Gather the medical, social, and all other relevant facts of the case.
2. Identify all relevant values that play a role in the case and determine which values, if any, conflict.
3. List the options open to you. That is, answer the question, "What *could* you do?"
4. Choose the best solution from an ethical point of view, justify it, and respond to possible criticisms. That is, answer the question, "What *should* you do, and why?"

Suppose that your best friend calls you one evening and tells you that he is faced with a difficult ethical dilemma involving an intimate other. "I don't know if I should leave this relationship or try to work it out," your friend says. "Please give me some advice!" What will be your response—to make a recommendation right away, or to ask for more information? Most people choose the latter. This is because we recognize that good moral decision making begins with getting the facts straight. Thus, the *first step* for making ethical decisions, in the clinical setting or anywhere else, is *gathering the relevant facts*.[7] What are the relevant facts in the case concerning patient M.M.?

The most critical piece of information we have is that the patient has a history of orthostatic hypotension, that this is one of the major side effects of the drug that has been prescribed for her, and that there are other drugs available that do not commonly have this as a side effect. While not necessarily life threatening itself, orthostatic hypotension may place the patient and others at great risk of harm, since the condition may involve losing

---
[c] *The patient may be making a legal claim as well, because rights may be justified by an appeal to the law as well as to moral rules and principles. While it plays a role in the peaceable resolution of disputes between pharmacists and patients, the legal component of these issues will not be considered in this chapter.*

consciousness, and the patient may be operating machinery, descending a staircase, or holding an infant when this occurs. Since we have noted that legal obligations are morally relevant, the pharmacist also should consider what the law requires of him or her. Although there is a general legal duty to inform physicians and patients of the potential risks of drug therapy, the specific laws in a case such as this vary from state to state.

To resolve an ethical dilemma such as the one in this case, facts are necessary but not sufficient. Addressing moral problems differs from addressing mere technical ones in that the former involves a consideration of values as well as facts.[6] In addition to the relevant facts, an appropriate response to the question, "What should you do?," requires an account of the values that play a role in the case, and what moral guidelines or rules those values suggest. *Identifying values* is thus the *second step* of ethical analysis. Certainly one important value suggested by the case is the welfare of the patient, which gives rise to the moral rule, "Protect others from harm." Pharmacist P.L. has good reason to believe that filling the prescription for the guanethidine will result in harm, not only to her patient, who already has experienced one of the known side effects of the prescribed drug, but also possibly to others who may come into contact with the patient. Her moral commitment to do no harm justifies the feeling she has that it would be wrong to fill the prescription.

If avoiding harm to patients were the only important moral consideration in the case, P.L. would not be faced with a dilemma, since it would be clear that she should not fill the prescription. There are other values, however, that play a role here. One of them is the pharmacist-physician relationship. Pharmacists are rightly obligated to promote a good relationship with the physicians with whom they work, and this obligation includes a responsibility to fill the prescriptions the physicians provide. A third value is respect for patient autonomy, or more specifically the patient's right to have information that will enable her to make an informed decision about her health care. This value gives rise to the rule requiring both the physician and pharmacist to provide the patient with the relevant facts about the likely consequences of various drugs, as well as no drug therapy at all. The final value that plays a role in this case is respect for the law, which requires the pharmacist to do what is legally required of him or her. We now have the makings of a genuine ethical dilemma: the pharmacist is bound to avoid harming her patients and others, but she is also committed to promoting a professional relationship with the prescribing physician, as well as to counseling her patient. To which moral rule, and thus to which group of people, does she ultimately owe allegiance?

This brings us to the *third stage* of ethical analysis, *generating options*. In other words, we might ask, "What *could* pharmacist P.L. do?" In class, I emphasize that this is the creative step of our process, and not surprisingly, this step usually elicits a greater response from students than the previous step (though not quite as great as identifying the relevant facts). Among the options open to pharmacist P.L. are to 1) fill the prescription but counsel the patient about the risks of the medication; 2) refuse to fill the prescription and explain to the patient why; and 3) attempt to persuade the prescribing physician to change the prescription. There are other possible courses of action, but these are the most obvious ones and correspond most closely to the values presented earlier. Which option is best from a moral point of view, and why?

To answer this question, we take the fourth and final step of ethical analysis, *choosing an option and justifying it*. If it were the case that P.L. had to choose between competing loyalties, it would be difficult to hold that her final decision must be to respect the wishes of the physician. After all, the primary commitment to the welfare and rights of patients distinguishes pharmacy as a moral practice. Still, it might not be necessary for pharmacist P.L. to choose between these apparently conflicting responsibilities. She might call Dr. T.D. back and provide the justification for her belief that alternative antihypertensive medications offer fewer risks to the patient than does guanethidine. Sometimes ethical conflicts can be handled adequately by exercising personal skills rather than by having to make tough choices, and this may be one of those cases. Only if such an attempt is unsuccessful will P.L. have to decide whether loyalty to Dr. T.D. requires placing her patient and others at risk.

One conclusion we may draw from this case is that turning to the law will not always help us resolve moral quandaries. Even if it is legally permissible for a pharmacist to dispense the medication, the pharmacist still may ask, "What is the *right* thing for me to do?" The analysis also suggests that some approaches to ethical problems in the clinical setting are more ethically defensible than others, and that through ethical analysis one is able to distinguish better from worse approaches. It is sometimes the case that any option one picks will have unfortunate consequences (in this case, the patient may be extremely upset by the refusal to dispense the medication), but this is not the same as saying that there are no answers to ethical problems. Indeed, the circumstances pharmacists find themselves in often require *some* kind of decision or action, and thus in many instances it is impossible to avoid making moral choices. Through ethical analysis and reflection, as well as discussing the problem with others in a systematic way, one is more likely to achieve a reasoned and justifiable decision.

One might think that the process of ethical decision making is too time-consuming and complex to use in the clinical setting. Obviously in emergent situations, the moral mandate of the pharmacist is to save the patient's life or prevent irreversible harm from occurring. Such situations arise relatively infrequently in pharmacy. For troubling ethical problems, it is both prudent as well as ethically appropriate to take some time to reflect upon one's options and consider the best reasons for choosing some rather than others. As the second case will show, the ethical issues raised in patient care are often strikingly similar, even if the clinical details differ.

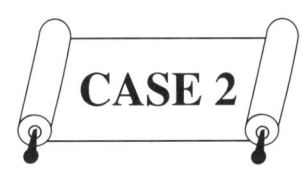

CASE 2

H.N., a pharmacist in a community drug store, recently created a program of patient counseling, featuring a pamphlet with 20 cautionary statements for pharmacists to make when appropriate. The program was well received by area physicians until Dr. G.M., a general practitioner, telephoned H.N. one day with a complaint concerning a prescription for phenytoin she had written for a patient with a convulsive disorder. The patient began consuming several ounces of alcohol daily after starting the medication and shortly thereafter experienced severe seizures. Dr. G.M. reprimanded pharmacist H.N. for neglecting to mention the danger of mixing alcohol and the prescribed drug, and added that the pharmacist had failed in his ethical responsibility to the patient. Is Dr. G.M. correct?

Case Discussion

We recall that good ethical decision making begins with getting the facts. The relevant facts in this case are that the chronic use of phenytoin and alcohol induces an increase in microsomal enzymes, which in turn may lead to a decrease in serum phenytoin levels. This decrease may be sufficient to induce seizures in persons who are predisposed to them, so

Dr. G.M. is correct in suggesting that alcohol presents a danger to patients taking the anticonvulsant drug phenytoin.

Facts are necessary but not sufficient to determine whether pharmacist H.N. failed to fulfill a moral obligation to his patient. First, one might ask where a pharmacist's obligation to counsel patients comes from. Because H.N. developed a patient counseling program, he is identifying himself as one who is willing to assume the responsibility for ensuring that patients are given the necessary information about the drugs prescribed for them. The duty, then, is self-imposed, and Dr. G.M. appears to be justified in reprimanding the pharmacist.

Pharmacist H.N. might claim that he was taking on a responsibility that belongs with the physician to begin with. According to this position, it is the physician, and not the pharmacist, who is morally (and legally) responsible for obtaining informed consent for medical interventions, including medications. The first element of informed consent is the disclosure of information a patient would need to make a decision based on their preferences and values. Because most patients would wish to avoid seizures, it is important to warn them about potential interactions with the drug the physician wants to prescribe.

Dr. G.M. could show that pharmacist H.N. failed to act in an ethically responsible manner if she were to appeal to the following moral rule: "When one is in a position to prevent harm to another without assuming a great risk of danger, one should do so." A pharmacist, Dr. G.M. might say, ought to know that alcohol consumption is contraindicated for patients taking phenytoin. Neglecting to mention this to such patients thus fails to fulfill the pharmacist's responsibility to protect others from harm. However, Dr. G.M. herself must realize that she too ought to know such basic pharmacology, and must accept some responsibility for failing to ensure the safety of her patients.

Rather than arguing about who ultimately has the obligation to disclose relevant information to patients, Dr. G.M. and pharmacist H.N. might agree to be more aware of their shared responsibility to protect patients from harm and to promote their health.

CONCLUSION

Even though the cases involve different patients with different kinds of problems, the general ethical question is the same: What should the pharmacist do? To be more specific, the *values* that play a role in the case are the same. This chapter has suggested that being a pharmacist involves more than possessing certain skills or having clinical knowledge. If pharmacy is understood to be a moral practice, then pharmacists have moral obligations, including, but not limited to, promoting the welfare of patients, protecting them from harm, and respecting their right of self-determination. Still, being technically competent and respecting patients rights are *necessary* but not *sufficient* conditions of being a good pharmacist. Developing the professional virtues of kindness, compassion, and a sense of justice, among others, also plays an important role in the moral life of the professional.

According to the protocol presented in this chapter, one may systematically approach ethical problems in clinical pharmacy by 1) gathering the relevant *facts* pertaining to the case, 2) clarifying the *values*, 3) *generating options* open to the pharmacist, and finally 4) *picking an option and justifying it*. Nevertheless, ethical analysis is only a tool for the conscientious pharmacist. It is up to the practitioner to fulfill the moral responsibilities that give pharmacy its distinctive character as a profession.

Discussion Questions

1. Someone sees you carrying this book and says, "Pharmacy ethics? I've heard about medical ethics, but what's an example of an ethical issue in *pharmacy*?" How would you respond?

2. Sometimes we finding ourselves saying, "If only I had known X, I would have made a different decision!" While there is only so much information we can reasonably collect, what does this suggest about the importance of beginning our analysis of moral problems with getting the facts?

3. How have you typically approached ethical problems in your life? Has this approach been satisfactory? What would you like to keep, and what would you like to change about this approach?

4. Use the protocol described in this chapter to identify and reflect upon an ethical question you have faced in pharmacy practice. In what ways is a systematic approach to ethical problems more useful than other kinds of approaches (for example, using your intuition or asking a friend)? In what ways is it less useful?

5. Consider the following statement: Pharmacists have no moral obligations to anyone other than themselves. Pharmacy students have to make a lot of personal sacrifices to get through pharmacy school. By the time they graduate, they're entitled to the good life.

Applying the Process of Ethical Decision Making

Robert A. Buerki
Louis D. Vottero

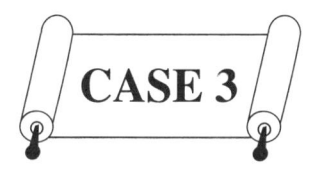

CASE 3

As a hospital pharmacy director and chair of the Pharmacy and Therapeutics committee, it is your responsibility to assist this committee in deciding which drugs should be in the formulary. Physicians want the hospital to have available a new drug that has been shown to be efficacious in reducing mortality from infection among cancer chemotherapy patients. Placing this drug in the formulary and stocking it for anticipated use will require 15% of your total budget and requires elimination of some other more frequently used medications. What should you do?[8]

Case Discussion

As pharmacists share the expanded decision making and accountability associated with providing good pharmaceutical care, they often become embroiled in making decisions that go beyond therapeutics. This case makes it clear how pharmacists can influence the medical outcomes of patients under their care: the physicians on the P & T committee wish to make a new—and expensive—anti-infective medication available to cancer chemotherapy patients to improve the quality of their life. As pharmacist and chair of the P & T committee, you understand that setting aside

15% of your annual drug budget to purchase one expensive anti-infective drug to treat a small number of cancer chemotherapy patients will require you to look closely at your drug product selection process for the remaining 85% of your drug budget, necessitating choices that will affect a far larger number of patients who not only have less serious medical conditions but also who have a better chance to survive and live a fruitful and productive life. This case presents an ethical problem because it involves the difficult challenge of allocating health resources to some and denying them to others.

The question "What should you do?" suggests a broad range of preliminary questions that must be addressed. Are there other less expensive therapies that would be equally efficacious? Are there methods for securing this life-saving drug for these patients other than placing it in the hospital formulary? Should both the cancer chemotherapy patients and the other patients who may be denied other drugs be part of the dialogue? Will all cancer chemotherapy patients have a right of access to this new drug, or will the indigent be excluded because of cost? Do all members of the medical staff, or only the oncologists wish to include the new drug in the formulary? What will be the effect on those patients who may be denied other medications if the new anti-infective is added to the formulary? Who is responsible for protecting the rights of those patients who may be denied access to other medications? How will the pharmacist-oncologist relationship change if the new drug is not included on the formulary? How will the oncologist-patient relationship change if the cancer chemotherapy patients are denied access to the drug? Some of these questions address clinical concerns that fall outside of any ethical dilemma: some others raise serious questions about behavior that can have a direct impact on the rights and welfare of others. Still others look at human relationships and the possibility of change that may ultimately affect patient welfare. These questions provide the framework for a complex series of interwoven events involving patient rights, patient welfare, and professional relationships, all of which combine to build an ethical dilemma.

At the heart of this dilemma is the difficulty of balancing benefits for a few cancer chemotherapy patients on the one hand, and for a large group that will use other, more frequently prescribed medications on the other. The institution's physicians supposedly are willing to restrict their freedom of choice of therapy for the vast majority of their patients in order to provide some added benefit to a small minority of severely ill patients. Expensive, high-tech pharmaceuticals present a special challenge to pharmacists, for there is no distinct reimbursement strategy in place for the use of these drugs from insurance companies and other third parties. Insurance companies that do not accept claims for the use of these expensive drugs effectively shunt this expense to the patient, or—if the patient is unable to pay—to the hospital itself. Moreover, the management strategies of pharmacoeconomic analysis, which are aimed at the safe, cost-efficient, and cost-effective use of all drugs through careful formulary management, may restrict access to such expensive pharmaceutical products. Finally, if drug prices and total costs for drugs on the hospital formulary are capped, should the sole responsibility for drug product selection rest with pharmacists and physicians, or should administrators, hospital board members, and patients have representation?

Let us make some factual assumptions before considering what you ought to do in this case. We assume that the pharmacist has legal permission to choose one—or none—of the options. Furthermore, we assume that this hospital is a typical acute-care institution, confined by finite resources, serving a typical mix of patients, not a comprehensive cancer treatment center. Similarly, we will suppose that this hospital is located within a culture that values individual rights more intensely than community rights. Finally, we assume that the other drugs on the formulary also make significant contributions to the quality of life of the institution's patients.

Justice or fairness is the central moral value that plays a role in this case. Although the concept of a right to health care is still being hotly debated, American society is committed to the ideal decent minimum of health care, and that pharmacists, physicians, and others have a duty to provide that care. In this case, conflict exists because of finite resources forcing allocations that may ultimately be unfair, that is, affecting a specific level of care. What criterion or criteria should society use in making health care allocations fairly? Some have proposed using the criteria of social worth and social contribution. Accordingly, one would look at the socioeconomic status of the patient, the patient's role in his or her family, the likelihood of success using the expensive anti-infective, the probable life expectancy of the patient, the patient's family role, the prospect of his or her future contributions to society, and the patient's previous record of service. Thus, a debilitated patient with a proven record of success, albeit a low life expectancy, would qualify for an expensive therapy.

Instead, we support using the criterion of equal opportunity for making health care allocations. With this standard, all patients should have equal opportunity to receive the best possible drug, perhaps by using some sort of random procedure whereby each individual selected to receive an expensive drug has an equal chance of being chosen to receive it. What *could* you do to fulfill your role as advocate for the welfare of all patients? You could include the new drug on the formulary, delete a corresponding number to balance the budget, and provide suitable information concerning the change to patients and physicians who are affected. A second option is not to include the new drug on the formulary, but still provide suitable information to affected patients and physicians. A third option is to allow patients access to the drug through a private payment process. Which option is best, ethically, and why?

The third option is the least justifiable. Most hospitals are community-supported institutions that proclaim they provide just, decent, and humane treatment to all patients, regardless of their ability to pay. As such, hospitals have a moral obligation to be fair and just to patients, and this option would violate that duty. Both the first or second option have unfortunate consequences. Without having specific information about the patient mix or the number and age of the cancer patients, the first option—denying the inclusion of the new drug onto the hospital formulary and providing reasonable information to all involved—would be most defensible. This action would no doubt be viewed by the oncologists and their patients as mean-spirited and harm-ful, but a cost-benefit analysis of the clinical results would justify this selection.

Unfortunately, there are no blueprints available for guiding the pharmacist on a course of equity and superior medical outcomes: it is difficult or impossible to compare the benefits of "reduced mortality" versus "improved quality of life." Nevertheless, the amount of funds needed to provide this benefit to cancer chemotherapy patients appears recklessly excessive when compared to the harm that may be inflicted to a larger number of other patients. This decision may be justified on the grounds of benefiting the greater number of patients within a medical context. Moreover, within the larger context of the total hospital community, the comparative cost-benefit analyses of these two groups of patients and the responsibility of the P & T committee to maintain the integrity of the hospital's drug budget adds credence to this decision.

This case is an example of the kind of ethical problems that pharmacists face in their expanding roles in health care delivery. As we have shown, resolving such ethical conflicts through reflective analysis may not provide easy answers, but it will assist the conscientious pharmacist in rising to the challenge of moral professional behavior.

REFERENCES

1. Clouser KD. Bioethics. In: Reich WT, ed. Encyclopedia of Bioethics. New York: Free Press; 1978:115–27.
2. Emmanuel E. Do physicians have an obligation to treat patients with AIDS? N Engl J Med. 1988;318(25):1686–690.
3. Beauchamp TL, Childress JF. Principles of Biomedical Ethics. 4th ed. New York: Oxford University Press; 1994:11.
4. Callahan JC, ed. Ethical Issues in Professional Life. New York: Oxford University Press; 1988.
5. Veatch RM. A Theory of Medical Ethics. New York: Basic Books; 1981.
6. Veatch RM. Generalization of expertise: scientific expertise and value judgments. Hastings Cent Stud. 1973;1:29–40.
7. Ackerman TF et al., eds. Clinical Medical Ethics: Exploration and Assessment. Lanham: University Press of America; 1987.
8. Adapted from Becker E. Ethical issues arising in biotechnology. In: Haddad AM, ed. Teaching and Learning Strategies in Pharmacy Ethics. Omaha: Creighton University Biomedical Communications; 1992:29.

Chapter 5

The Counterside Conversation: Application as Narrative in Pharmacy Ethics

Dawson S. Schultz
David S. Ornes

Several of the preceding chapters have discussed the role that ethical principles play in the moral life of the pharmacist. Although principles may help the pharmacist to respond to ethical challenges, they are not sufficient. In this chapter, we will discuss the role that *narrative* plays in giving meaning to the patient-pharmacist relationship. We will use a case study to suggest that the "counterside" conversation has all of the elements of a good story, and that a narrative approach to thinking about ethical issues in pharmacy will supplement or enrich a principle-based approach.

TOWARD AN "ETHICS OF RESPONSIBILITY" FOR PHARMACY

What does it mean to be a responsible pharmacist? More specifically, how can the pharmacist best achieve professional responsibility in his or her practice at "counterside"? These issues, which pertain to the task of defining the main standard for pharmacy ethics, give rise to what we will refer to as the "responsibility question" in pharmacy: *What is responsibility in pharmacy?*

Generally speaking, professional responsibility in pharmacy, as in other areas of health care, has been understood on the basis of an appeal to bioethical principles. While a number of principles are implicated in this appeal, two in particular have been most influential in defining the standard of professional responsibility. First and foremost, responsibility has been understood as helping the patient and avoiding harm to him (the principles of beneficence and nonmaleficence). More recently, however, the meaning of responsibility has been understood as treating the patient as an "end" in himself or herself, rather than as a means only (the principle of respect for autonomy). This newer standard, which often has been construed in terms of the patient's right to determine which health care she believes is in her own best interest, represents an important change in the meaning of responsibility in pharmacy.

According to this so-called "principled approach," the pharmacist or other health provider is best able (some would say *only able*) to understand and resolve moral issues and quandaries in health care settings on the basis of appeals to bioethical principle(s) (which are deduced from underlying ethical theories). This approach, sometimes described simply as "principlism," is the bioethical method or orientation originally formulated by Tom L. Beauchamp and James E. Childress in *Principles of Biomedical Ethics*.[a]

While some accounts of principlism are problematic, Bruce Weinstein in Chapter 4: Ethical Decision Making, makes constructive use of this approach by stipulating that pharmacy ethics "is an *application* of ethical rules and principles to the practice of pharmacy," (our emphasis). Although Weinstein emphasizes the role played by the application of principles in establishing the pharmacist's obligations and duties, still he does not give an account of how these principles are to be applied. In particular, he stops short of considering what we call the "question of application" in pharmacy ethics: *"How can the pharmacist best apply bioethical principles and rules at counterside, when engaged in the task of understanding and responding to the patient's medication needs and desires?"*

Our claim, generally speaking, is that the outcome of application in pharmacy ethics—the outcome of appeals to principle—is influenced not only by the *techniques or procedures* involved, but by the *type of process* in which the pharmacist anchors, and through which he conducts, the "appeal to principle" as well. That is, the task of responsibly understanding

---

[a] By "principlism," we refer to the so-called "principled approach" that is characteristic of "applied biomedical ethics." This approach was originally formulated by Tom L. Beauchamp and James F. Childress in Principles of Biomedical Ethics. *In our view, this approach presupposes a view of moral knowledge that is theoretical and technical in nature, rather than practical. This theoretical understanding of moral knowledge has dominated pharmacy ethics. For example, it is presupposed by Courtney S. Campbell and George F. Constantine in "The Normative Principles of Pharmacy Ethics" (Chapter 2).*

and responding to the patient's medication needs and desires is influenced by the formal knowledge and procedures of the *pharmacist as professional* (used as a means of realizing the desired purposes and goals of care). This task, however, also is affected by the complex experiential factors, including emotions, values, and interests, that influence how the *pharmacist as person* approaches and conducts the process wherein the purposes and goals of pharmaceutical care are chosen.

Our thesis, first, is that the appeal to principle or rule in pharmacy ethics is a narrative process that involves *writing* and *interpreting* a story—in this instance, the story of "this" patient's medication needs and desires. And second, we suggest that the type of process through which the story of "this" patient's medication needs and desires is constructed is conversational in nature, rather than formal or intellectual. While the story of these needs and desires is told "at counterside," the construction of this story is complex. It is shaped by multiple other narratives and interpretations, including, for example, the *biomedical narrative* involving certain pharmacological and medical considerations; the *autobiographical narrative* reflecting the life and experience of both the patient and the pharmacist as persons; and the *socioeconomic narrative* pertaining to the larger cultural and financial forces that influence the commercial transactions at the counterside. The actual dialogue that transpires between patient and pharmacist modulates and transacts these "hidden texts" in ways that produce the story of "this" patient's medication needs and desires. The *pharmaceutical narrative* is therefore written and interpreted through what we refer to simply as the *"counterside conversation."* The pharmacist's appeal to principle is not only an intellectual or technical procedure, but also a narrative event that is realized through the transactions of speech and language that comprise this conversation.

If the counterside conversation establishes the concrete significance of the pharmacist's obligations and duties in specific instances, it follows, therefore, that pharmacy is in need of a "dialogue ethics." That is, pharmacy is in need of an ethic that focuses upon and articulates the ethical requirements of fully responsible counterside conversation. This ethic is important, since it is through this conversation that the appeal to principle or rule is primarily realized and implemented when attempting to become a responsible pharmacist.

Before reflecting on the significance of the above claims, we will first present a brief pharmacy narrative that exemplifies some of the features of our approach. We will then examine some of these features in greater detail, in order to show the ethical significance of "counterside" conversation for the task of becoming a responsible pharmacist.

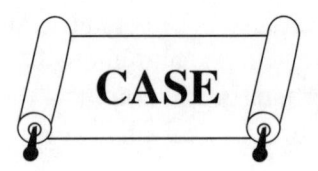

CASE

The Case of M.R.

A 33-year-old Hispanic woman, M.R., is at Safebet Pharmacy, Inc. requesting medication because her foot hurts. The pharmacist, H.B., knows M.R.'s family well because she has filled the family's prescriptions for the last several years. M.R. is the mother of three children (ages 12, 10, and 2). The pharmacist recommends that M.R. use one of the over-the-counter (OTC) antibiotic ointments that are currently on sale. M.R. picks up a small tube of triple antibiotic ointment and some sugar-free cough drops and then moves toward the front of the store after thanking pharmacist H.B. for her help. As M.R. moves past her, H.B. notices a distinct odor.

M.R. is accompanied by her 70-year-old mother-in-law, T.R., who lives with the family and often cares for the children. T.R. has complained to her daughter-in-law and now to pharmacist H.B. about her bowel habits; she is no longer as regular as she once was. H.B. remembered that T.R. has a history of hypertension, and gastrointestinal upset, witnessed by the two bottles of antacids she carries. T.R. reports dizziness when she strains at the stool and has come to the pharmacy with M.R. to see if she can get some quick and inexpensive medical advice from the pharmacist. H.B. recommends a stool softener for T.R.

After the family leaves the prescription counter area, H.B. decides to look at the family's medication profile. The pharmacy's patient medication history for 33-year-old M.R. reveals prescriptions for insulin, hydrochlorothiazide for mild hypertension, and birth control pills. H.B. notes that the prescription for insulin is not filled regularly and the birth control pills have not been filled at all for the past six months. The medication profile for T.R. shows that she also has been less than compliant with her furosemide prescription.

Pharmacist H.B. looks up from her computer and sees that both ladies are still in the store. She then looks over and sees that she has two other patients waiting for their prescriptions. She thinks to herself, "Now what should I do?"

The Role of Narrative and Dialogue in Interpreting the Pharmacist's Professional Responsibility

Pharmacist H.B. in this case may or may not have had the opportunity to participate in a formal study of bioethics while engaged in her pharmaceutical education. Consequently, her understanding of professional responsibility may not have been formed on the basis of an intellectual or reflective grasp of the concepts of beneficence, nonmaleficence, and patient autonomy (together with a variety of other bioethical concepts, principles, and rules). Her understanding, aspirations, and beliefs concerning what it means to be a responsible pharmacist may have been shaped instead by the web of examples and stories of responsibility that she encountered during her years of professional training, as well as by her upbringing and experience.

Although this pharmacist's concept of professional responsibility may not have been formed by an intellectual grasp of bioethical theory and principle, H.B., like many other fully responsible health professionals, nonetheless relies upon a "narrative understanding" of responsibility, that is, an understanding derived mainly from moral examples and stories in her background. This is not to suggest, however, that she might not have benefited from a more formal study of bioethical concepts, principles, and rules. Indeed, we believe that this type of study can be very beneficial in helping the student of moral education to develop various conceptual skills and competencies that will better enable him or her to sort through the moral complexities and ambiguities involved in patient care. This counterexample (to principlism) nevertheless raises the following question: Is there more to the moral life than ethical principles?

Most pharmacists and other health professionals do not have the benefit of a formal training in bioethical theory. Nevertheless, they succeed, more often than not, in providing fully responsible patient care. This fact suggests that the standard approach to bioethics—principlism—may be limited or inadequate in certain respects.

Principlism is limited, we suggest, because it wrongly assumes that the kind of moral or bioethical knowledge involved in responsible pharmacy practice is mainly or solely theoretical or technical in nature (knowledge logically deduced from bioethical principles). As mentioned above, however, the fact that many pharmacists lack this type of deductive knowledge, yet succeed in providing fully responsible care, calls into question how we can best understand the role played by theoretical bioethical knowledge in the formation of pharmaceutical responsibility.

In particular, it is not fully clear whether this "universal moral knowledge" supposedly derived from bioethical theory and principle *shapes—or is shaped by—the narratives and interpretations that tell the story of "this" patient's medication needs and desires*. It is, therefore, arguable whether this type of knowledge is at all necessary for the pharmacist to understand and resolve moral dilemmas at the counterside. If such knowledge were necessary, then, since expertise in ethical theory is required for attaining such knowledge, it would seem that most pharmacists (and other health professionals) would be incapable of engaging in responsible professional practice, because so many have not had the benefit of formal bioethics training (wherein such knowledge is supposedly acquired).

The idea that theoretical, deductive bioethical knowledge may not be an essential aspect of responsible pharmacy practice does not mean, however, that bioethical principles or rules are unimportant or play *no role* in the achievement of pharmaceutical responsibility (or in clinical decision making generally). At the same time, the role played by principles in the formation of the pharmacist's sense of professional responsibility is undoubtedly different than that often assumed in the "mainstream" approach of applied biomedical ethics. If the pharmacist's appeal to principle plays a narrative role as well as a technical role—if bioethical application is shaped by how the story of the patient's medication needs and desires is told as well as by the formal decisional procedures employed—at least two things are clear. First, the application process in bioethics is far more complex, and undoubtedly richer, than previously acknowledged by the mainstream approach. And second, it is imperative that we give greater attention to understanding how language, especially narrative and dialogue, shapes and influences "what is going on" in bioethical application.

In our view, bioethical principles can play a useful didactic role in moral education. They can be helpful in calling attention to the cognitive or intellectual dimension of ethics, thereby alerting pharmacists to, and heightening their awareness of, certain common moral considerations that pertain to many different types of situations at the counterside. But, although principles enjoy a certain universal grandeur, still, in and of themselves, their significance is shaped and formed through application comprised primarily by the linguistic interplay between patient and pharmacist, as well as among pharmacists themselves—the counterside conversation. This interplay is dynamic, in that it both reflects and, at the same time, shapes the patient and pharmacist's "stock of knowledge" which is inherited from their past examples and stories of responsibility. In this way, the counterside conversation not only "expresses" the sense of bioethical knowledge that guides responsible pharmacy practice, but "constitutes" this knowledge as well.

What is said in this conversation, as well as how and when it is said, and by whom, are not the only influences on bioethical application. The dynamics of this process, both literally and figuratively, comprise this application as well. The pharmacist's appeal to principle unquestionably involves technique. Still, application is always more than a mere technical production, because what gets applied in this process, first and foremost, is the pharmacist as a person.

Case Discussion

H.B. is fully alert to the importance of both establishing and maintaining effective, respectful, truthful communication with her patients: an exchange in which a "fusion of horizons" is formed between the parties involved, which potentially can leave them changed. By taking the time to enter into counterside conversation when other patients are waiting and when a backlog of prescriptions need to be filled, this pharmacist makes use of the opportunity to engage both M.R. and her mother-in-law, T.R., in a process of "question and answer." This dialogue, rather than the prescription and/or H.B.'s technical knowledge and expertise *per se*, on this occasion will largely determine how she understands, evaluates, and responds to M.R. and T.R.'s medication needs and desires. The events and interactions involved in this conversation will shape H.B.'s particular knowledge of how best to help the family, as well as how best to understand and respect their preferences or desires.

Of course, it would be very easy for H.B. simply to recommend the OTC products and to continue filling the other prescriptions that are awaiting her attention. H.B., however, senses a duty to these patients that no responsible pharmacist can ignore. Through her training and experience, she knows that something needs to be done for both of these women. M.R. may have a serious peripheral vascular condition, manifested through the foot problem, as a result of her diabetes. The distinct odor H.B. noted on M.R.'s breath could be an indication of ketoacidosis, and her diabetes may be out of control. There needs to be dialogue about these possibilities.

T.R. may be creating her own problems by taking antacids that cause constipation. She may not need more drugs at all, but merely need to alter her current regimen. The straining at the stool that causes dizziness may be a warning that her hypertension is not under control. Does she realize the seriousness of the disease and the consequences of her noncompliance? Does she wish to know? These questions need to be addressed through the counterside conversation because their answers bear directly upon H.B.'s ability to understand and to appropriately respond to T.R.'s medication needs and desires. In short, a dialogue between all the interested parties is needed to inform and help H.B. sort out T.R.'s problems and misconceptions.

Medical triage is frequently performed and health care advice given at the pharmacy counterside. This is the place where the patient and pharmacist meet to understand and negotiate various needs and desires associated with the delivery of health care. Each side brings something to the conversation that helps to shape and influence the unfolding story that defines these needs and desires.

Since there are two sides to the dialogue, the patient must be involved. The pharmacist must always remember that the patient is an integral part of this discussion. The *patient's* medication needs and desires, more than the pharmacist's personal preferences, directly influence not only his or her bodily chemistry, but, more importantly, the patient's *life,* and sometimes *death,* as well. Consequently, the patient's life (or death), not simply her chemistry, is the *subject matter* of pharmaceutical care. And so the patient's life must not only be a factor in this conversation, but must define what the conversation is about as well.

If the patient is not vested in the process at this point, she is not likely to appreciate the medication sufficiently to realize its optimal benefit. Such noncompliant behavior can negatively affect the patient's health status, as well as waste precious health care dollars. By the artful use of counterside conversation, the pharmacist can fulfill both the clinical and the ethical obligations of the profession.

This narrative illustrates a type of ethical dilemma faced every day by practicing pharmacists. In this particular case, there are many questions the pharmacist needs to ask herself. How much time do I have to spend with this family? What are my ethical obligations to these patients and how should I carry them out? Should I be doing something more for the family?

In general terms, answering the question, "How much time should I spend?," would be easy if one takes the pragmatic approach and answers, "Well, it depends." It is, of course, true that health care delivery is dependent in some ways upon the type of health care setting in which the pharmacist is practicing. A large chain pharmacy is or can be different than a small independent pharmacy, while both are different than a pharmacy in a community health clinic, doctors' office building, or hospital setting.

Is it, therefore, correct to say that the pharmacist who is practicing in the busy chain/grocery setting is not required to fulfill his or her obligation to the patient because there are too many prescriptions to fill? We think not. The pharmacist who is practicing in the "busy" chain pharmacy in an urban setting is obligated to take the same amount of time with the patient and to engage his or her patient in meaningful dialogue as the independent pharmacist practicing in a small town.

The ethics of M.R. and T.R.'s narrative make it clear that H.B. is obligated to take the time necessary to explore their level of understanding concerning their medical conditions and, where necessary, to fill in the gaps in their knowledge regarding their medication needs. In order to facilitate their recovery, however, a meaningful dialogue must be established that accomplishes several things: to ascertain how these patients actually understand their medical condition, and to explore and interpret their desires concerning the use of medication that is both "medically-indicated" and "pharmaceutically-correct." In short, this conversation is required in order to fulfill H.B.'s—or any pharmacist's—responsibility to the patient.

The narrative also raises the question about the pharmacist's comfort level with and/or knowledge level concerning the Hispanic culture in general, and this particular family's attitude toward individual wellness in particular. There could be knowledge deficits based on long-held family/cultural beliefs and traditions. Should the pharmacist do anything other than "fill and bill?" As implied by our thesis, he or she should engage the patient(s) in dialogue to find out what is going on in their situation of illness.

Another dimension of the narrative that affects the pharmacist's willingness to engage the patient in conversation, and that therefore impacts the quality of pharmaceutical care, concerns the following question: "What are the business interests versus the professional interests served with this interaction?" The theory that business interests and professional interests are not always congruent, and often are at odds, is held closely by many in pharmacy and often is used to rationalize questionable ethical behavior. This issue is contentious, not only in pharmacy, but throughout the entire system of health care.

From the business perspective, the predominant, current view is that firms that act in the best interest of their customers (patients) will realize the greatest amount of profit and prosperity—the idea that corporate flourishing can reflect the human flourishing of its members/employees. Applying this maxim, would it not be in the best interest of the pharmacy business to permit, even to encourage, pharmacists who are employees to engage in rational discussions with business managers about the "ethics of care" for their customers? Are pharmacists any longer able to justify decisions that are split by conflicts between the interests of business versus the interests of professionalism? Is not the most enlightened business decision to act in a thoroughly professional manner?

At yet another level, the narrative raises questions about the ethical implications concerning the pharmacist's professional responsibility. Should the family leave without receiving some type of intervention? Both of these women could have serious problems. What should the pharmacist do about them? Allowing these women to leave unassisted will amount to abandonment of one of the golden opportunities in health care service: the opportunity to make a positive contribution to a patient's health. On the negative side, allowing them to leave without proper pharmaceutical care will increase the potential for harm to one or both of them. On the positive side, however, the pharmacist has the opportunity to make a dramatic impact on the health of these two patients, since much could go wrong with either or both.

Finally, something left to speculation here is the need for, or frequency of, other health care services for these women. Why do we see a pattern of noncompliance on the part of both patients? Are they more concerned about their family's health than their own? Are there money problems associated with their health care and/or are there transportation problems associated with obtaining health care? Are there transcultural issues that affect the delivery of health care to these patients? Whatever the answers to these and other questions, it is certain both that the issues they raise are relevant and important to the health of the women, and that if answers are forthcoming, they will come only through a form of health care delivery that incorporates meaningful dialogue between pharmacist and patient as an integral aspect of care.

NARRATIVE ETHICS: THE EXPANSION OF "PRINCIPLE-BASED" ETHICS

As the story of these women illustrates, the role played by bioethical principles, such as beneficence and patient autonomy, in the formation of obligations and duties is more complex than often supposed. What is different about our view is that principles, alone, we think, do not *constitute* moral understanding and obligation. In one sense, these principles mainly *mirror or reflect* deeper issues that the pharmacist brings to counterside. In another sense, however, talk about ethical principles, even when conducted at a conceptual level, is or can become part of our everyday language (even though we might once have learned this language through the study of ethical theory).

Moral discourse involving reference to ethical principle, like moral stories, can motivate the pharmacist, but it also can help to illuminate his or her understanding of moral issues and problems as well. When the pharmacist's more abstract knowledge reflecting moral discourse does not appear to agree with his or her narrative understanding that is embedded in the moral story, the abstract knowledge derived from ethical principle sometimes can be informative. That is, this abstract knowledge can help to complete and even correct the pharmacist's narrative understanding, which may be incomplete, inchoate, or even wrong.

Even when this happens, however, the abstract knowledge derived from ethical principles is neither separated from, nor, at least on most occasions, opposed to the deeper moral understanding already embedded in the pharmacy narrative. The pharmacist's abstract knowledge and his or her narrative understanding, even when they appear to disagree, are not really different kinds of knowledge, but only different facets of the pharmacy narrative. The pharmacist's ability to complete, and even correct, his or her narrative understanding of the patient's medication needs and desires partly depends upon his or her rational capacities. In summary, narrative understanding, and the moral knowledge resulting therefrom, is neither distinct from nor opposed to rationality, but, in fact, exemplifies the form or type of practical rationality that we make use of in our mundane experience of the everyday world.

The unfolding of the narrative within M.R. and T.R.'s story—in particular, the force of the ensuing dialogue—"shakes and stirs" certain deeper sources within H.B. in ways that evoke within her a sense of practical wisdom. It is, we suggest, this practical wisdom, more than her intellectual knowledge of beneficence or respect for patient autonomy (however learned), that primarily moves her on this occasion to responsible pharmacy practice. Of course, this does not mean that her understanding and response to the women's medication needs and desires was not partly influenced by her knowledge of bioethical principles.

Nevertheless, if principles played a role in H.B.'s sympathetic engagement with and response to the women, narratively speaking, that role pertained to what was going on within the *process* that constituted the application of the principles. It had little or nothing at all to do with the sheerness of the principles themselves, prior to, or apart from the moment of application.

While the appeal to principle necessarily involves technical knowledge and skill, application itself, as earlier suggested, is essentially a dramatic or historical event or process, rather than an intellectual or technical production only. In other words, the process, through which the appeal to principle is conducted, is like the activity of *writing or telling a story*, more than it is like the technical procedures in a court of law involving formal appeals to rules of evidence. Good storytellers can make creative use of what philosophers call "formal" or "hypothetical-deductive" reasoning when spinning their tale, even though the process through which the tale is written has an essentially narrative structure. That is, the process is narrative, in the sense that the events that comprise the story *happen* or *unfold* in dramatic fashion through the "interplay of characters."

To summarize, application in pharmacy ethics (involving the "appeal to principle") is narrative, rather than technique (i.e., applied science or applied ethics), although this process makes use of technical knowledge both from the biomedical science of pharmacology and from biomedical ethics. It is the process through which the patient and pharmacist join together in writing and interpreting the story of "this" patient's medication needs and desires.

By way of further specifying and clarifying our thesis concerning the narrative significance of application in pharmacy ethics, we have suggested that the process through which the story of "this" patient's medication needs and desires is written and interpreted is essentially conversational in nature, rather than formal or intellectual (in the sense specified earlier).

The task of narrating and interpreting the story of "this" patient's medication needs and desires, like other aspects of pharmaceutical caregiving, is, itself, an essential aspect of, and is therefore governed by, this ethic of responsibility in pharmacy. Inasmuch as narrating and interpreting these needs and desires comprises application in pharmacy ethics, this activity or process, we think, should become the primary focus or task of pharmacy ethics. It is primary because how the story of this patient's medication needs and desires is told and interpreted shapes the significance of ethical principles and rules and thus, constitutes the meaning of the pharmacist's obligations and duties in specific cases.

If the purposes and goals of pharmaceutical care are affected by the type of process in which the application of principles and rules is anchored and conducted, as well as by the technique(s) employed in achieving the desired ends, then this brief outline of what is going on in the application process may help to illuminate the significance of responsibility in pharmacy ethics. Our working assumption is that the dynamics involved in the application of principles in pharmacy ethics—what we will refer to simply as "ethical process"—affect determination of the pharmacist's obligations and duties in specific instances. A greater appreciation of these dynamics also should help to illuminate what is meant by Weinstein's idea that the pharmacist's obligations and duties are *established* by the *application* of ethical principles and rules (rather, we would add, than by the sheerness of principles themselves).

If pharmaceutical care is affected by the application of principles and rules as Weinstein and others claim, and if, as we claim, this application is influenced and shaped by the type of process in which it is anchored and conducted, as well as by the technique(s) employed in achieving the desired ends, then more attention is needed as to how this process happens. In particular, what is needed is a complete description or account of this process in which appeals to principle are anchored and conducted. Such an account, we believe, will help us to better understand in more specific ways how it is possible to become a responsible pharmacist.

Discussion Questions

1. What are some ways in which it might be possible for patients to establish more communicative relations with their pharmacist at the counterside?

2. In what ways can dialogue between the patient and the pharmacist help to influence and shape a better understanding of the patient's medication needs and desires?

3. If application shapes the significance of bioethical principles and rules in specific instances, is it possible that a principle like beneficence (helping the patient) could mean different things under different circumstances (different applications)?

4. If counterside conversations between patients and pharmacists contribute an important ethical dimension to responsible pharmaceutical care, should we try to change the physical environment of pharmacy counters (to promote better communication)?

Chapter 6

Relationships with Patients and Physicians

Stuart G. Finder
David M. DiPersio

The first section of this book focused on several theoretical ethical foundations that may be linked to pharmacy practice. The second section turns to specific ethical considerations associated with being a practicing pharmacist. These concern the rights and responsibilities with which pharmacists must contend, individually and collectively, in their work.

What is the best way to address these practical, ethical considerations? This question is the subject of much debate. Many books on ethical issues in health care have followed the typical academic form of exposition and analysis of concepts, but it is becoming more widely accepted that narrative, rather than didactic, approaches better attend to the richness and continuity of actual moral experience.

We will follow this approach as we explore some of the ethical questions that arise in the relationships that pharmacists have with patients and physicians. For instance, although it is indisputable that pharmacists have ethical obligations to both patients and physicians, given the specifics of the circumstances in which patient-pharmacist-physician interactions occur, it is not always clear to whom the pharmacist is most obligated in a particular circumstance or what actions should be pursued to meet that obligation in that circumstance. To illustrate, we use a short story about two pharmacists who recount experiences that are characterized by this kind of ambiguity. One pharmacist works in a community pharmacy, and the other is based in a hospital setting. Both appreciate the ways in which the context of their interactions with patients and physicians reflect and shape what they believe and how they act.

Following the story, we provide a brief comment about how attending to the context of the pharmacist's interactions with patients and physicians is necessary for clarifying which values are present and how they operate in a given situation. Because the uniqueness of each situation influences how, and even if, it is possible to be so attentive, we acknowledge that being attuned as we are calling for may be extremely difficult. Nevertheless, we believe it is important to make this effort so that pharmacists can successfully meet the ethical challenges they face in their relationships with patients and physicians.

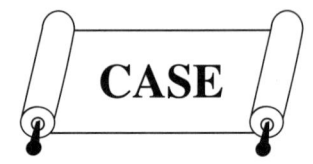

CASE

Two Pharmacists—A Common Story

Towards the end of the month, I was checking my inventory when the phone rang. Janet was calling from the hospital. I wasn't surprised to hear from her. Since we met 12 years ago during our pharmacy training at the University, we've developed a close professional friendship despite our different career choices. I own and operate a pharmacy in one of the more well-to-do suburbs in town. Janet, on the other hand, works as a clinical pharmacist in the medical intensive care unit (MICU) at University Hospital. I actually think that's why we get along so well—our daily professional lives are, in most ways, totally distinct and yet based in a shared profession. For instance, I'm not only a pharmacist, but a small business owner, and I have to be intimately familiar with any proposed legislation in our state and at the federal level that will affect both my ability to run a business and practice pharmacy. Unless I tell her about it, Janet rarely knows even when new legislation has been passed, let alone proposed. On the other hand, I'm slightly ashamed to admit, I don't keep up with the latest research; it's just not my interest. Janet, on the other hand, is often participating in that research, both in its laboratory as well as clinical phases. Janet keeps me informed about research and hospital-based pharmacy practice, and I keep her informed about the "real world" of pharmacy and business, patients and profit. I guess you could say we keep each other aware of the multitude of issues in and related to our profession. If there's one thing that both Janet and I share about pharmacy, it's a solid commitment to it. After all, one of the things that drew me to Janet back in school (in addition to the fact that her husband and I had been friends in elementary school) was the way she talked about being a pharmacist. I always wanted to be a pharmacist, and once in school, I thought everyone else in the program would be similarly passionate and committed. Unfortunately, there were many students who were interested only in the business prospects or the employment possibilities, who saw being a pharmacist merely as a job. Janet, on the other hand, shared my sense of pharmacy as a vocation, not because it was a means to something else, but because, in providing a service, there is a sense of fulfillment that extends beyond simply helping others. I guess that's what I mean by being committed to it.

Anyway, we shared that, and it was some consolation to find a soul mate. It's this philosophical bent that has served as the basis for many conversations, both in school and now years later, as we both follow our own particular interests in the field. And it is due to our mutual interest in some of the more philosophical questions associated with pharmacy that motivated Janet to call me today.

Janet's Tale

As part of her daily routine in the MICU, Janet rounds with the MICU team. The team is a big group. It is composed of an attending physician trained in intensive care medicine; a Fellow currently training in ICU medicine; two residents and two interns from internal medicine; occasionally a fourth-year medical student; the MICU clinical nurse specialist; the various nurses caring for the patients in the MICU; and occasionally a medical ethics consultant. At times, Janet also has a Pharm.D. student who is rotating through the MICU as part of his training. "Sometimes rounds are pretty unwieldy," Janet has told me, "both in terms of the space we take up in the hall, and in terms of the time for any real discussion." As I recall from my own training, this is especially true at the beginning of the month when the new attending physician and the new residents and interns all come onto service. I remember it seeming like the whole first week of the month was a period of reorientation. That is, unless there's a particularly dynamic case, which means a case that the physicians are really excited about. The end of the month wasn't necessarily better, since by then the residents—after having been on call every other night—and the attending—who only does this three times a year—are pretty burned out. By the last several days of the month, most talk is about getting out of the unit and back to a normal life.

The Fellows rotate in and out of the intensive care unit over six-week periods, so their comings and goings don't cause too much disruption, at least for Janet. And of course the nurses are like Janet: they are always there (although like everywhere else in the hospital, there's a high turnover rate for nurses, so in any given week, chances are good that there'll be a new nurse in the unit).

Having been around the unit for close to seven years now, Janet knows most everybody—and if she doesn't know you, she'll take some time to try to get to know you at least well enough to get a handle on your clinical practice. Even though Janet works in the high-tech world of a major medical center, she's still what you might call a "people person." She's a firm believer that for her to do her job effectively, as much as she needs to be up-to-date on the latest pharmaceutical thinking, she needs to have a good sense of how all of the different participants in the unit work and think. In this way, when she's asked for advice or to give some input, she's better able to anticipate others' responses—both medically and politically. There are certain personnel mixes (e.g., this attending and that nurse, or this resident and that Fellow) that are like paper and fire. Even when not working directly together—they're simply in the same proximity with one another—things can get pretty heated. Janet tells me she tries to avoid getting in between these occasional eruptions, which means paying attention to individual personality as much as anything. As a fact of institutional life, those personal interactions influence the workings of any unit in subtle yet significant ways. To tell you the truth, it's one reason why I chose not to work in such a setting. That things don't always run smoothly is also one of the reasons Janet sometimes calls me, and today was no exception.

Janet told me that during rounds today discussion was particularly spirited. This was in part due to the activity in the unit last night. "Up until about 8 or 9 o'clock last night," Janet said, "things were pretty slow. But I gathered from talking with the residents and nurses when I first got on the unit this morning, that starting around 10 p.m. it was nonstop action. First, a patient who's been in the unit for over three weeks, and who is 193 days out from a bone marrow transplant, started having runs of V tach (ventricular tachycardia) and needed to be cardioverted five times. Another patient, a man with COPD (chronic obstructive pulmonary disease) who developed pneumonia and then ARDS (acute respiratory distress syndrome), arrested and required a full code. He's now on full ventilatory support, but he doesn't look good. While that was going on, another oncology patient was transferred to the unit from the heme-onc (hematology-oncology) ward after being resuscitated there. And if all of that wasn't enough, beginning at 5:30 this morning, a patient who everyone thought was improving hemodynamically suddenly dropped her pressures. So, by the time rounds started this morning, the team was pretty wound up."

The atmosphere of an intensive care unit is itself different from other parts of the hospital—and for that matter, different from anything else in life! In itself, that makes one's time there unforgettable. When there's a lot of action of the sort Janet was telling me about, well, it's like being in a foreign country that has just experienced some horrendous natural disaster. And, Janet told me, so it was for her this morning as rounds proceeded in the midst of the electricity flowing through the unit.

Janet started giving me the details.

It started when one of the residents reported during his review of the particular patient under discussion that the patient had been admitted last evening before things started getting crazy. The patient was confused and disoriented—in view of a negative toxicity-screen for benzodiazepine, hepatic encephalopathy was thought the most probable cause—and there was some concern that the team might want electively to intubate him. No family could be contacted, however, so there was some concern about getting consent; after all, this was not clearly an emergent situation in which you could claim medical necessity, like they do down in the ER, and, the resident continued, hadn't the ethics consultant told them about the need to talk with patients, to establish that their choices were consistent with previously expressed values? So, they gave an infusion of flumazenil, to "wake" him up so that they could talk with him and get his informed consent, which they did. The flumazenil was DC'd (discontinued), he became stuporous again within an hour, and did end up getting intubated.

"As you know," Janet went on, "flumazenil is approved as a reversal agent for benzodiazepine class drugs.[1] However, a common side-effect is that patients with hepatic encephalopathy experience temporary reversal of the encephalopathy.[2-5] Explicitly using flumazenil for this purpose, however, is not approved,[1] although in practice, it's sometimes used for just this purpose."

Janet had told me about this before (she actually had participated in the last phase of clinical trials before FDA approval and had met with some of the researchers who reported flumazenil's effect on encephalopathy) so I wasn't surprised to hear that flumazenil was, in fact, being used for this purpose. I told her I remembered her telling me that flumazenil sometimes is used that way. I knew Janet well enough to be blunt. "So what was the problem? I mean, it's not like you haven't seen this before. So, what did you say to the resident?" Without realizing it when I said it, I had hit the nail right on the head.

"I didn't say anything," Janet replied, "because of what the attending said after the resident finished his report; or rather, what he didn't say." Janet then told me that the attending, Dr. Sherman, one of the more senior members of the group who provides attending services, as well as someone who has historically been open to having Janet participate on rounds but hasn't enthusiastically embraced her presence even after seven years, asked a question about blood gases and chest films, and then asked the resident about the next patient. "And in that moment of transition from one patient to the next, it was quite clear that there would be no opportunity for me to say anything."

I asked her why.

"Because of the way he glanced over at me, and then looked away, while asking the resident about the next patient. You see, he and I have talked about the use of drugs for nonapproved purposes in the past, and he has told me to speak up during rounds if I see residents using drugs for other than their stated purposes. In this patient, using the flumazenil was clearly not right, and I know that he knows that, but he didn't say anything and he didn't give me a chance to say anything."

I could tell from Janet's tone that she was greatly bothered by the attending's actions. I even had a sense, as I listened to her, that her concerns were less prompted by the use of the flumazenil than by the character of the interaction she had with the attending.

"The funny thing is," Janet continued, "the whole thing took maybe thirty seconds, was rather routine in appearance, and seemed to be a reasonable decision given what had occurred in the unit last night. Prolonging rounds any longer than they had to be wasn't a good idea today. It wasn't until after rounds, when I approached the resident to tell him that flumazenil isn't approved for this use, that I began to feel the pinch of the moment."

When I asked her to explain what she meant by "the pinch of the moment," she said, "Well, I was walking down the hall and I saw the resident sitting at the nurse's station looking at a chart. I didn't see any other residents there with him, so I figured now would be a good time to talk with him. I didn't want my telling him about the flumazenil to come off as punitive. That's what I was thinking as I reached the desk, and that's when it struck me: it's just not a matter of "correcting" the resident, of helping him learn something about the appropriate use of drugs; it was about the character of our interaction—at this point as well as in the future. I mean, I could tell him that the use of flumazenil was inappropriate for this patient in a variety of ways. But the differences between these various ways of conveying that information had to do with how I see myself in the unit: am I an authority, an expert, a consultant, a teacher? And it occurred to me that when Dr. Sherman both turned towards me but then allowed for no input from me, a similar question about my role was at stake. I was reminded of all those discussions you and I have had about our role as pharmacists and how we should understand our relationship with physicians."

I was beginning to see her point since we often have talked about this question over the years. And what we've always come around to is how the real force of this question, no matter what we conclude in our discussions, the real weight is realized in a moment, when we are reminded that the "normal" understanding we work from is in tension with the particular circumstances in which that moment occurs. And in that moment, everything seems to be out of kilter. And even if there is a restabilization in the very next moment, so that the "normal" understanding is again present, the disruption of that moment does not immediately disappear.

"You know," Janet said after a short pause, "I keep asking myself if I should have interrupted Sherman. Since I didn't do it this time, will I do it the next time he's attending and I hear something that I know needs to be addressed?"

Once again, I thought as Janet said this, a favorite philosophical question we have discussed numerous times over the years was being transformed into a practical concern. Janet has to decide how she ought to comport herself in the face of the actual circumstances of the MICU. It's the fundamental ethical question: "What do I do now?"

Janet knows, as do I, that there are no simple answers out there. Oh sure, we both are familiar with the textbook and academic answers, those that begin by talking about the American Pharmaceutical Association's Code of Ethics, general principles and Western ethical theories, standard models of professional-patient relationships, and the like. We also know there's a big difference between deciding what to do in the abstract and figuring out what's right then and there with that attending, let alone actually *doing* the right thing in that particular situation.

"The funny thing about this," Janet continued somewhat ruefully, "is that at the recent APhA conference I saw some of our old classmates, and this question about what to do when physicians don't seem responsive to our input came up. Some of the stories I heard were unbelievable, especially when they added in the way all of these decisions we make also affect, or potentially affect, patients. At least I was only dealing with Sherman and not the patient as well."

"That's right, I forgot you went to that meeting." I hardly ever go to these professional gatherings. Like this last one.

"There was a lot of talk of trying to get the profession to attend more directly to the ethical issues facing us," she said. "The emphasis was mostly on the practical side. Most of the people I talked to agreed that there are no universal answers out there. It's a matter of making judgments in light of the circumstances."

On that note, Janet reflected on APhA's 1994 Code of Ethics for Pharmacists. "Who can argue with this document?," she asked, and then quoted from it: "A pharmacist places concern for the well-being of the patient at the center of professional practice. In doing so, a pharmacist considers needs stated by the patient as well as those defined by health science." Janet felt these kinds of statements were virtually meaningless, since they failed to explain what a pharmacist ought to do in a particular situation, especially when the needs as defined by the patient and "health science" differed.

This wasn't news to me. As a small businessman as well as a pharmacist, I've never turned to the Code for guidance. It isn't that I don't believe that we pharmacists have certain moral obligations; it's just that I don't think an eight-point code of ethics could come even close to capturing the kinds of issues I experience in my store. Janet's situation, in fact, was but another example, as far as I was concerned, of this ambiguity between the Code and actual practice.

I told Janet that I was sorry to hear that she had found herself in this situation this morning. I felt bad because I know what it's like to feel caught between what we perceive our obligations to be towards patients and physicians and what we can actually do. Janet understood that. It wasn't that long ago that I was involved in a situation that raised similar questions and, in the end, reminded us of the ambiguity that often exists between our attempts to codify ethics and the actual moral dynamics in practice.

In fact, I told Janet that her predicament reminded me of my encounter those many months ago during which I too was engaged with the question of the obligations between pharmacists, patients, and physicians.

A Momentary Meditation: My Own Tale

It was a Thursday morning when Mr. Harris, a frequent customer, came into the store. I had known Mr. Harris as a customer for a number of years, both before and after he developed trigeminal neuralgia, a condition marked by excruciating episodic pain in the area supplied by the fifth cranial nerve. Initially treated with carbamazepine (Tegretol), Mr. Harris was one of those patients who no longer responded to its effect.[6] Furthermore, as with most patients suffering from trigeminal neuralgia, the extent and severity of pain associated with his condition were difficult to measure by the use of objective means. Different patients have different experiences. The standard treatment, in the face of such pain, is thus to prescribe moderate-strength class III pain relievers (those containing hydrocodone, such as Lorcet, Lortab 5, or Vicodin) to be used as needed during the episodes in which pain occurs.

While hydrocodone-type drugs aren't the most effective pain control substances, they are the preferred medication for patients like Mr. Harris. The reason is that not only do these kinds of drugs provide adequate—if not optimal—pain relief, they are class III drugs, which means physicians can write prescriptions for them without concern for scrutiny by the government. This is not the case with class II drugs, such as Percocet and Roxicet, which may be considered more potent but which cannot be prescribed without filling out regulatory forms and opening oneself up to review. In addition, to write prescriptions for class II drugs, physicians in some states need to use special blanks that cost more to buy than standard prescription pads. As with many patients whose physicians don't want to deal with the bureaucratic mess associated with class II drugs, Mr. Harris has been taking Lorcet, a class III drug, for his pain.

For nearly two years, I had been filling Mr. Harris' prescription, and until that day several months ago, I wasn't concerned about his use of the Lorcet. I had learned in conversation with him that on occasion, when his pain was even more severe than usual, he had taken one or two additional doses. In other conversations he had told me that his episodes of pain rarely last more than several days. Hence, I was not troubled by his occasional overuse. On that Thursday morning, however, Mr. Harris brought in a prescription not for Lorcet but for Lorcet 10 which, while still a class III pain reliever, is considerably more powerful. The prescription was written for one every four hours, or six tablets per day.

When I saw the prescription, two thoughts ran through my head at the same time. On the one hand, I was immediately concerned about the acetaminophen level; whereas a single dose of Lorcet has 500 mg of acetaminophen, a single dose of Lorcet 10 has 650 mg of acetaminophen. If he took even two extra tablets for several days, that extra 150 mg of acetaminophen per dose could raise the total daily dose of acetaminophen to a possibly dangerous point; if over 4 gm, the risk of hepatotoxicity is significantly increased.[7] On the other hand, I was concerned that the reason for switching from the Lorcet to the Lorcet 10 might be reflective of a known possible side-effect of using Lorcet chronically: Mr. Harris had become dependent on, had developed an addiction to, the hydrocodone. After all, Lorcet has only 5 mg of hydrocodone in it whereas Lorcet 10 has 10 mg. With both thoughts in mind, I began to feel uneasy.

I tried not to display my uneasiness to Mr. Harris as I accepted his prescription, and as I always do when working behind the counter, told him it would be 10 or 15 minutes, and suggested that while he was waiting, "you can pick up any other items you need." I had learned years ago, during my internship at Discount Drug Store, that you always tell customers that "as long as you're here, look around the store and see if there are any other items you need." At Discount Drug Store, there had been great emphasis placed on the fact that unlike the hospital setting, where the people you service are patients, in the community setting, they are customers. Hence, as my supervisor drilled into me, I needed to remember "the business side of the profession." Of course, we never talked about what that meant beyond the obvious; I was not only responsible for filling their prescriptions, I was also responsible for getting them to buy things in the store that would bring profit to the store. The most complex issues we ever discussed regarding this "business" side of pharmacy concerned the differences in profit margins when comparing generic and label drugs. The more complicated issues such as the implicit power residing within my role as a pharmacist—even if I think of them as mere "customers," my customers are still patients, and as such are coming to me because of the health care service I provide and which they need—and whether I ought to use my professional position, with its implicit power, as a means for generating profit for the store were not addressed. Nor did we ever discuss issues such as price fixing within sales districts, the influence of pharmaceutical representatives on what drugs we routinely stock, and other "business" related topics that I've encountered since I began working in my own store.

Like I always do, I told Mr. Harris it would be a few minutes, and like he always has, he said "OK" and walked over toward the magazines. In some sense, it was because of his always acting the same whenever he came into the store—the way he never seemed to be in a hurry, his politeness, how he always bought a *Science Digest*—these regularities in his behavior are what "tipped me off," so to speak, that something wasn't right with this prescription. Mr. Harris was nothing but predictable as a customer; nothing ever seemed to change with him. And as far as I could tell from our interactions over the years, the same was true in other parts of his life. Any noticeable change was thus significant. Hence my concern when I saw his prescription.

As I told Janet later, it was a strange moment when Mr. Harris turned and walked over toward the magazine rack. Filled with questions about the prescription, I felt an immediate sense of paralysis; "What should I do now?" I asked myself, with no clear answer in mind. However, a number of options did start to come to mind, although in retrospect, they did so in no particular order. What I began to think was that I could:

- fill the prescription as if it were any other, and not think another thought about it;
- fill the prescription and ask Mr. Harris how he was doing, with the intent of raising with him the question of why his prescription had been changed, although if he didn't "bite," I wouldn't force the issue;
- don't fill the prescription and tell Mr. Harris that I didn't have any of this drug in stock;
- call Mr. Harris' physician, and ask him about the change;
- call Janet and ask her what she thinks I should do;
- fill the prescription and simply tell Mr. Harris the risks associated with this new dosage;
- call Mr. Harris back to the counter and talk to him about the new prescription and then determine whether to fill it or call his physician, Dr. Blander.

At the same time I was thinking about what to do, I also knew that I had to do *something now*, that I couldn't just stand there thinking about what to do. But what do I do?

As Janet later told me, "I've actually talked with the ethics consultant who rounds with us in the unit about this very thing, of how you feel the need to do something but don't really know what that something is. He said that this sense—of not knowing what to do but knowing that something must be done—which occurs in the flash of a moment is a kind of marker of what he likes to call 'moral disequilibrium.' That is, when we feel compelled to act, and at the same time feel constrained at that moment from doing anything other than simply noting that we must do something, that moment presents the possibility for some moral sense of whatever it is we are doing."

Luckily for me, while I was trying to figure out what to do, Janet wasn't in my store telling me all that! After all, I needed to do something fairly quickly—three minutes had already passed since I told Mr. Harris that I'd be done in ten or so minutes—and there wasn't time to be philosophizing!

It didn't take long, however, before I did begin to recognize what I needed to do. The reason was that in recognizing that I wasn't sure what to do, I further recognized that I was already seeing the situation as being problematic in a certain way or in a certain light. Any attempt to resolve it would have to be similarly oriented, so that the proposed solution would actually address my concerns. After all, it's hard to solve a problem if you don't see that there is a problem! And in this situation, I knew what was troubling me.

When I first saw the prescription, two thoughts ran through my head, both of which were focused on the Lorcet 10 and its effect on Mr. Harris, and both of which brought on my unease. First, there was the concern regarding the total daily dose of acetaminophen and the risk of hepatotoxicity. Second, there was the concern that Mr. Harris may have developed an addiction to the hydrocodone in the Lorcet. While the first is a very serious concern, in Mr. Harris' situation, the concern about acetaminophen only arose because of the switch from Lorcet to Lorcet 10, which itself only seemed to have arisen in light of inadequate pain relief from the Lorcet. I was thus struck by the possibility that Mr. Harris had developed an addiction to hydrocodone, thereby requiring more hydrocodone—as found in Lorcet 10—to produce the same palliative effect as Lorcet. The prospect that Mr. Harris might be becoming dependent on the hydrocodone concerned me.

Why I was concerned was something I had to address, for in being able to account for the basis for my concern, I would then get even clearer on what in particular I found problematic, and hence what in particular I might do to resolve this tension. Of course, at the time, none of this was clear to me beyond the recognition that I had to attend to what it was that I perceived to be problematic. And here I knew: it was the issue of addiction more than anything.

As a community-based pharmacist, the issue of addiction is one of those things with which I am familiar. I have to be. While it might not be as prevalent in my community as in other towns—or at least, that's the culturally biased picture we all seem to hold—narcotic abuse through the abuse of prescription drugs is a real problem, and one with which pharmacists have to deal. As stated in the Uniformed Narcotic Act, pharmacists have an explicit legal responsibility regarding Schedule II drugs: their dispensing must be in line with normal dosing requirements, and suspected abusers should not be given these drugs.[8] Likewise, most states' Board of Pharmacy Rules of Professional Conduct have explicit statements about pharmacists' responsibilities to make every reasonable effort to prevent abuse of drugs they dispense. In addition to these legal concerns, I also was worried about Mr. Harris. Given my impression of him over the years, I couldn't believe that if he's been needing more medication to control his pain, that he hadn't been noticing that he's been needing more drugs to control his pain. He's a smart guy. If he's even had the thought that he maybe is becoming dependent on the Lorcet, well, that's a hard self-recognition to have given our societal view towards drug use and drug dependence. And as is always the case, this possibility raises more questions.

For instance, if Mr. Harris was thinking these thoughts, had he been able to talk to anyone about them? And in particular, had he talked with Dr. Blander? If so, how had Dr. Blander responded? Unfortunately, I've encountered a lot of health care professionals—both pharmacists and physicians—who do not want to talk about this issue. They'll go out of their way, in fact, to avoid even acknowledging that patients like Mr. Harris might develop addictions. I guess this issue, like that of death, is just one of those topics we have difficulty with, and hence seldom openly address. To tell the truth, I wasn't so comfortable with it either. But in Mr. Harris' case, well, I felt the need to overcome my reluctance. After all, I had developed a relationship with Mr. Harris over the years; he was more than a "customer," more than a patient who frequented my store. If I didn't at least attempt to talk about this, I felt like I'd be deserting him.

Another minute had gone by, and although I was getting a bit clearer on what I ought to do, I also was aware that the clock was ticking. Not only for Mr. Harris, but for the store too. Another one of those "business" concerns I had encountered was the issue of time allocated for working through issues such as those I was now addressing. Most customers come to a pharmacy expecting service that is quick and efficient. That means that if the pharmacist has to take additional time to contact physicians or other pharmacists because of questions, the customer may interpret the delay as indicative of inefficiency and hence, a poor reflection on the store. Customer satisfaction can go down, and that customer is lost. Furthermore, in taking that time, new customers are forced to wait or be delayed, so that a chain effect becomes likely. This is another reason for telling customers to look around the store while they wait: it buys time not only for that particular customer, but also for others whose prescriptions may require more than the allotted time.

So far, since Mr. Harris had come into the store, no other customers had arrived. While I generally like to have customers, in this instance I was hoping things would stay slow for a bit longer. Although I wasn't yet settled on what to do, things were getting clearer. The next decision, of course, was the hardest, for I needed to decide whether to talk with Mr. Harris about my concerns, or call Dr. Blander. I wasn't sure. So I paged Janet.

When I learned to drive a car, my parents grilled into me that when I was unsure of what to do, then I at least knew what not to do, namely, something rash. Uncertainty, they told me, was a sign that further thought was needed. That bit of wisdom has stuck with me. I had figured out what was concerning me, but I still was unclear how to proceed. I needed to talk to someone—as much to provide the possibility for another perspective as to "hear myself," to give myself a chance to say explicitly what I was thinking, and hence better perceive my own commitments. In addition, although not the final action in this situation, actually talking about my concerns would be the first active step beyond my thinking about them, and I needed to start acting.

Janet and I seldom talk in the mornings or afternoons during working hours unless there's something important happening; if we do talk during the day, it's at lunch time, or toward the end of the day. I thus felt Janet would call me back immediately if she was available. In the meantime, I checked my inventory just to be certain that I actually did have Lorcet 10 in stock. I don't keep a lot of it around since, if it becomes known you're stocking these kinds of drugs, a store may become more prone to robbery; these kinds of drugs sell well on the street, even in suburban areas. The phone rang. It was Janet.

I quickly thanked her for calling back, and then gave her an overview of the situation. "A customer I've known for years who's been on Lorcet to control pain secondary to trigeminal neuralgia brought in a new prescription for Lorcet 10. I'm a bit concerned that the reason for this change may be that he's developing a tolerance for the hydrocodone, and so his physician is simply increasing the amount instead of directly addressing the issue of possible addiction. I'm thinking of calling the doc and using the acetaminophen level as a means for raising this issue of addiction. What do you think?"

My report didn't completely capture my thoughts about Mr. Harris' situation, but in this kind of moment, the report usually doesn't. I had to trust that Janet knew that, that over the years of our conversations, she had learned how to listen to me.

"OK, hold on a second, let me get this straight." Janet began to review. "The patient's hydrocodone dose has been increased secondary to the switch to Lorcet 10, and you're concerned that this increase reflects a growing need for more hydrocodone to control the pain, which itself might mean the patient is developing an addiction. Maybe the patient is having worsening pain. So what are you concerned about? Do you think the patient might be abusing his medication, or using other drugs as well? Are you worried that since you don't regularly keep a large supply of Lorcet 10 in stock, you'll have to order more, which might make you more prone to state inspection, or if the word gets out that you have Lorcet 10 in stock, robbery? And why aren't you explicitly concerned about the acetaminophen level?"

As always, I was immediately struck by how difficult it is to respond when asked the kind of question I just laid on Janet. You can't just walk into the situation and instantly "see" the complexity and texture of what's going on. That's why I think talking about it is so important; conversation provides the opportunity for the other to gain access to whatever the concern is.

I replied to Janet, "The acetaminophen level concerns me in the sense that since the physician apparently isn't concerned that he's prescribing a drug that, if even slightly more than the recommended dose is taken, is possibly toxic, he must be attending to something else. This physician sends a lot of business my way, and I think I've come to learn a lot about him. He doesn't miss these kinds of things. And so, the only reason for the switch to the more potent drug I could think of was the hydrocodone level, and that raised the issue of addiction, which as we both know, is not a favored topic of discussion among physicians."

Janet must have "seen" what was going on, because she then asked me to say more about the sort of relationship with Dr. Blander I had beyond his "sending a lot of business my way." In this simple question Janet provided me the opportunity to question my relationship with Blander, and in so doing, again raise the question of my motivations. After all, Blander did send a number of patients to the store, and many of these subsequently became regular or semi-regular customers. I couldn't deny that some of my hesitation in calling him was based on this.

"And," Janet went on, "why haven't you asked your customer about this change? I think that if you really believe that there's more at root than a simple oversight, you need to determine which relationship—that with your customer or that with the physician—you believe capable of withstanding the implications of your questions concerning the increase in hydrocodone. And if neither can, which one you're willing to risk. But remember, all of this is premised on your acceptance that addiction is the issue. I think you need to find out if that's accurate or not, so I recommend you call the physician and give him a chance."

Janet knew that I was in the middle of this—both in terms of the time and the relationship between Mr. Harris and Dr. Blander—so she ended by saying that I could call her back later to talk this through some more. I thanked her and hung up. Seven minutes had gone by since Mr. Harris had walked over to the magazines. I saw that he was leafing through the *US News & World Report*. I still had some time, so I dialed Blander's office.

I had actually only spoken to Blander several times in the years he'd been sending patients to the store. From his patients who were my customers, I gathered that he was a very personable physician. Still, I was a bit unsettled as I dialed. Would he think I was barking up the wrong tree? What if I've misinterpreted the situation? Moreover, what if I'm correct in my assessment and he doesn't *want* to address it—with Mr. Harris, with me, with himself? Am I ready for all of this?

"Hello, Dr. Blander's office."

I told the receptionist who I was and that I had a question about a prescription. She asked me to hold, and thirty seconds later, Blander was on the phone.

"How can I help you?"

"Dr. Blander, a patient of yours, Mr. Harris, brought in a prescription for Lorcet 10 one every four hours, and I'm a bit concerned. With that dosage, if he takes any additional doses—even though he's not supposed to—the acetaminophen level could be problematic."

I didn't say anything about the hydrocodone, figuring that this was the best way to open the subject—it didn't directly present a confrontation, but it did raise a concern. I'd have to determine while he was responding whether to raise the other issue.

"Hmm...what was that dosage again?"

I told him. There was a pause. It seemed to last a bit too long. Then,

"Let's change the script to Tylenol No. 3 (Tylenol with codeine). If you don't mind, tell Mr. Harris that I decided to switch his medication because I was a bit concerned with the acetaminophen level. Thanks for calling." And he hung up.

"What do I do now?" I thought as I hung up the phone. In using the acetaminophen level as a means to engage Dr. Blander, I had completely failed to address the issue of the hydrocodone level. And what's more, in now switching to the Tylenol No. 3, I couldn't raise it; Tylenol No. 3 doesn't contain hydrocodone, and the amount of narcotic in it—in the form of codeine—is less than the amount of hydrocodone in Lorcet 10. And having just called Dr. Blander, it wouldn't have been a good idea to call him again, or at least not now. To do so would present an appearance that I'd rather not have: of looking over his shoulder and antagonizing him.

However, even if unintentionally, Dr. Blander had set the stage for me to talk directly with Mr. Harris about his prescription. Not only did he ask me to talk with Mr. Harris about the switch to the Tylenol, but in making the switch, I would have to tell Mr. Harris that a side-effect of now taking codeine is that too much causes severe stomach upset. Hence, the opportunity was there for me to address the issue of addiction with Mr. Harris—giving him the opportunity to talk with me as well—should I recognize it and then take it. As it often goes, at each point, to choose one option excludes another, but gives rise to yet a third. Yes, I had failed to speak directly on the issue of addiction with Dr. Blander—had even failed to establish whether, in fact, this was a concern for Dr. Blander at all. However, in so doing, a new opportunity was provided for me to talk with Mr. Harris. And this opportunity, I told myself, I would not lose.

When I later called Janet to fill her in on what had transpired, she too remarked how often it is that every choice we make leads us toward further choices previously unavailable or untenable. "Moreover," she said as our conversation concluded, "The sort of thing you underwent this morning in your thinking about it, in your calling me, in your calling the physician, and finally in your discussion with the patient demonstrates how gross a misunderstanding it is to think that the moral dimensions of our relationships with patients and physicians can be captured in a standardized Code of Ethics or theoretical discussion of ethics and pharmacy."

Janet's Tale: A Slight Return

"Yeah, I remember," Janet said when I told her that her situation this morning reminded me of my encounter with Mr. Harris. "Maybe someday we'll find a way to avoid these situations." I told Janet that I could only think of two ways to avoid them: work toward getting more dialogue about these issues out into the profession as well as cross-professionally—have pharmacists, physicians, and other health care professionals actively engaged in these discussions—or, as has become a joke between us, "We could become farmers." Janet laughed, and then told me that I really ought to consider getting more involved with the APhA. I needed to think on that one. Over the phone I heard Janet's beeper. "Oh, gotta go now. Thanks for listening. Tell Cindy I said 'Hi.' Talk to you soon."

I hung up the phone and returned to my task of checking the inventory. Nothing was really different, but for a moment, I felt refreshed.

Case Discussion
A Comment on Relationship: Moral Features of Health Care Contexts

It may be surprising to think of health care as a moral enterprise—historically, health care and health care professions have not been talked about in the same terms as has been ethics. During the past 25 years, however, as critical attention has been focused on the moral dimensions of, and ethical ramifications associated with, such issues as health care distribution, delivery, education and research, and the use of high technology, the linkage between ethics and health care has become more widely acknowledged. The link between ethics and health care, of course, is not itself new: Aristotle suggests in *Nicomachean Ethics*, written over 2300 years ago, that a central question for ethics is not how ethics may help medicine and its pursuit of health, but rather how medicine, which is subordinate to ethics, is useful in the pursuit of ethics.[9]

Along with the recognition that health care and ethics are intimately linked comes further recognition that those who engage in health care professions need to attend to the moral and ethical facets of their professions as much as they need to attend to the scientific, economic, sociological, and political factors which are present in their daily practices.[10,11] But recognizing these facets raises a number of important questions. First and foremost is the question, *"How* can health care professionals actually attend to these facets in the midst of engaging in their professional practices?" Closely related to this first question is a second: *"How well* do health care professionals actually attend to these facets?"

Attempts to answer these questions often are made by turning to the theoretical foundations on which a particular health care profession rests; much of the literature in medical ethics thus concerns itself with theoretically-derived ethical principles and values and how these might serve as a basis for clinical practice.[12–14] This is the approach, in fact, suggested in Chapter 2: The Normative Principles of Pharmacy Ethics, and Chapter 4: Ethical Decision Making, of this book. However, there has been a shift in the literature and among those interested in health care ethics to recognize that imposing ethical frameworks developed external to the actual contexts in which health care occurs is problematic.[15–18] Essentially, this is because it is within the clinical setting—with all of its complexity and nuances—that we encounter the moral significance of situations, and it is in light of such encounters that we seek resolution to problems. Janet's and the narrator's tales clearly display this.

It is thus vitally important when addressing questions about the moral and ethical aspects of health care that critical attention be paid to the practical setting in which health care professionals engage in their daily activities and practices. The actual dynamics associated with health care distribution, delivery, education and research, and the use of high technology, in other words, must be explored because it is within such a context that the moral dimensions and ethical ramifications of health care arise and are defined, realized, and acted upon.

It is in the attempt to describe this context that the notion of relationship emerges. The reason is that, in general, the health care context is defined by a multiplicity of relationships.[19] This context may, therefore, be best understood by considering the different layers and kinds of relationships present in the health care setting.

One way of viewing relationships in the health care setting is to attend to the different kinds of individuals present in that context. We all are familiar with the most obvious cast of characters: in terms of explicitly health care-oriented professions and occupations, there are allopathic and osteopathic physicians, dentists, nurses, pharmacists, podiatrists, chiropractors, and the various therapists (physical, occupational, respiratory, speech) and technicians (laboratory, x-ray)—many of whom may be further distinguished in terms of specialties and subspecialties—who are present in any health care setting. There are also the numerous support personnel whose roles in general are not specific to the health care context although their roles in it are tailored so as to fulfill specific supportive functions—administrators, administrative assistants, chaplains, dietitians, legal counsel, insurance processors, nurses aides, orderlies, patient advocates, secretaries, and social workers. And finally, there are the patients and their families.

Relationships in the health care settings also may be viewed in terms of specific institutional considerations, in which the specific sets of guidelines, rules, and norms of the differing institutions become prominent. In attending to these institutional considerations, however, it must be noted that the term "institution" may be understood in at least two ways. The facility in which health care is provided—health maintenance organization (HMO), community hospital, or public nursing home—is one form of institution; professions, with their particular forms of training, local and national organizations, standards of practice, and so on, are another form of institution. For any institution, there are both written and unwritten institutionally defined criteria that establish who ought to be doing what, when, and how.

A third way of viewing relationships found in the health care setting is to attend to the political considerations that serve to shape and define professional and institutional responsibility, accountability, and function. These political aspects may be seen in terms of various immediate microlevel considerations: policies of particular facilities; local professional organizations' standards and protocols; and community norms. There are also the various macrolevel political bounds: state and federal laws and regulations; national and international professional organizations' standards; and cultural and religious norms.

Finally, relationships found in the health care setting may be attended to in terms of the innumerable personal considerations: the particular religious, ethnic, social, and economic beliefs and values that any individual within the health care setting—be they one of the professionals, support personnel, or patients and families—brings with him- or herself.

At any given time, individuals thus wear a variety of hats—pharmacist, intensive care team member, Catholic, middle class, married, mother, and so on—each of which draws the individual toward different kinds of understandings about who one is, for what one is responsible, to whom obligations are owed, what counts as good in these circumstances, what is at stake in this context, and what is a "problem" at any given time. In short, the health care context may be defined in terms of a variety of individuals, all of whom have their own particular personal backgrounds, traditions, histories, and religions, and some of whom also are immersed in particular professional and institutional roles. In addition, the interactions among all of these people occur within a penumbra of (written and unwritten) rules, codes, regulations, policies, federal and state procedures, and numerous legal decisions found within, and resulting from, the different professions, traditions, histories, and religions of all participants. And all of this occurs at some time in our particular society, with its particular history, tradition, norms, social values, mores, and folkways. The health care setting, in other words, is an exceedingly complex array of interpersonal, professional, institutional, and cultural relationships.

In some very obvious sense, this picture of the complexity of relationships should be familiar since, for the most part, every aspect of life involves much the same complexity and dynamics (e.g., I am a son, a brother, a father, a friend, a Democrat, college educated, musically inclined, active in city politics). What sets the particular enterprise called "health care" apart from other similarly complex contexts is this fact: there is an explicit focus on caring for ill individuals who are, for the most part, strangers to the health care providers, and where the interactions between providers and patients require multiple forms of unavoidable trust given the various inherent uncertainties associated with health care and illness.[16,20]

Given this complexity of relationships that revolve around the care for ill individuals, deciding what to do, and then actually doing it, is what gives health care its moral character. The relationships between any particular individuals within the health care context—including the relationship between patients, pharmacists, and physicians—is thus fluid and dynamic. It is within this complex of relationships that pharmacists, like all health care professionals, find themselves; the previous story displays this with exquisite detail. To whom pharmacists are obligated—patients, physicians, the institutions in which they work, the profession of pharmacy—and in what way such obligations may be actually acted upon in a particular moment are thus not easily answered since every particular situation in which questions of obligation and responsibility arise brings with it its own unique blend of overall complexity.

For Janet, this means having to attend to a different set of concerns than does the narrator. Even though both are pharmacists, both find themselves in situations in which they have to decide what kind of interaction with a physician is "appropriate." Likewise, in both situations, the medications prescribed have direct effects on patients. Each must decide what to do. Each decision must be attentive to the fact that decisions are made *in a moment*. In addition, each decision must be attentive to the fact that the choices leading up to the decision are directed by those specific relations within a fluid network of concerns. Thus, each decision must also be attentive to the specific network of concerns that help define *that specific moment*.

The character of the relationships pharmacists have with patients and physicians both exemplifies and is defined by the network of concerns that arise in the contexts of those relationships. As a result, any questions about pharmacists' responsibilities and accountability to patients and physicians, much less questions about how these concerns arise and might be balanced, must therefore be addressed in the specific contexts of their occurrence.

Discussion Questions

1. If you were the narrator in the story, given what occurred during the ten minutes since Mr. Harris gave you his prescription, how would you approach Mr. Harris once it becomes clear that Dr. Blander has left the door open for you to raise the issue of addiction with Mr. Harris? How might you explain the extent of your responsibility to Mr. Harris?

2. By the story's end, it appears as if Janet is not going to talk with Dr. Sherman about the incident this morning in the MICU. If she decides to approach him, will that make any difference, and to whom? For instance, how might this influence future interactions between Janet and Dr. Sherman?

3. In Chapter 2: The Normative Principles of Pharmacy Ethics, Campbell and Constantine propose five normative principles for pharmacy ethics that, they suggest, "establish duties and give action-guides." How would knowledge of these principles be useful for either Janet or the narrator in those moments in which they must make their respective decisions?

4. Janet and Dr. Sherman, the narrator and Dr. Blander, the narrator and Mr. Harris, and the narrator and Janet have all known each other for varying lengths of time. For each of the pairs, how do the histories of their interactions influence the character of their relationship?

5. If Janet and the narrator followed the four-step process for ethical decision making discussed in Chapter 5: The Counterside Conversation: Application as Narrative in Pharmacy Ethics, would they experience a similar resolution in each of their situations? How could we tell?

REFERENCES

1. Roche Laboratories. Romazicon package insert. Nutley, NJ: 1993 April.
2. Scollo-Lavizzari G, Steinmann E. Reversal of hepatic coma by benzodiazepine antagonist (RO 15-1788). Lancet. 1985;1:1324.
3. Grimm G et al. Improvement of hepatic encephalopathy treated with flumazenil. Lancet. 1988;2:1392–394.
4. Meier R, Gyr K. Treatment of hepatic encephalopathy (HE) with the benzodiazepine antagonist flumazenil: a pilot study. Eur J Anaesthesiol Suppl. 1988;2:139–46.
5. Grimm G et al. Effect of flumazenil in hepatic encephalopathy. Eur J Anaesthesiol. 1988;2(Suppl. A):147–49.
6. Voorhies R, Patterson RH. Management of trigeminal neuralgia (tic douloureux). JAMA. 1981;245:2521.
7. Analgesics and antipyretics. In: McEvoy GK, ed. AHFS Drug Information. Bethesda: American Society of Hospital Pharmacists; 1993:1247–253.
8. Simonsmeier LH, Fink JL. Laws governing pharmacy. In: Gennaro AR, ed. Remington's Pharmaceutical Sciences. Easton: Mack Publishing; 1990:1921–927.
9. Owens J. Aristotelian ethics, medicine, and the changing nature of man. In: Spicker SF, Engelhardt HT, eds. Philosophical Medical Ethics: Its Nature and Significance. Dordrecht: D. Reidel Publishing; 1977:127–42.
10. Pellegrino ED. Humanism and the Physician. Knoxville: The University of Tennessee Press; 1979.
11. Rothman DJ. Strangers at the Bedside. New York: Basic Books; 1991.
12. Veatch RM, ed. Medical Ethics. Boston: Jones and Bartlett; 1989.
13. Graber GC, Thomasma DC. Theory and Practice in Medical Ethics. New York: Continuum; 1989.
14. Beauchamp TL, Childress JF. Principles of Biomedical Ethics. 3rd ed. New York: Oxford University Press; 1989.
15. Pellegrino ED, Thomasma DC. A Philosophical Basis of Medical Practice. New York: Oxford University Press; 1981.

16. Zaner RM. Ethics and the Clinical Encounter. Englewood Cliffs: Prentice Hall; 1988.
17. Cassell EJ. The Nature of Suffering. New York: Oxford University Press; 1991.
18. Hunter KM. Doctors' Stories. Princeton: Princeton University Press; 1991.
19. Zaner RM. Voices and time: the venture of clinical ethics. J Med Philos. 1993;18:9–31.
20. Pellegrino ED, Thomasma DC. The Virtues in Medical Practice. New York: Oxford University Press; 1993.

Chapter 7

Relationships with the Pharmaceutical Industry

Carol Bayley
Jeanine K. Mount

The pharmacist's role in contemporary health care is deeply tied to the role of the pharmaceutical industry and pharmaceutical manufacturers. This fact has diverse effects on pharmacists and pharmacy practice and raises new ethical dilemmas for pharmacists.

We highlight two roles played by the pharmaceutical industry. First, as mass producers of prefabricated medications, manufacturers are the source of virtually all drug products dispensed by pharmacists. Second, because of their work in drug development and testing, manufacturers also are a major source of drug information.

Thus, the pharmaceutical industry is a significant element in the pharmacist's evolving role as a health care system manager. Pharmacists have become more involved in evaluating and selecting drug products, and many pharmacists now hold formal responsibility for managing drug purchasing and distribution systems. The pharmaceutical industry also plays an important part in the pharmacist's role as a clinical professional; pharmacists have assumed greater influence in the drug use process, particularly in their evolving role as providers of pharmaceutical care.

SUCCESS OF THE PHARMACEUTICAL INDUSTRY

By any yardstick, pharmaceutical manufacturers comprise one of the most successful industries in the world. Achievements in new drug development, in drug product manufacturing and in drug marketing have firmly established the pharmaceutical industry's influence in the health care system. These achievements have altered both the context and the practice of pharmacy.

Pharmaceutical manufacturers experienced remarkable growth between 1940 and 1970 as industrialization of drug production processes grew. During what Hepler[1] calls the "scientific era" in pharmacy, development of prefabricated dosage units resulted in availability of products that were more uniform, pure, convenient and economical than extemporaneously compounded medications. Prefabricated products now account for over 98% of all prescribed medications[2] and manufacturers are the source of virtually all drug products.

Similarly, recent developments in molecular biology, pharmacology and other sciences have led to new treatments for many diseases. Of particular note is the creation of completely new drug classes or "new chemical entities" (NCEs). Most of the work involved in drug development and testing is carried out by researchers employed by pharmaceutical manufacturing companies. Consequently, manufacturers have come to serve as a major source of drug *information*, particularly for newly marketed products.

Pharmaceutical manufacturers' industrial and scientific successes have been met or surpassed by their financial success, making this one of the most profitable industries in the world.[3] This success relies, at least in part, on efforts of sales and marketing: marketing specialists plan strategies for profiting from scientific discoveries and sales personnel promote the drugs to health professionals who hold the key to a drug's success (or failure) in the marketplace. Thus, sales and marketing are as crucial to the pharmaceutical industry as they are to any other business enterprise.

TRANSFORMATIONS IN PHARMACY

The pharmaceutical industry's success has had far-reaching effects on pharmacy. Two important effects relate to the growth of pharmacists' roles as system managers and as clinical professionals. Let's look at each of these. Traditionally, pharmacists saw manufacturers simply as sources for products that the pharmacist stocked and dispensed. And traditionally, pharmacists played little role in deciding which drug products to stock or dispense. Today, though, as costs, complexities and risks associated with drug therapy escalate, pharmacists have become more involved in evaluating and selecting drug products, both for individual patients and for health care organizations. In fact, many pharmacists now hold formal responsibility for managing large drug purchasing and distribution systems, particularly in health maintenance organizations (HMOs) and other managed care settings, in hospitals, and in chain pharmacies.[4,5]

A parallel change has been expansion of the pharmacist's role as a clinical professional involved in direct patient care. The pharmacist's "job" has shifted from simply *dispensing* drug products decided upon by physicians and other prescribers to *advising* patients and health professionals regarding drug therapy and *participating* in actual treatment decisions.[6] Thus, the pharmacist has assumed greater influence in the drug use process. We see this clearly reflected in growth of the ideal of pharmaceutical care provision.

Expansion of pharmacists' managerial and clinical roles creates novel bases for pharmacists' relations with the pharmaceutical industry. These relations with the pharmaceutical industry (in general) and with individual manufacturers (in particular) present pharmacists with a new array of ethical challenges. The two cases presented below illustrate some of the ethical dilemmas that can develop. The case of J.D. (Case 1) identifies the quandary that a pharmacist can experience when, as a system manager, he must make difficult resource allocation decisions that affect the availability and use of medications. The case of M.H. (Case 2) points out that conflicts of interest may arise when the pharmacist's professional need for up-to-date information for treatment of patients is coupled with the pharmaceutical manufacturer's need to promote its product. After analyzing these cases, we will discuss their implications for patient care and pharmacy practice as they relate to the provision of pharmaceutical care.

In analyzing any ethical dilemma, there are at least two methods for proceeding. In the first method (described in Chapter 4: Ethical Decision Making), the beginning step is to gather the facts. Next, we try to identify the various values that seem to be in conflict. From there, we move toward resolution of the dilemma by generating possible ways of addressing the conflict and then by selecting one and justifying it as better than the alternatives.

An alternative, but similarly structured, method for ethical analysis questions the separation of the first two steps in the standard method. Proponents of this thinking hold that facts and values, at least for the purposes of ethical analysis, are not as clearly distinguishable as we would like them to be. Behind every bit of information we label as "fact" there is a host of evaluative choices that helped construct that fact. This is not to say that there is nothing to be gained from searching for relatively objective information that can affect an outcome. Nor is it to say that scientific observations, even if shaped by the categories of the observer, are not helpful in deciding what to do. Rather, facts and values are too tightly entwined to be separated usefully. In the analyses that follow, we will use this second method of analysis, to emphasize all the value considerations, or choice points, that are embedded in the decisions that pharmacists must make.

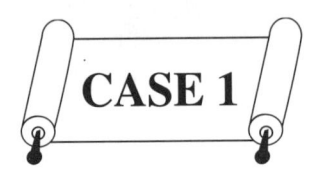

CASE 1

Safety, Efficacy, and Cost

Health Mark is a health maintenance organization (HMO), a system of health care that provides or ensures delivery of an agreed upon set of comprehensive health maintenance and treatment services for an enrolled group of persons (members) under a prepaid fixed sum. Health Mark limits payment for therapies based on the effectiveness of the therapy, both to safeguard its members and because it has limited resources to make available for all members. Pharmacist J.D. is a member of the formulary committee at Health Mark, the group that decides which therapies will be paid for by the HMO. J.D. has been asked to research the therapeutic effectiveness of transdermal nicotine patches (used to help smokers break their addiction to nicotine and stop smoking) and to make a recommendation as to whether Health Mark should pay for them when prescribed by Health Mark physicians.

J.D.'s research shows that nicotine patches are effective in helping a person stop smoking in about 35% of cases, and that figure applies only to patients who simultaneously are enrolled in behavior modification programs. Nicotine patches alone have little effect on smokers trying to quit. In addition, smokers who use nicotine patches and continue to smoke experience increased risk of cardiac arrest. J.D. wonders whether Health Mark should foot the bill for the nicotine patches if the patient requesting them is not enrolled in a behavior modification program.

S.H., the regional sales director for one of the manufacturers of nicotine patches, learns that Health Mark's formulary committee is deciding whether to include nicotine patches as a covered therapy. S.H. assumes that the product's price will influence Health Mark in the discussion. He contacts J.D. to suggest that Health Mark solicit bids from manufacturers for purchasing various nicotine patches. S.H. adds that he is certain his company will submit a drastically lower bid than what is indicated in their list prices.

Case Discussion
Analysis

An important feature of this case is that J.D. is a pharmacist for a health maintenance organization. In this role, J.D. is asked to make decisions, not just for the welfare of individual patients, but for whole groups of patients. The two main moral questions he must answer in this role are:

1. Should I recommend that nicotine patches be a Health Mark benefit, that is, should Health Mark pay for nicotine patches, and if so, under what conditions?

2. If I decide Health Mark should cover or provide nicotine patches, from whom should I purchase the patches, that is, should I use bidding procedures and (how) should I consider S.H.'s company?

Each of these questions involves making a moral judgment about what is good or right to do. In the following analysis we will see that neither question has a simple answer.

When J.D. gathers the information he must have before he can make an ethical evaluation of the first question above, he must gather information about both the safety and the efficacy of the patches. Let us look at each consideration separately.

Safety

Safety seems like a straightforward concept. Something is safe (or safer) when it carries a smaller risk of harm than the alternative. For example, riding in a car is safer when we wear seat belts. Should we sustain a collision while in a car, if we are wearing a seat belt we are likely to experience less harm than if we collide wearing no seat belt.

In order to assess the safety of a particular therapy, two separate evaluations are necessary. First we must decide on what the harm of undergoing the therapy could be; second we must assess the likelihood of that harm occurring. Safety, then, is really the product of the kind of harm and its probability of happening. A therapy with a very small chance of a very minor side effect probably would be considered quite safe. An example here might be a drug that causes mild dryness of the mouth in one person in 10,000. A therapy with even a much greater chance of a minor side effect (for example, a drug that causes mild dizziness in one of every 100 persons) might still be considered safe. Less safe, though, are drugs with even a low probability of a very substantial harm. A drug that can kill even a tiny percentage of those who take it is considerably less safe than either of the previous examples. Finally, the obviously unsafe therapy is one that carries a great likelihood of substantial harm.

The safety of a particular drug or therapy is subjective and depends upon how an individual evaluates how bad a particular harm would be to him or her. For example, many persons would probably consider a drug that carried a 1 in 100 chance of causing mild dizziness to be safe; on the other hand, a tightrope walker or an electric line repair worker, to whom an acute sense of balance is exquisitely important, may come to a different conclusion.

J.D.'s assessment of the safety of the nicotine patches has mainly to do with the increased risk of cardiac arrest a person sustains who is using the patches while continuing to smoke. In a person who is not smoking, the nicotine patch supplies a (steadily decreasing) volume of nicotine to the body, which usually begins by approximating the "dose" of nicotine he or she had been getting through cigarettes. If the person also smokes, he or she would receive excessive amounts of nicotine, which could trigger cardiac arrest. Even if the likelihood of a person smoking while using the patch is low and the likelihood of cardiac arrest in a person using the patch is low, the harm is still great, resulting in what J.D. might consider an unsafe situation. If the evidence shows that those enrolled in behavior modification programs are less likely to smoke while using the patch, J.D. might be justified in attempting to raise the overall safety of using the patches by recommending that they be a covered benefit only for those enrolled in behavior modification programs.

Efficacy

Safety is never the sole evaluation to be made. As J.D. considers any particular therapy or drug for inclusion in the formulary, how well it works—its efficacy—also is evaluated. [Note that there is a technical difference between efficacy (i.e., the level of benefit achievable under ideal conditions) and effectiveness (i.e., the level of benefit achievable under ordinary conditions); we need not consider it here, though.] In scientific studies of how well a drug works, researchers try to control various factors that can alter the drug's effects and then evaluate the results by comparing the drug under study to a known efficacious agent, a placebo, or to no drug at all. This kind of research yields useful results, even if all confounding factors are never completely controlled or are not entirely known. This messiness of the real world is what causes one decongestant to be more effective in one person than in another. At the same time, attempting to compare therapies for their effectiveness also allows us to say that this decongestant works at opening stuffed up noses better or more often than say, hot tea.

Efficacy, in shorthand, is "what works." As with evaluations of safety, efficacy is not as straightforward a concept as it might initially appear, however. What "works" is always tested in a particular population under certain conditions, which may not approximate the population and/or conditions in which the therapy is later used. In addition, "working" needs to be carefully defined, so that it can be measured. If the goal of using nicotine patches is to make it possible for a person to stop smoking because smoking is hazardous to one's health, has the patch worked if it helps the smoker go from three packs a day to one? Has it worked if the person ceases to smoke for eight months, and then resumes smoking occasionally?

The conditions of clinical research are not always presented fully to the public. For example, some clinical trials showing that nicotine patches helped people quit smoking achieved this result only in groups that also underwent behavioral modification programs. The appeal of a speedy solution, especially to a challenge such as smoking, sometimes overshadows the details. It then falls to a clinician familiar with the scientific literature, such as a pharmacist, to interpret that literature in a way that is likely to be of real help.

J.D.'s determination of the safety and the efficacy of nicotine patches seems to be strictly factual assessments but also involves conflicts of value. What is the relation between safety and efficacy in J.D.'s rendering of a decision about whether nicotine patches should be included in the benefit package? Some believe that safety should always be the cardinal consideration: unless a product is safe, its efficacy should not play a role in the decision to make the product available to the public. In contrast, others believe that simply because a small group of scientists decided a product is not safe enough, this is not sufficient moral justification for withholding the product from the public. Because safety and efficacy are subjective concepts, a person may legitimately decide to elevate safety concerns over efficacy (or vice versa), depending upon the risk tolerance of that individual.

J.D. is in the challenging position of having to make a recommendation about nicotine patches to the entire Health Mark organization. Rather than simply consider whether safety, efficacy or personal choice is of greatest value in a particular patient's situation, he must look at the aggregate good. There are several methods by which he could make this determination. One method is to poll a representative sample of Health Mark consumers to see if they are more or less risk-averse. He can then make a decision about which value to promote based on the aggregate desires or interests of Health Mark's constituents. Another method, one that is more common in HMOs' decisions about what therapies to pay for, is to poll payers such as other insurance carriers or HMOs to determine the health insurance industry's standard in such cases. A health maintenance organization's long-term interest in remaining price-competitive might justify this choice. J.D. also could perform a traditional cost/benefit analysis to examine whether patch users who were *not* engaged in a behavior modification program were ever successful in stopping smoking. He also could examine whether the cost of providing patches to these patients matched the money saved through a reduced need for the treatment of ailments such as emphysema, cardiac arrest, pneumonia, or lung cancer. This analysis would not be easy to do, however; smoking is only one risk factor for any particular disease, smoking-related diseases can take many years to develop and treat, and calculating "money saved" can be difficult to determine.

Purchasing

The other moral question J.D. must answer concerns from whom he should purchase the patches if he decides that they will be covered by Health Mark. If J.D. were the buyer of widgets for a company that used widgets in production, his choice of supplier might not pose any moral problem. As a pharmacist, however, J.D. is involved in decisions about purchasing drugs and other pharmaceutical therapies that are understood to be *medical goods*. The ramifications of his decision make it a moral one, as we shall see.

Pharmaceutical manufacturers, like other producers of goods, often reduce prices to customers who purchase the goods in large quantities or to those who are able to generate physician support for a particular product. Because the pharmaceutical company for which S.H. works sets particular financial targets, it cannot simply give the patches away to Health Mark inexpensively. The cost of the price break to Health Mark either will be made up by the manufacturer's volume of sales (the more persons who use nicotine patches, appropriately or inappropriately, the better for the company) or the cost will be passed on to the consumer of nicotine patches purchasing them in another way—at a neighborhood pharmacy, for example. The ethical issue raised for J.D. by this situation is one of fairness. Is it fair for Health Mark to purchase the nicotine patches at a lower cost?

On the one hand, the less expensive they are, the less money Health Mark will have to shift from other services to pay for the patches. Further, if the patches are less expensive, they may be more likely to be prescribed and used by Health Mark members (although whether they are used under conditions that make them safe and effective remains a question). In this view, the better the deal J.D. can arrange, the more the patches will be available to Health Mark members who might benefit from them. Under one conception of "fair," a seller has the right to set any price for a particular good; if a buyer pays the price and gets what was paid for, fairness has been served. If this is what constitutes fairness, S.H.'s strategy of contract bidding with J.D. to get Health Mark's business for his company is fair.

A different conception of fairness dictates that if a price is set for a particular product, then anyone who wishes to purchase that product should get it for that same price. In this view, fairness exists only if S.H.'s company charges the same price for nicotine patches to any purchaser, so that the rate Health Mark pays is the same as what the neighborhood pharmacy would pay. Under this "equal charge for equal product" definition of fairness, if S.H. is substantially discounting the patches in order to secure Health Mark's business for his company, and if the company makes up the "lost" profit by marking up the price of the patches to other buyers, then J.D. might consider the deal unfair. Some persons (not members of Health Mark) who need the nicotine patches will end up bearing the increased cost of the patch if Health Mark gets a good deal.

Part of J.D.'s decision may turn on his attitudes toward himself as a professional. If J.D. understands his professional commitment as dedication solely to Health Mark and its members, he may judge that doing business with S.H. in order to get the patches at a good rate for Health Mark will be the best course of action: the more cheaply Health Mark can purchase the patches, the more readily they may be made available to members, and the more likely members are to quit smoking. The more members who quit smoking, the healthier they will be and the more effective Health Mark will be in accomplishing its mission. If, on the other hand, J.D. understands his professional commitment more broadly, as dedication to society at large (including those with poor or no health insurance), J.D. may believe that what he purchases for Health Mark comes at a price for other smokers wishing to quit, and that for the sake of fairness toward those who are not Health Mark members, he should not take advantage of S.H.'s implicit offer.

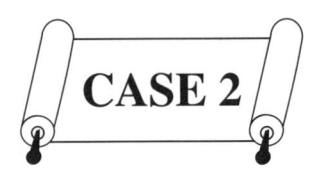

CASE 2

Educational Benefits For Pharmacists

M.H., a 30-year-old pharmacist, works at Community Hospital, a 350-bed teaching hospital in the Midwest. Most of M.H.'s duties involve working as a clinical pharmacist in a cardiology unit. On a part-time basis, she also assists in managing clinical drug trial activities in the hospital.

M.H. recently received a newsletter from the state hospital pharmacists' association, stating that it was organizing a special continuing education seminar focusing on development and use of new drug technologies. The newsletter noted that the seminar would be underwritten by an educational grant from PharmaQuest, a pharmaceutical manufacturer involved in developing novel drug delivery systems for antihypertensive medications. Based on the topic and overall objectives of the seminar, M.H. decided that she would like to attend.

A few weeks later, L.L., a district sales manager from PharmaQuest, met M.H. when she visited Community Hospital. L.L. asked M.H. whether she heard about the seminar. M.H. said that she had heard about it, was really excited about it and hoped the hospital would be able to pay for her to attend. L.L. said that PharmaQuest had decided to sponsor several pharmacists' participation in the seminar and offered to make arrangements for M.H.'s registration and travel costs to be picked up by her (L.L.'s) company.

Case Discussion
Analysis

The corporate sponsorship by pharmaceutical companies of lectures, seminars and workshops on new treatments and technologies poses a host of ethical questions. Some of these are questions about whether it is right to pass on marketing expenses (a "cost of doing business") to the consumer. Others concern truth-telling (i.e., whether the planned seminar will report on independent research or will promote a particular product in the context of research-like information). Whether these are ethical practices from the standpoint of the industry is a separate question from what we will examine in this section. Our main focus here is on the ethical issues that marketing by the pharmaceutical industry raises for the *pharmacist*.

Two main ethical questions face M.H.:

1. Should she attend an industry-sponsored seminar?
2. If she does attend, is it right for her to accept the offer of PharmaQuest, the sponsor of the seminar, to pay for her attendance?

These questions present themselves as ethical dilemmas because there are values in conflict. To think more clearly about how M.H. might resolve them, we need to look carefully at the values involved. There also may be relevant factual information, for example, about the existence of codes of conduct or other guidelines, that can help M.H. place her decision in the proper context. What values are at play in this case?

Information For the Welfare of Patients

An obvious value is the new information about drugs, delivery systems or other technologies M.H. is likely to learn at the seminar. Depending on the actual subject of the conference, this might manifest itself in different ways. For example, a pharmaceutical company may have discovered or developed a new, unique drug. That company might sponsor a seminar specifically to introduce and promote its new product and educate physicians, pharmacists and other clinicians in its appropriate use. After all, it is these clinicians who will determine whether the new drug penetrates the market and accomplishes the good it is intended to.

Another possibility, however, is that the pharmaceutical company sponsors a seminar on a broader spectrum of topics in which the company has an interest. A manufacturer of heart medications, for example, might sponsor a conference on the management of coronary artery disease. In this case, the purpose of the information communicated is less straightforward. In the case described above, M.H. would *expect* to hear about a specific product that the company makes. She is more likely to get promotion of a particular treatment modality (such as a drug the company makes) embedded in a more general discussion of the clinical problem of coronary artery disease. For example, a pharmacist or physician knowledgeable about the product may describe his or her experience with it. It may be difficult for M.H. in a situation like this to distinguish outright marketing from clinical experience of her peers. Recognizing how common and how confusing such situations are, the U.S. Food and Drug Administration recently established rules requiring that seminar participants be informed when speakers at medical meetings are compensated by a specific company.

Even if such a disclosure is made, however, a conference sponsored by a particular business (a pharmaceutical manufacturer) is likely to emphasize those aspects of the subject that are important to that business. In the coronary artery disease example, for instance, one might expect to hear little about the relative merits of lifestyle changes (such as diet, exercise or meditation) over the merits of pharmaceutical intervention. Nevertheless, information of this kind is essential for evaluating any intervention's overall risks and benefits to patients. We might be inclined to dismiss these concerns by saying that it is the responsibility of the seminar participant to recognize and consider the source of the information and to form his or her opinions as objectively as possible. Although we might expect that clinicians base their views on independent examination of the scientific literature, various studies have shown that their views are often highly influenced by marketing literature from manufacturers.[7]

In summary, the value of the information M.H. can expect to gain at the seminar depends on the context. M.H. should try to learn as much as possible about the subject, the speakers and the sponsor's interests in order to evaluate the likelihood that the seminar will provide balanced clinical information versus slanted marketing information.

Professional Integrity

Another value that deserves consideration in the dilemma M.H. faces is that of professional integrity. When L.L. offers to have her company pick up the tab for the expenses M.H. incurs, as well as when she gives her notepads, mugs or pens, she is in fact offering M.H. a gift on behalf of her company. The purpose of gift-giving often is to engender friendly relations. But even when gifts have no apparent "strings" attached, they remain gifts. In our culture, gifts (particularly gifts between strangers) generally establish some sort of reciprocal obligation. That is, we anticipate that one who receives a gift will return a gift or favor at some time, whether in the near or distant future.

When L.L. approached M.H. to extend PharmaQuest's offer to pay M.H.'s way to the seminar, she likely came as a professional acquaintance with whom M.H. had previous, probably positive, contact. Her offer to pay for M.H. to attend the seminar was neither a bribe, to manipulate M.H. to do something she did not want to do, nor was it a secret offer made only to her. It was part of the usual relationship of a pharmaceutical sales representative with a pharmacist. For decades, such relationships have taken place with no oversight, regulation, or even professional organizational guidance.

That situation has begun to change, however. A number of professional organizations [e.g., American Society of Health Systems Pharmacists (ASHP)] have written ethical guidelines for the conduct of health professionals' relationships with the pharmaceutical industry.[8] Some aspects of these guidelines are designed to protect the clinician from the appearance of impropriety or bias; others attempt actually to limit the influence pharmaceutical companies have on clinicians by restricting gift-giving, by limiting companies' control over the content of continuing education programs and by prohibiting direct payment to clinicians to attend conferences.

Obviously, the size of the "gift" will make a difference in the perceived propriety of the gift. When a pharmaceutical company offers to pay for a pharmacist to attend a conference, the location of the conference and whether the gift covers registration only or includes room, board, and entertainment may affect the pharmacist's decision. The pharmacist may have more misgivings if the conference is to be held in a luxurious resort with all expenses paid than if it is held, say, in the doctor's dining room over cold cuts and soft drinks. The guidelines from ASHP, however, do not permit such discretionary decisions. They prohibit a pharmacist from accepting *any* direct offer from a company to pay his or her costs for seminars or other educational opportunities.

Pharmaceutical companies have questioned whether such restrictive policies might negatively affect continuing education in the long run.

After all, if the seminar is worthwhile, and the pharmaceutical company can afford to subsidize the attendance of clinicians, why shouldn't clinicians take advantage of the opportunity and save themselves, their departments or their hospitals money? One creative response (also endorsed by ASHP) has been to offer the pharmaceutical companies the opportunity to contribute, not to any particular conference or seminar, but rather to a continuing education fund from which scholarships or attendance at conferences can be paid. That way, the hospital or department retains control over the content of the meeting as well as who attends.

In choosing a response to L.L.'s offer, M.H. will need to consider seriously the statements made by her professional organizations, such as ASHP, to see if they comport with her assessment of the present situation. If M.H. has not been active in her organization, she may want to explore further its guidelines governing this situation, who wrote them, in response to what situations, and evaluate the degree to which the situations cited in the guidelines are similar to her own. The corporate culture of M.H.'s organization also may affect her perceptions about the importance of guidelines or codes. There may be an unwritten rule that "everybody does it" that could amount to a certain degree of peer pressure if M.H. opts for another response.

When M.H. is satisfied that she has obtained the relevant factual information and assessed the importance of the relative values involved, she needs to choose a course of action that will best honor the values she believes are most significant in this case. In comparing her options, M.H. also must project what the consequences of her various choices could be. For example, if M.H. chooses not to accept L.L.'s offer of a subsidy from PharmaQuest, she still must decide if the seminar itself is worth attending. If she chooses to go, her department director may help her secure other funds to pay for her attendance. If she chooses not to go, she will need to evaluate what kinds of information she may miss and how important that information is to the development of her skills. She also will need to find other means (such as reading various drug compendia, accessing professional journals via MEDLINE, or attending a different seminar) for obtaining this information.

DISCUSSION: CASE 1 AND CASE 2 PRINCIPLES

Pharmacists must address diverse ethical considerations when attempting to reconcile their multiple roles or to balance various interests that compete for their attention. In this chapter, we focus on the fact that relations with the pharmaceutical industry and with specific pharmaceutical manufacturers have numerous ethical implications for the pharmacist. These implications can be direct, such as when an employee of the pharmaceutical manufacturer attempts to manipulate its relationship with a pharmacist (or a group of pharmacists). Alternatively, these implications can be indirect, such as when actions of the pharmaceutical industry alter the context in which a pharmacist engages in professional decision making.

The Patient-Professional Relationship

Thus far, our discussion has focused primarily upon whether and how the *pharmacist* can be affected by his or her relationship to the pharmaceutical industry. We now turn to address questions of the greatest ultimate importance: is the *patient* affected by the pharmacist's relations with the pharmaceutical industry? If so, in what way(s) is the patient affected and how can this occur?

Like all health professionals, the pharmacist's relationship with the patient can be described as a covenant or social contract: in exchange for being granted special trust by society, the pharmacist assumes particular responsibilities. Many of these responsibilities relate to the pharmacist's role in patient care and to meeting the needs of individual patients whom the pharmacist serves. We refer to these as the pharmacist's "duties to the patient" and, as a professional, the pharmacist has a moral obligation to fulfill these duties to the best of his or her ability. What are the pharmacist's duties to the patient and how are they fulfilled? These questions are addressed in depth throughout this textbook. In general, though, we recognize that the pharmacist is committed to promoting the welfare of the patient, respecting the autonomy of the patient, and acting with honesty and integrity in the patient-professional relationship. The pharmacist manifests these commitments in a wide variety of everyday acts and contexts.

The Pharmaceutical Care Model

The pharmaceutical care model[9] provides a framework for characterizing the practices employed by the pharmacist in carrying out duties to the patient. We acknowledge, of course, that this model reflects an *ideal* system of patient care but note that it is to this ideal that the profession aspires. The pharmaceutical care process begins with the pharmacist establishing a unique relationship with the patient. Thus, the pharmacist recognizes the individuality of that particular patient and makes a deep commitment to the patient. This commitment is essential for securing and fostering the patient's trust. Further, honoring the patient's individuality calls upon the pharmacist to place primary importance on the personal values, preferences, and desires held by that patient.

In the second stage in the pharmaceutical care process, the pharmacist applies (as objectively as possible) expert knowledge to analyze the patient's situation and recommends means for preventing or ameliorating drug- or other health-related problems. Carrying this out requires two general competencies. First, the pharmacist must possess or be able to access expert information about drugs and diseases. Second, the pharmacist must be able to apply this information in a manner that is fitting and proper, as judged from both technical and humanistic perspectives.

The third stage in the pharmaceutical care process involves the pharmacist following up with the patient to determine whether selected therapies and/or actions have advanced the patient's welfare. Fulfilling this responsibility again requires that the pharmacist and the patient share an understanding of the situation: here, their need is for agreement on desired outcomes. Conducting appropriate follow-up and evaluation of patient outcomes requires that the pharmacist has access to extensive information regarding the patient's drug regimen, other treatment regimens, biomedical condition, and psychosocial condition.

The Pharmaceutical Industry's Impact on the Patient-Professional Relationship

Having outlined the general stages in pharmaceutical care provision, we now are able to explore whether and how relations with the pharmaceutical industry can affect the pharmacist's ability to carry out duties to the patient. The cases presented above again serve as useful illustrations. In the case of J.D., a pharmacist is asked to make recommendations as to whether and when an HMO recognizes nicotine patches as a covered benefit for its members. His primary concerns are the high cost (regardless of whether under traditional or lower-cost bid pricing) and the equivocal effectiveness of this smoking cessation therapy. This case illustrates one way in which the actions of a pharmaceutical manufacturer can decrease the likelihood that an individual patient's interests are recognized or held to be of greatest importance. The reality of resource scarcity and finite budgets causes the interests of a given patient to be viewed in the context of the interests of the larger group.

The case of M.H. focuses on a pharmacist's involvement in an educational seminar sponsored by the manufacturer of a new drug product. It shows that a pharmaceutical manufacturer's actions can affect the pharmacist's ability to fulfill duties to the patient both positively and negatively. In a positive light, the educational seminar may present the pharmacist with scientifically rigorous, clinically valuable information regarding a new therapy. If the pharmacist then cares for a patient who is a good candidate for the new therapy, the pharmaceutical manufacturer-sponsored seminar can materially assist the pharmacist in promoting the patient's welfare.

We must recognize, though, that a new therapy most likely is appropriate for only a limited number of patients. In cases where the new therapy actually is inappropriate, it may be difficult for the pharmacist to dismiss subtle influences of the seminar; the temptation to apply a new therapy can be intellectually exciting and enhance the pharmacist's professional status. Further, it may be impossible for the pharmacist to determine the extent to which information presented in the seminar is factual, complete, and unbiased. If he or she relies on information of uncertain accuracy, the pharmacist's neutrality could be undermined; biased, incomplete, or otherwise faulty information might serve as the basis for subsequent treatment recommendations. Thus, the pharmacist's ability to provide relatively objective, expert advice could be compromised and his or her ability to fulfill duties to the patient damaged.

CONCLUSION

The relationships between pharmacists and the pharmaceutical industry are indeed complicated. In this chapter we have highlighted some of the ethical aspects of that relationship and have seen that no matter what the context of practice, the pharmacist is challenged to adhere as closely as possible to the ideals of good pharmaceutical care. We also have seen that the power of the pharmaceutical industry to negotiate prices and underwrite educational opportunities can be a mixed blessing: the industry can contribute to the goals of pharmaceutical care for patients, but this contribution comes with trade-offs for both the pharmacist and patients whom the pharmacist serves.

Discussion Questions

1. Imagine that J.D.'s (from our first case) formulary committee has decided to include nicotine patches in the package of member benefits offered by Health Mark, only on the condition that their use is simultaneous with enrollment in a behavior modification program for smoking cessation. Consider a patient who, due to a scheduling conflict with work, is unable to attend such a behavior modification program. Should her situation receive special consideration in evaluating her request for nicotine patches? Perhaps a patient simply prefers not to go through a behavior modification program. Does that patient warrant special consideration?

2. Imagine that you are a pharmacist with Pharm-Aid, a drugstore chain. A patient comes to you for a refill of a prescription for nicotine patches. She is smoking as she waits to have her prescription filled. In your conversation with her, she tells you that she knows it's wrong to smoke, especially when she is paying so much money for the patches to help her stop. She has never heard of behavior modification. Later, when you talk to her physician about the situation, he insists that he gave her a brochure on a smoking cessation program and told her not to smoke while using the patches. But, he insists, if she smokes anyway, "that's her choice." What do you do when she comes in for her next refill?

3. Your brother has tried to quit smoking twice but has only succeeded for a week or two at a time. He now has gone to his family physician who tells him the nicotine patches might help, but only if he enrolls in a behavior modification program. Since he is very serious about wanting to quit, your brother comes to your pharmacy to have his prescription for the patches filled and enrolls in a smoking cessation program through the hospital that seems to have a good reputation. He attends class faithfully, practices the prescribed exercises at home and takes up jogging to deal better with stress. You know he is really trying. Shortly after he closes on a big deal at work, he resumes smoking. If he decides to try again to quit, should you refill his patch prescription?

4. After taking their antihypertensive medications, patients commonly experience hypotensive episodes that result in problems with dizziness. PharmaQuest has been working to complete development of the "NormoTens" system, a novel drug delivery system that is intended to reduce the frequency of this troublesome side effect. PharmaQuest is conducting clinical trials to test the NormoTens system and has made arrangements with Community Hospital to study patients treated in its cardiology unit. M.H. (from our second case) is asked to assist in recruiting patients for the study. She is told that she will be paid $400 for each patient she recruits. Should M.H. assist in recruiting patients for this study? If so, under what conditions?

Continued

Discussion Questions continued

5. Imagine that M.H. has been responsible for supervising Community Hospital's trial of the NormoTens system. PharmaQuest anticipates that the first drug product using the NormoTens system will receive governmental approval soon. L.L. is developing an educational program focused on the use of the NormoTens system. The program will be broadcast to physicians statewide. Knowing that M.H. is familiar with its use, L.L. asks her to serve as one of the three main speakers in the broadcast, for which she will be paid $750. Should M.H. agree to participate?

6. Imagine that the drug product using the NormoTens system has received governmental approval and that marketing is beginning. L.L. would like to present information about the product to physicians at Community Hospital. She asks M.H. to assist her in arranging a casual luncheon seminar to do so. Should such a luncheon be permitted by the hospital? If it is, should M.H. provide assistance to L.L.?

REFERENCES

1. Hepler DC. The third wave in pharmaceutical education: the clinical movement. Am J Pharm Educ. 1987;51:370–71.
2. Smith MC, Knapp DA. Pharmacy, Drugs and Medical Care. 3rd ed. Baltimore: Williams and Wilkins; 1992:116.
3. Braithaite J. Corporate Crime in the Pharmaceutical Industry. London: Routledge and Kegan Paul; 1984.
4. Lipman AG. Drug use management. In: Brown TR, ed. Handbook of Institutional Pharmacy Practice. 3rd ed. Bethesda: American Society of Hospital Pharmacists; 1992:63–7.
5. Allen SJ. Purchasing and inventory management. In: Brown TR, ed. Handbook of Institutional Pharmacy Practice. 3rd ed. Bethesda: American Society of Hospital Pharmacists; 1992:73.
6. Keith TD, Foster MT Jr. Drug therapy monitoring. In: Brown TR, ed. Handbook of Institutional Pharmacy Practice. 3rd ed. Bethesda: American Society of Hospital Pharmacists; 1992:273–74.
7. Silverman M et al. Prescriptions for Death. Berkeley: University of California Press; 1982.
8. Anon. ASHP guidelines on pharmacists' relationships with industry. Am J Hosp Pharm. 1992;49:154.
9. Strand LM et al. Pharmaceutical Care: An Introduction. Kalamazoo: Upjohn Company; 1992:14–22.

Chapter 8

Is There a Right to Medication?

Robert L. McCarthy
James D. Richardson

One of the most intense debates in our society today concerns the right to health care. Some argue that health care is a commodity, just like cars or shoes. If we are able to purchase these things, we ought to be free to do so, but if we are poor, then we simply have to go without them. People in this camp say that health care is a privilege, not a right.

Others argue that health care is essential to our existence and it should, therefore, be considered a right, not a privilege. There is a great deal of disagreement, however, about how much health care we are entitled to receive if we are not able to pay for it.

We will attempt to bring some clarity to this debate by making some important distinctions, and by applying this conceptual analysis to a realistic case study. We will examine the distinction between rights and privileges, moral and legal rights, positive and negative rights, and rights and responsibilities. Understanding these distinctions may not resolve the debate, but it will help us to see what is at stake and how one can support one's position rationally, rather than through mere emotion or rhetoric. Consider the following situation.

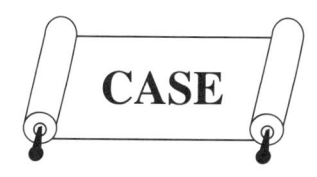

CASE

T.G. is a 36-year-old widower, the father of two children ages three and seven, and has insulin-dependent diabetes. T.G. is able to work only on a part-time basis because of the need to care for his children and the severe nature of his illness (half of his left foot has been amputated). His limited income allows him to be eligible for state assistance including Medicaid.

One day, in late summer, T.G. stops by his local pharmacy to replenish his diabetes supplies. T.G., a long-time patient of Miller's Pharmacy, is well known to pharmacist J.M. Unfortunately, today J.M. has some bad news for T.G. He informs his patient that because the state is near the end of its fiscal year and expenditures for health care have been exceeded, the Medicaid program is out of funds. As a result, J.M. tells T.G. that he will have to pay for his medication until the start of the new fiscal year, several months away. T.G. protests that there is no way that he can afford to pay for his medication. Further, he suggests that J.M. should, considering T.G.'s long patronage, provide the medication to him at no or minimal cost.

J.M. responds that he cannot do this because if he did so for T.G., he also would have to do the same for his many other Medicaid patients. T.G. claims that he has a right to his medication and since the state won't provide, J.M. will have to.

This illustrates a problem frequently encountered by many health care professionals: how to care for patients who cannot afford the care they need. Those who deliver such care are confronted by patients who contend that they have a right to health care even when the responsibility for payment falls upon others.

In this chapter, we will attempt to provide a conceptual framework within which such debates can be carried out. We will address the question of whether health care is a right or a privilege. If a right, what kind of right—positive or negative, legal or ethical? Are ethical rights parasitic upon ethical principles? What societal and ethical questions must be addressed if one accepts the assumption that health care is a right? Should there be universal access to health care?

The last portion of the chapter will speak to the issue of right to medication. Do patients have a right to medication as they do to other forms of health care? Does society have the obligation to provide medication to those unable to afford it? If society has this obligation, does the obligation fall upon the pharmacist if society fails to meet it?

RIGHTS AND PRIVILEGES

The case discussed above raises many issues, not the least of which is whether patients have a right to medication or whether access to medication is a privilege. T.G. claims that he has a right to his diabetes supplies, whether he can or cannot pay for them. If having his diabetes supplies is a privilege, then no one is obligated to provide them; no one is obligated even to make them available to T.G. for purchase.

To decide whether T.G. is correct in asserting that he has a right to medication, we must first clarify what is meant by "rights" (i.e., just claim) and "privileges" (i.e., benefit or favor). As might be expected, attempting to make this distinction is difficult largely because of problems involved in characterizing what is meant by a right. This task is even more difficult when one wishes to clarify what is meant by a right in the context of health care. When rights to health care are claimed, they are asserted in terms of moral rights, a much more problematic type of right than legal rights.

What Is a Right?

What does it mean to have a right? We begin our discussion by examining several common uses of claims for rights. People differ in what they perceive to be a right, and what those claims to rights are. The political philosopher Thomas Hobbes defines *"natural rights"* as those "which all men possess in virtue of being human beings and which in some cases cannot transfer by agreement, even if they want to."[1] The English philosopher John Locke asserts

> that men have certain rights...merely because they are God's creatures. ...These rights include the right to life (hence no man can justly be destroyed by another), to freedom (hence no dictatorship is legitimate), and to property."[1]

If Locke's assertion sounds familiar to Americans, it is because he was a primary influence on those individuals who drafted our founding documents. In the United States, we often think of rights as those stated in the Declaration of Independence or constitutionally guaranteed. Freedom of speech, assembly, religion, the right to bear arms, due process, and suffrage—all represent those rights that are well known by Americans but not always completely understood. In addition, there are other rights people claim but are not in our founding documents. Examples might include education, privacy, and the right to have basic needs met, including food, shelter, and medical care.

There is some uncertainty as to what constitutes a right, and also who possesses such rights and how such claims are to be justified. Because of the range of claims to rights, there is tremendous difficulty in trying to give a single definition of rights. Hence, a good starting point might be to contrast rights and privileges.

The Distinction Between Rights and Privileges

A fancy sports car, a house by the shore, and European vacations twice a year are things many people may want; however, most agree that these are things they do not have a right to. These are classified by rights theorists as privileges—that is those things that people may want and get, but do not have an absolute claim to. Rights, on the other hand, are the sorts of things that individuals legitimately can lay claim to. These include trial by jury, right to counsel, and, most recently, the right of access to buildings by the handicapped. More controversially, health care also is considered by some to be a right. But if it is a right, what kind of right?

To answer this question, we will need to make some distinctions among the different types of rights. We will begin our taxonomy with an easy question: If health care is a right, is it a positive or a negative right?

Positive and Negative Rights

Rights are classified as either positive or negative. *Positive rights* require someone or some entity to do something if someone asserts that right. For example, if health care is indeed a right, it is a positive right because it requires some individuals, or a government, to take positive action for that right to be exercised (e.g., provide an antibiotic for a bacterial infection). On the other hand, a *negative right* prohibits certain actions by individuals or governments. The right to privacy requires someone not to do something for that right to be exercised (e.g., not tap telephones).

Legal and Ethical Rights

Potential rights to health care also may be classified as legal or ethical. Purtilo and Cassel explain that:

> Traditionally, a distinction has been drawn between moral [ethical] rights and legal rights. A *moral right* entitles a person to possess or perform something, but one's moral entitlement may or may not be supported by law. If it is, one speaks of a legal right. However, to speak of a *legal right* presupposes that a moral right exists and is being recognized or protected.[2]

Although such a distinction appears plausible, it ignores the fact that some legal rights may have no moral basis. Yezzi describes that differentiation more accurately by contending,

> If rights are asserted to exist separately from specified governmental or institutional guarantees, then they are moral [ethical] rights; if they are asserted to exist within a system of such guarantees, then they are legal rights."[3]

With this as a guide, let us examine legal and ethical rights more closely.

What Is a Legal Right?
What Are the Types of Legal Rights?

A person has a legal right if, and only if, that right is granted by the legal system. As one might expect, there are legal rights that are constitutionally granted (e.g., free speech), others that are the result of judicial interpretation (usually of the Constitution such as the right to legal counsel to defend oneself in criminal proceedings), and still others that may be conferred by law or regulation (e.g., T.G.'s right to Medicaid assistance). Usually, legal rights confer on the person given these rights an enforceable claim. That is, the person will have legal backing if he or she wishes to assert a claim against the party or parties responsible for assuring that right. Unfortunately, because of one circumstance or another, legal rights may not always be enforceable—sometimes the result of a lack of funds as in T.G.'s case, and sometimes because responsibility for assuring that right has not been assigned. One of the ways in which this latter type of situation may arise is under the condition of the assertion of an ideal, an assertion that takes as its aim the promotion of a direction which public policy in the future should take, or an assertion of a societal value (e.g., U.N. Declaration of Human Rights).

What Is an Ethical Right?
How Does It Differ from a Legal Right?

This last sense of legal rights, in fact, seems to be a misnomer since one of the essential characteristics of a legal right would seem to be its enforceability. However, such rights clearly are not legally enforceable and to that extent might be better classified as ethical rights. That is, rights that can be asserted on the basis of ethical principles, but not legal ones.

As it stands, this is somewhat misleading because it seems to imply that legal rights have no ethical basis. With this caveat in mind, a more accurate definition of ethical rights might be those rights that are justified by ethical principles, whether or not they also are grounded in the law. When we are talking about ethical rights that do not have legal grounding, we shall refer to them as "simple ethical rights."

In theory, T.G. has a legal right to his medication, but due to financial demands, he finds it unenforceable. His demand that J.M. has a duty to provide him with his medical supplies is an example of an assertion of a "simple ethical right."

The Relationship Between Ethical Rights and Ethical Principles
How Are Claims to Ethical Rights Argued For or Rebutted?

Respect for autonomy and social justice (especially fair opportunity and distributive justice) are the principles most often appealed to when one attempts to justify the assertion of an ethical right. The principle of respect for autonomy, in its most basic form, asserts that "a person's liberty of thought, choice, or action is not to be interfered with."[4] This principle suggests that, generally speaking, individuals know what is best for them, and hence others have a duty not to interfere with their independent decisions about their own lives. Clearly, the principle of respect for autonomy also provides the foundation for negative rights, as discussed earlier in this chapter, since negative rights guarantee the right of the individual not to be interfered with. The principle of respect for autonomy is the primary ethical justification for what often are called liberties (freedoms to), since it prohibits interference with anyone wishing to exercise these liberties.

Social justice concerns itself with the treatment of individuals within a society, particularly in terms of fairness or getting what one deserves. The starting point that essentially everyone agrees with is Aristotle's classic definition of justice, "treat equals equally and unequals unequally," sometimes called the *formal principle of justice*.[5] Part of the reason for the unanimity is that it says so very little, only that, in effect, one must have grounds for treating people differently. For justice to have a greater degree of specificity, one needs to turn to material principles of justice, a much more controversial and complex topic. For our purposes, we will focus on the concepts of fair opportunity and distributive justice in an attempt to minimize this complexity. The *principle of fair opportunity* asserts that individuals ought to have a "fair opportunity" to achieve the goods of life (i.e., that people ought to have a level playing field in the "game of life"). *Distributive justice* concerns itself with how the benefits and burdens of society are allocated among its members.[5] Together, these principles play a major role in the ethical justification of positive rights, including health care.

For instance in the case of T.G., who thought he had a legal right, one could argue that there is an ethical obligation to provide care on the grounds of fair opportunity. Without this care he could not even attempt to have a minimally decent life since life for him is impossible without insulin.

RIGHTS TO HEALTH CARE

As mentioned previously, health care remains controversial in how it is to be designated; a right, a privilege or, perhaps, partially a right and partially a privilege. It is this dilemma that represents the fundamental question that plagues the American health care delivery system. This issue is quite long-standing and was addressed in the Preamble to the Constitution of the World Health Organization published in 1958. It states, in part, "The enjoyment of the highest attainable standard of health is one of the fundamental rights of every human being without distinction of race, religion, political belief, economic or social condition."[6] However, as Mappes and Zembaty so aptly point out, "A citizen of the United States, for example, cannot walk into a hospital, demand and receive treatment simply on the basis of the claim that the U.N. Declaration proclaims his or her right to such care."[6] This implies that, at best, health care in the United States is an ethical right, not a legal one.

Is Health Care an Ethical Right or a Privilege (Private Consumption Good Based on Ability to Pay)?

If health care, in the American perspective, is considered to be a right, whether ethical or legal, then on grounds of social justice (i.e., fairness) it should be universally available. As a result, accessibility to health care, as a right, would not be restricted based on ability to pay. On the other hand, if it is merely a privilege, which might be referred to as a private consumption good, then as with other such goods it is available only on a free-market basis.

On What Grounds Is Health Care as a Privilege Claimed?

Those who argue that health care is a privilege, rather than a right, do so based upon both legal and ethical considerations. Although the United States' Constitution and Bill of Rights guarantee a number of rights (e.g., free speech, assembly, religion), there is no explicit right to health care. Since such a right is not constitutionally mandated, some contend that classifying health care as a legal right places government in an area rightly the province of the private sector. This strict constructionist approach to interpreting the Constitution is consistent with that used to oppose other governmental "interferences" in the marketplace, such as environmental and safety regulations. Additionally, there is a long-standing tradition in this country of being highly suspicious about the efficiency and fairness of "big government."

An ethically based argument depends strongly upon the principle of respect for autonomy: claiming that making health care a positive right would impose significant restraints upon health care providers and patients alike. In the more extreme versions of this argument, claims are made that physicians would be told where, when, and how to practice; who their patients would be; and what compensation they would receive. Likewise, patients would be told who they would use for their health care, in what setting, and with what limitations. Even more extreme is the argument that a legal right to health care would produce such high costs and such limitations on autonomy that no rational person would prefer it to our present system.

Unfortunately for these lines of argument, Canada, Great Britain, and most other Western democracies have implemented a system of universal availability of health care. In fact, the United States is the only industrialized nation, other than South Africa, without national health care. Unlike other nations who have established health care as both a legal and ethical right for all its citizens, the United States, as we have discussed, is still unsure of whether it has a similar obligation, except perhaps for the oldest and very poorest of its people.

On What Grounds Are Rights to Health Care Claimed?

Generally speaking, claims to health care as a right are based on the perception that health care, in contrast to commodities such as automobiles and television sets, is a *fundamental need*. What then is meant by a fundamental need? Further, why do fundamental needs give rise to rights? Fundamental needs include at least those things without which a person cannot live. Food, water, and some form of shelter are among the most obvious examples. Clearly, some forms of health care do not qualify as meeting fundamental needs—cosmetic surgery and some drugs (e.g., oral contraceptives) quickly come to mind. Others, however, including drugs such as insulin, cardiac medications, and antibiotics, very well may be classified as meeting the criteria for fundamental needs.

Beauchamp and Childress[5] contend that there are two moral arguments that may be used effectively to support the premise that health care is a right. The first concerns "collective social protection." This argument equates health care with other societal needs such as protection against crime and pollution that require a collective public response to deal with them effectively. This position is strengthened further when one considers society's "investment" in educating medical professionals and developing biomedical equipment to deliver health care to members of society. This collective "investment" by society requires a "return" (i.e., access to medical care). The second contention is based on the "fair opportunity rule" as discussed earlier in the chapter. This argument is consistent with the previous discussion of fundamental needs. The principle of justice demands that the members of society are treated the same—treat equals equally—and if they are not because of circumstances they cannot control, society has an obligation to ensure they are treated justly. Illnesses are unpredictable and do not discriminate based on an individual's ability to pay for its treatment. Justice demands that all individuals of a society, regardless of socioeconomic status, have access to medical treatment.

However, a case can be made that a number of medical conditions are not out of the individual's control. For example, cigarette smokers who develop lung cancer, alcoholics who develop liver cirrhosis, motorcyclists who refuse to wear helmets, or mountain climbers who take risks, all contribute by their actions to their medical conditions. Hence, an argument can be made that society, even a just one, ought not to be held morally responsible for the costs associated with the treatment of these conditions. One must, however, be careful in ascribing culpability to the individual since many conditions formerly regarded as the result of voluntary actions now are viewed as less than voluntary (e.g., alcoholism, severe obesity).

How Is an Individual's Right to Health Care Affected by Resources Available?

Heart transplants provide an instructive example of a medical treatment that does seem to address a fundamental need (i.e., life), but it does not follow that every patient who needs a heart transplant has a right to one, even if there were enough hearts available. The issue is not solely one of meeting fundamental needs, but also of allocation of resources, for no society has an unlimited amount of resources available. As Beauchamp and Childress point out, health care is but one of a number of "values" a society holds:

> The most general question for a society committed to providing a decent minimum of health care to all citizens is how much of its budget should be allocated for health care and how much for social goods, such as housing, education, culture, and recreation.[5]

Therefore, at the "macro" level, society must decide how large a piece of the valued commodities pie health care will receive. This may be accomplished in a number of ways, both governmentally or through the private sector. Who makes those decisions, and how, underlies many fundamental differences among those who disagree about how health care is to be delivered.

As Howard Hiatt[7] has argued, a society must choose how it will allocate its scarce resources. He refers to the amount of such resources a society chooses to spend on health care as the "medical commons." He further asserts that this finite amount of resources must be suballocated within health care. That is, money spent on neonatal intensive care units (NICUs) is not available to spend on prenatal care, and it also is a societal decision how this will be done. Allocation of scarce resources, therefore, must be carried out at two levels. The first includes all the valued commodities held by a society, and the second involves microallocation of expenditures within health care. Consequently, an individual's right to have a fundamental need met by the society is not an unrestricted right. However, fairness dictates that these decisions should not be arbitrary. But then, how should we decide?

How May a Society Justify Its Allocation of Its Scarce Resources?

Although some medical conditions involving fundamental needs may arise from conditions over which the individual had control (e.g., lung cancer from cigarette smoking, liver cirrhosis from alcohol consumption), the vast majority of serious medical problems do not. If most conditions are not self-inflicted, how then might resources be allocated in such a way that prevents discrimination? It seems to follow that justice demands that we treat all; however, resources may not permit us to do so. At times, we have attempted to accomplish this seemingly impossible task by setting varying criteria to use for deciding who will, and who will not, be treated. Age, cost-benefit ratios, and, ironically, even ability to pay have been invoked as criteria.

Yezzi suggests that allocation of scarce resources occurs at several different levels:

> On the first level, are situations where critical, but temporary, conditions demand decisions about allocation of scarce resources. Natural disasters provide a good example. On the second level are those situations where long-term conditions of limited resources demand a procedure to make decisions when demand continually exceeds supply. On the third level are situations where people must decide what allocation of a society's total resources should go toward providing medical needs.[3]

It is the third level that Hiatt refers to in his "medical commons" model (i.e., deciding the health care share of the total allocation available to meet societal needs). It is these constraints at the third level that cause constraints at the second level.

We suggest adding a fourth level to the three described by Yezzi. This fourth level deals with how resources within health care are allocated among competing programs. For example, money allocated to Medicare (for the elderly) cannot be spent on funding Medicaid (for the poor). T.G. and his pharmacist (introduced to us earlier in the chapter) are faced with a crisis, not simply because of society's decision about its total allocation to health care, but also because of society's fourth level decision about how much money to allocate to Medicaid.

Rationing of Health Care

Once one accepts the reality that a finite amount of resources is available to support the delivery of health care, the idea of rationing must be dealt with. American health care policy makers have tried to avoid this approach because it represents a contradiction with a long-standing implicit belief that all that can be done for each patient ought to be done. Medical insurance, both publicly and privately funded, has attempted to support this ideal. But without cost-containment, this has resulted in rising insurance rates which drive individuals out of the health insurance system and threaten the viability of governmental programs. The consequence of this policy is seen in both increasing numbers of individuals, who are unable to afford health insurance, and increasing restrictions on who qualifies for public programs. Therefore, fewer people have access to health care (approximately 38 million without either private or public health insurance), or at the very least have decreased choices of where they can receive health care (e.g., municipal hospitals, free clinics). As a result, the United States currently may not have *de jure* rationing of health care, but certainly has *de facto* rationing.

Should the United States decide to adopt a formal rationing approach to health care, then several questions must be addressed. As Beauchamp and Childress suggest,

> Both procedures and outcomes need attention in rationing health care. 'Who should make the decisions?' is a procedure-oriented question, whereas 'What should the criteria be for decision making?' is a substance-oriented question.[5]

The second question posed by these authors suggests that rationing may take several forms.

The first method is to ration by establishing a maximum per capita expenditure (e.g., $2000 per person per year) on medical care. Should one's expenses exceed this limit, any additional costs must be met by the patient or care is not provided. Currently, essentially all forms of public or private health insurance use this type of rationing, setting a maximum annual cap per person for at least some forms of health care.

Rationing also may mean denial of care for a segment of the population based on such criteria as age, cost-benefit ratio, or likelihood of success. For example, the state of Oregon has begun a program where rationing of health care services is based on the disease state or medical condition as they relate to both the cost-benefit ratio of treatment and the total budget allocated to health care.

If society should decide that the first two methods of rationing are unacceptable because of issues of fairness, then what seems to be the only alternative is to provide care to all, but at a substantially lowered level of quality shared by all. This societal mandate might, for example, limit length of hospital stay, cap laboratory tests, or severely restrict the use of emerging biotechnology and highly qualified health care practitioners. Opponents to the Canadian health care system have argued against the United States adopting such a plan because they envision it as involving this type of rationing.

For at least the present, American health care planners have determined that rationing of care, in any manner, is not a viable alternative for dealing with our current crisis. At the same time, however, there is a shared determination by the government and the public at large that reform is essential and, further, whatever changes are made must ensure universal access to health care while controlling costs and reducing fraud.

RIGHTS TO MEDICATION

Up to this point, we have been talking about health care in general. We now will focus our attention on the right to medication. It should be obvious by now that any right to medication that a patient might have comes about as part of the right to health care.

Do Patients Have a Right to Medication? All Medication or Some Medication?

As we suggested earlier in this chapter, whatever rights patients have to medication are not unlimited. First of all, not all medications treat fundamental needs; and, hence, society is not obligated to provide them as a right. For example, most people do not believe that acne or hair loss products treat fundamental needs. Second, society may disagree about whether a drug meets a fundamental need. Examples of such drugs include psychotropics and medicinal uses of marijuana and heroin. Third, even if society agrees that a medication does treat a fundamental need, it does not follow that society has an obligation to provide that medication as a right because of limited resources. Orphan drugs (i.e., those drugs whose development and marketing a drug company may not choose to pursue because of a limited market) provide an example of drugs that meet fundamental needs, but for only a few individuals. Another example is the hospital or HMO formulary that prohibits, based on the availability of less expensive substitutes, the use of certain drugs to treat fundamental needs.

Determining which medications treat what we have referred to as fundamental needs, is no trivial task. Even a class of medications such as oral contraceptives might prove to be problematic. For example, if by providing oral contraceptives to a poor woman receiving public assistance and already overburdened with child care responsibilities, society can prevent further pregnancies and their accompanying problems, might such an allocation be justified, even if most members of society consider birth control to be a privilege, not a right? In such a case, the justification, as public policy, would be in terms of containing costs, here taken more broadly than health care costs.

If Patients Have a Right to Medication, Who Has an Obligation to Provide It?

In the best of all possible worlds, society would meet fundamental needs for medication. However, even if society was willing to provide medications to treat fundamental needs, any real world system will have flaws so that worthy individuals will not have their needs met. If society fails in this responsibility, then either the responsibility is not met or it must be met by individuals or groups of individuals. Because of the history of failure by American society to meet these needs, a varied number of other sources have emerged. These include not-for-profit hospitals and clinics, charitable organizations, pharmaceutical manufacturers (compassionate use programs and samples to physicians), physicians and other prescribers, and pharmacists.

Do Pharmacists Have an Ethical Duty to Provide Medication?

Pharmacists find themselves in the peculiarly sensitive position of being the first and the last group of persons to which patients can turn. First, because they are often the resource for referral of patients for health care, and last because they are the group that receives prescriptions, dispenses them, and must be reimbursed for them. So, if patients and society have avoided addressing the issue of cost up to this point, it is no longer avoidable. This leaves pharmacists in a dilemma of what to do. Should they refuse to dispense medications without payment? In extreme cases, such refusals may place the patient's life at risk. On the other hand, pharmacists who regularly dispense prescriptions for free to patients who cannot afford them are likely to go out of business.

This dilemma is even more acute when one considers community pharmacists who practice in a poor urban or rural setting. These practitioners have a patient mix that is far more likely to need assistance in paying for their medications. Further, they may have a disproportionately small number of patients on the higher end of the socioeconomic spectrum with which to lessen the financial impact of nonpaying patients. This suggests that depending upon pharmacists to provide medications to patients when the government is unwilling to do so, places an unfair burden on at least those individuals willing to serve the poor.

Still, the absence of action by the government does not necessarily free individual pharmacists of their obligation or fidelity to their patients, even when their financial viability may be at risk. After all, to let a patient suffer, and perhaps die, for lack of money to pay for their medication seems to be blatantly immoral. It may be that pharmacists must decide each individual situation as it presents itself and not hope to establish a general rule of action.

CONCLUSION

What then of our patient, T.G.? Is he to die because society has chosen not to provide enough resources for him to meet a fundamental need that already has been labeled by society as a legal right? Legal rights of this type are hollow because they are unenforceable. Does then the responsibility for providing T.G.'s medication fall upon the pharmacist J.M.? If so, whose responsibility is it to ensure that J.M. does not go out of business? We have argued that to ask individuals to meet the responsibilities that are properly those of society at large is neither to solve the problem nor is it fair to those practitioners who care for the poor. But in this imperfect world, what is J.M. to do? Let T.G. sink into a diabetic coma? Ship him off to the emergency room at the local hospital? The answer may depend upon factual matters such as the possibility of alternative resources (e.g., charity, compassionate use programs), the number of patients needing life-saving medication, and the financial strength of the pharmacy. Further, adopting a political activist approach to ensuring that such crises do not happen may be the best long-range approach if it is consistent with wise choices in the allocation of scarce resources.

Discussion Questions

1. In a desperate attempt to put a cap on AIDS-related health care costs, it has been proposed that Medicaid reimbursement for treatment (except for comfort measures) for this condition cease for anyone 15 years of age or older who contracts the virus three years after this regulation goes into effect. Is this a fair proposal? Why or why not?

2. Imagine that you are the owner/manager of a small independent pharmacy located in a low-income area, in fact the only one in that area. Because of your location, many of your patients (at least 25%) are on Medicaid, and the rest are low income. You are satisfied with the quality of care you are providing and your patients are appreciative. Unfortunately, you have just received a letter from Medicaid stating that, due to a budget crisis, reimbursements will be delayed indefinitely. A few quick calculations convince you that this will result in a major cash flow problem. What ought you to do? Why?

3. A patient comes into your pharmacy to have her prescriptions filled. One is for a psychotropic and the other is for an antibiotic. The patient realizes that he does not have enough money to pay for both prescriptions, and he lacks insurance coverage of any kind. Since he can only afford one of the medications, he asks you which one he should have filled. What ought you to do? Why?

4. You are the owner or manager of a community pharmacy that provides both professional and convenience services (e.g., free delivery). Because of rising costs, it appears you cannot maintain the same level of service. A consultant recommends, as part of a plan to cut costs while maintaining as much service as possible, that you not provide convenience services for patients covered under third party plans while continuing to do so for cash customers. Should you follow the consultant's advice? Why?

5. Imagine you are a pharmacist in an HMO and on a committee setting institutional policy. A member of the committee, concerned about escalating parenteral nutrition costs, has suggested that the HMO cease providing parenteral nutrition (or at least the very expensive amino acids component) to patients who, at the time of decision about whether or not to initiate parenteral nutrition, have a life expectancy of less than one month. Is this suggestion fair? Why or why not?

REFERENCES

1. Stroll A, Popkin RH. Introduction to Philosophy. New York: Holt, Rinehart and Winston; 1979.
2. Purtilo RB, Cassel CK. Ethical Dimensions in the Health Professions. Philadelphia: WB Saunders; 1981.
3. Yezzi R. Medical Ethics: Thinking About Unavoidable Questions. New York: Holt, Rinehart and Winston; 1980.
4. Richardson JD. Pharmacy Ethics. Unpublished.
5. Beauchamp TL, Childress JF. Principles of Biomedical Ethics. 3rd ed. New York: Oxford University Press; 1989.
6. Mappes TA, Zembaty JS. Biomedical Ethics. New York: McGraw-Hill; 1986.
7. Hiatt HH. Protecting the medical commons: who is responsible? N Engl J Med. 1975;293:235–41.

Chapter 9

Do Pharmacists Have a Right to Refuse to Fill Prescriptions for Abortifacient Drugs?[a]

Kenneth Mullan
Bruce D. Weinstein

With the possibility that the abortifacient drug RU-486 will become legally available in the United States and elsewhere, pharmacists who believe that abortion is immoral are beginning to wonder whether they would be entitled to refuse to fill prescriptions for this drug. We will present a scenario that raises the question, "Does the pharmacist have a right to refuse to fill the patient's prescription for an abortifacient drug?" We then analyze the question from both a legal and an ethical perspective and show that the answer from both points of view is, "It depends."

Some pharmacists who believe that abortion is immoral are troubled by the thought that they might be required to fill a prescription for abortifacient drugs. Do pharmacists have the right to refuse to fill such prescriptions? As discussed in Chapter 3: The Relationship between Ethics and the Law and Chapter 8: Is There a Right to Medication?, questions about rights have both legal and moral dimensions. We begin by considering what the law has to say before moving to an ethical analysis of the question. We do so by way of examining a fictitious case study.

---

[a] A portion of this chapter appeared in "Do Pharmacists Have a Right to Refuse to Fill Prescriptions for Abortifacient Drugs?" Law Med Health Care. 1992;20(3):220–23. Reprinted with permission from the American Society of Law, Medicine, and Ethics.

CASE

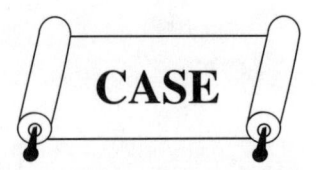

S.S., Pharm.D., works as an employee pharmacist in Main Street Pharmacy, an independent, community pharmacy located in Small Town. There is no other pharmacy within a 20-mile radius. One afternoon M.P. enters the pharmacy and presents a prescription to the pharmacist. The prescription is for mifepristone, an antiprogestin drug, which may be used to treat breast cancer, inoperable meningioma, Cushing's disease, and some forms of hypertension and diabetes. It also is used to end early pregnancies. Women have a legal right to obtain an abortion.

S.S. studies the prescription and a puzzled look appears on her face. She asks M.P. to explain the use and purpose of the medication. M.P. responds with indignation, indicating that such information is personal. Dr. S.S. persists, asking whether M.P. is pregnant and intends to use the drug as an abortifacient. M.P. indicates that she is feeling very uncomfortable and regards Dr. S.S.'s actions as being very unprofessional; she then asks for the medication.

S.S. indicates that she is sorry but cannot fill the prescription if it is to be used to end a pregnancy. She tells M.P. that such an action would be contrary to her own religious beliefs. She says that if M.P. intends to take the drug for a legitimate medical reason and indicates that reason to the pharmacist, she will be happy to dispense the medication. M.P. responds that if she does not get the drug from this pharmacy then she will not be able to get it at all. Her car is not very reliable and she cannot get to a bigger town.

Case Discussion
A Legal Perspective

Does Dr. S.S. have the *legal* right to refuse to dispense the prescription that has been presented to her? The answer to this question is that it depends on a number of factors. These factors are found in four main areas of the law: 1) Pharmacy Law, 2) Employment Law, 3) Abortion Law, and 4) Antidiscrimination Law.

Pharmacy Law

The granting, denial, suspension, revocation, or renewal of a license to practice pharmacy is controlled by individual states. State legislation usually delegates power to a State Board of Pharmacy to control licensing in the manner described above. The legislation that controls licensing also may delegate a power to make regulations detailing standards of pharmacy practice and rules of professional conduct. When such regulations are made, they have the force of law and deviation from them may have significant legal implications.

State legislation may include a requirement that the pharmacist may not refuse to dispense a prescription unless there is a valid reason for that refusal. Such is the case, for example, in West Virginia:

> No pharmacist shall refuse to accept and fill, or cause to be filled, for payment thereof any prescription order presented to him [or her] unless there is a valid reason for his inability to fill such prescription order.[1]

S.S., in deciding whether to refuse to fill the prescription presented to her, will have to consider the legal implications of the decision to refuse under pharmacy law provisions such as these. The rule in West Virginia is prescriptive, the pharmacist shall not refuse, thereby suggesting that there is no right to refuse to fill a prescription except where Dr. S.S. can show a valid reason for her refusal to fill such a prescription.

A refusal to fill a prescription in the absence of a valid reason may be sufficient grounds for a State Board to revoke or suspend S.S.'s license to practice pharmacy or even to fine her. Whether declining to fill such a prescription because to do so is contrary to religious belief qualifies as a sufficient reason to refuse to fill a prescription would be a matter for the State Board of Pharmacy to decide—although a decision to revoke or suspend a license on this basis would likely be judicially reviewed. Much is, therefore, going to be based on the exact wording of the particular state's rules and regulations.

It is important to note that the pharmacy profession *does* require pharmacists to refuse to fill prescriptions in certain defined circumstances (e.g., where the prescription is not in the correct form). If the pharmacist believed that a prescription was not in the correct form, was forged or fraudulent or contained some other error, he or she would have the legal right to refuse to fill it whether it is for an abortifacient or any other drug.

There are important legal justifications for the maintenance of such a rule. It ensures that the supply of drug substances—which may have harmful effects if abused—is strictly controlled.

It is a general principle of contract law that individuals are bound only by the contract that they freely negotiate with each other. As such, the law would reflect a notion of freedom of contract and hold that a pharmacist has the right to refuse to enter into a binding contract with anyone— physician or layperson. The typical arrangement is such that a layperson presents a prescription to a pharmacist and requests the pharmacist to fill that prescription in return for payment—a contract in the eyes of the law that would give rise to the legal right, on the one hand, to have the goods supplied and, on the other, the legal right to be paid. Is the right to refuse to enter into that contract a legal right? It is to the extent that there is nothing in law to coerce the pharmacist to act. Many pharmacists abrogate their legal rights by agreeing to provide all prescriptions under a certain scheme or agreeing to dispense all prescriptions in a certain area within a certain time period.

It also has been suggested that pharmacists, in their role as monitors of prescription drug therapy, might refuse to fill a prescription where the monitoring process has allowed the pharmacist to determine that the medication, as prescribed, has a potential harm for the patient.[2]

Employment Law

The facts outlined in the case described above indicate that Dr. S.S. is an *employee* pharmacist. As an employee, S.S. will have certain legal rights that derive from employment law. In particular, S.S. may exercise the general employment right to bring a wrongful discharge action against her employers if she believes her dismissal to be unfair. One of the grounds for bringing such an action is where an employee believes that the discharge was contrary to a clear mandate of public policy.[3] What this means is that an employee may argue that a refusal to carry out an employer's instructions is vindicated on the basis that the employee was acting consistently with established public policy on the issue.

An employee, particularly a professional employee, may act contrary to his or her employer's instructions where he or she is acting in conformity with the recognized professional code of ethics of his or her occupation[4] and could expect to found a wrongful discharge action on the grounds of public policy. However, it appears to be the case that where an employee acts contrary to the employer's wishes, on grounds that are motivated by individual conscience with the result that he or she is then discharged from employment, any claim that the discharge is contrary to a clear mandate of public policy would appear to be ill-founded.[3]

Abortion Law

Specific legal rights have been afforded to certain health care workers who do not wish to participate in abortion procedures. Those legal rights are to be found in specific clauses in legislation, essentially at the state level,[b] that in some way exempt certain health care workers from participating in pregnancy terminations. The specific legal rights created by these clauses are in addition to the general employment rights described above. Because these clauses often are phrased as dependent on individual conviction or personal belief, they have been classified as "conscience clauses."

Conscience clauses create specific legal rights. They oblige employers not to discriminate against those who conscientiously object to participation in abortion procedures. However, the legal rights afforded by the state laws differ in their legal significance and impact. It is, therefore, essential to note these differences.

Most conscience clauses are framed with the specific intention of making unlawful discrimination against those health care workers who conscientiously object to participation in abortion procedures. Some clauses extend the scope of the protection to other medical procedures such as sterilization and artificial insemination. Some of the clauses give a general protection against discrimination for the duration of the period of employment. Others restrict it to protection at the point of hiring. Some clauses extend the scope of the protection to include training and education. Some clauses also seek to protect medical institutions that refuse to allow abortion procedures. Some clauses require that individuals express their objection in writing. Some clauses are dependent on an objection on moral, ethical, or religious grounds. Others give general protection without the specific grounding requirement. Some clauses give protection unconditionally while others seek to limit the protection to nonemergency situations. Some clauses specify the penalty for infringement of the clause that may include civil and criminal liability. Some clauses allow for the possibility of a change of view on the part of the objector. Importantly, some clauses restrict the scope of the protection to those who are directly

---

[b] *Federal legislation including conscience clauses does exist in 42 U.S.C. 300a-7 (1976 & Supp. III 1979). However, although it has appeared to grant specific legal rights to individuals, the state conscience clauses have been used more often by conscientious objectors as a possible form of protection. As a result, it is important to concentrate on those.*

involved in the termination of the pregnancy—essentially the consulting physician, other consultants, and the nursing staff—but do not include those indirectly involved such as clerical, technical, and administrative staff.

Each conscience clause has been interpreted by the relevant judiciary to consider the scope of its effect. Whether the conscience clause has been drafted in wide all-embracing terms or narrowly to restrict the legal effect, they do create specific legal rights for those individuals and situations covered by them. The legal system is granting those rights to those individuals and will allow them to enforce those rights, when violated, if they so choose.

As a result, Dr. S.S. will have to look closely at the state legislation on abortion. She will have to determine whether the legal rights outlined in those laws would extend to pharmacists in their role of dispensers of abortifacient drugs. That question will be dependent on a number of factors.

First, Dr. S.S. will have to show that she can be classified within the range of individuals granted legal rights by the conscience clause legislation and that the procedure she performs is a termination procedure within the meaning of the legislation. In truth, the question of the possibility of the granting of the legal right will depend on the exact wording of the relevant clause. As it presently stands, such a task may be onerous for the following reasons.

Many of the conscience clauses restrict the range of persons whom they cover to those who actively participate in the medical procedure that leads to the termination. Other clauses specifically name the classes of person to whom they will apply. Further, the clauses often contain other restrictions that limit their effect.

Importantly, the conscience clause legislation, when it was enacted, was designed to deal with terminations that involved specific medical (surgical) procedures. The dispensing of abortifacient drugs may have the same clinical effect, but does not involve the same direct (surgical) participation by the pharmacist. If anything, it is the wording that describes the medical procedures whereby the pregnancy is terminated that will have to be redefined to include the dispensing of abortifacient drugs if pharmacists are to be granted the legal right provided by the conscience clauses. This has happened in some cases but most conscience clauses are still worded to deal with surgical procedures.[3]

Antidiscrimination Law

We have seen that conscience clauses often do not give sufficient protection to those who feel that they have a legal right to that protection. The legal rights created by conscience clauses are specific—they extend only to those health care employees either named in them or judicially interpreted as being included within their scope. Further, the conscience clause may only extend to certain types of procedure.

Those deemed to be without the protection afforded by the clauses have sought to scan the range of rights granted by the legal system to see if they may claim other legal rights that protect their personal beliefs and convictions. In that much personal belief and conviction on the question of abortion is dictated by religious belief, the most appropriate location for those legal rights was the federal and state legislation that outlaws discrimination on the grounds of religion.

Federal[5] and state legislation[c] does render unlawful discrimination on the grounds of religious belief; thereby, creating specific legal rights. Individuals covered by the legislation—employees and potential employees—may seek to enforce their legal rights by, for example, bringing actions for breach of the legislation.

The legal effect of the specific legal right granted by the antidiscrimination law has been diluted by judicial interpretation of the scope and effect of the legislation.[6] The net effect of that interpretation has meant that employers have only a *de minimis* obligation to accommodate the religious beliefs of their employees.[3] What that means is that if any proposed accommodation of the employee—such as changing shifts or work assignments—creates undue hardship for the employer then the *de minimis* test is satisfied and the employer is justified in the discrimination.

The interpretation seems harsh and seems to leave employees or potential employees with little protection. However, the legislation does give specific legal rights in those limited circumstances and those rights may be (and indeed have been) enforced by employees.

A pharmacist, such as S.S., may argue that her religious beliefs preclude her from dispensing drugs that she knows will have the effect of terminating a pregnancy and argue further that she has a legal right not to be discriminated against on the ground of her religion. In this respect, pharmacists who refuse to fill prescriptions for abortifacient drugs, such

---

[c] *It is important to note that individual states also have enacted legislation outlawing discrimination on the basis of religious belief. As much of that legislation mirrors the federal requirements, we shall concentrate on analyzing the latter.*

as Dr. S.S. in our case, may fare somewhat better. S.S. may be able to show that her employers have failed to accommodate her religious beliefs; have, therefore, infringed her legal rights and be able to enforce that right accordingly.

Again, however, the caveats and limitations predominate. The protection extends only to employees and potential employees. The employee's legal right might in turn conflict with a duty to their employer to carry out the terms of the contract of employment. Self-employed pharmacists who wished to have their beliefs and convictions protected by law could not, naturally, rely on the antidiscrimination legislation.

Employers have only a *de minimis* obligation under the antidiscrimination legislation to accommodate the religious beliefs of their employees. Any employer pharmacist who shows that accommodation, such as the changing of shifts or the reallocation of dispensing tasks, causes undue hardship will not fall foul of the law. It may be possible for an employer to show that a substitute pharmacist is available to deal with what might be a minor amount of prescriptions for abortifacient drugs or that other reasonable accommodations have been made.[d]

A Moral Perspective
The Nature of the Professional-Layperson Relationship

From a moral point of view, the answer to the question of this chapter turns on the model of the physician-pharmacist-client relationship one holds. If one believes that physicians, pharmacists, and laypersons are bound only by the contract that they freely negotiate with one another, then the pharmacist has no moral obligation to fill a prescription for mifepristone (or any other drug for that matter), unless he or she has expressly contracted to do so. One might refer to this as the libertarian model of pharmacy practice.[7] If, however, the pharmacist is bound to do that which the profession requires of him or her (what Ozar calls in another context the "guild" model of professionalism),[8] then the pharmacist has a right to refuse only if the profession makes allowances for conscientious objection. In a third model, the pharmacist is a puppet of the physician and is morally bound to honor any prescription the physician writes. This might be called the "technician" model, similar to what Veatch calls the "engineering" model of the physician-patient relationship, in which

---
[d] *Again the accommodation need only be a reasonable one*—Brener vs. Diagnostic Center Hospital *671 F2d 141* (5th Cir 1982).

the physician's values do not play a role in decision making.[9] Finally, if society has a role in determining what the pharmacist's moral rights and obligations are, on the grounds that it is society that confers the status of professional upon the pharmacist, then the pharmacy profession does not have the sole authority to grant pharmacists the right to refuse to fill prescriptions they find objectionable. According to what might be called the "societal" model of professionalism, the only refusals a pharmacist can ethically make are those authorized by society. In this final metaphor of professionalism, the pharmacist has more autonomy than in the technician model, but less autonomy than in the libertarian or guild models.

The Role of Professional Codes

Whichever model one holds, it is helpful to consider the profession's official position on the issue of conscientious objection, as articulated in its code of ethics. At the very least, this will describe what organized pharmacy believes is the right and good thing to do, even if there is disagreement about the moral authority of the profession on such matters. Unlike other professional codes, however, the American Pharmaceutical Association's 1994 Code of Ethics for Pharmacists does not make explicit reference to what a pharmacist ought to do in particular circumstances. (The American Dental Association's Principles of Ethics and Code of Professional Conduct specifically states, for example, that, "A decision not to provide treatment to an individual because the individual has AIDS or is HIV seropositive, based solely on that fact, is unethical."[10]) Instead, the APhA Code offers eight general principles, one of which states that, "A pharmacist acts with honesty and integrity in professional relationships." The Code elaborates upon this principle by referring to a duty to "act with conviction of conscience." It is not immediately clear whether or how this duty applies to a pharmacist who is morally troubled by the thought of filling a prescription for an abortifacient drug.

The silence or ambiguity of a code of ethics with respect to a particular issue does not necessarily mean that a conscientious professional does not have a basis for making a morally justifiable decision, especially if he or she rejects the guild model of professionalism. One might argue from analogy and suggest that, if physicians are not ethically required to perform abortions, then consistency requires that pharmacists also should be free to refuse to fill prescriptions for abortifacient drugs. There are two reasons why one might make the antecedent claim. First, some physicians believe that abortion constitutes a harm to the fetus, and physicians have a moral obligation to refrain from harming others (as do the rest of us). Thus, one might appeal to the ethical principle of nonmaleficence in justifying the claim that physicians have a right to refuse to perform abortions.[11] Second, one can argue that physicians are entitled to have their autonomy respected, and those who believe that abortion is immoral should be free to exercise their right to self-determination and not perform the procedure. (Problems with this position will be examined subsequently.)

Morally Relevant Differences Between Pharmacy and Medicine

The profession of medicine rejects the model of the physician-patient relationship in which only the patient's values may be used to assess the rightness or goodness of the physician's actions. If the patient's values are the sole determinant about which kinds of actions are rightly considered harmful, or which kinds of behaviors are morally appropriate, then on the issue of abortion it is a moot point to appeal to the physician's duty to avoid harming patients because the patient does not consider the action harmful, on balance. Furthermore, it would be moot to appeal to the physician's right to self-determination because the patient is the only one in the relationship with autonomy. For the sake of discussion, let us assume that the patient's values are not the only ones that ought to play a role in health care decision making. We then may accept the claim that physicians have a right not to perform abortions, on grounds of both nonmaleficence and respect for autonomy. To hold that consistency requires pharmacists to be free to refuse to fill a prescription for an abortifacient drug presumes that there is no morally relevant difference between what physicians and pharmacists do with respect to abortion. Is this the case?

Probably not. Physicians have the authority to prescribe medications, and most pharmacists do not. To have more authority for an action or practice is to be more accountable for the consequences of that action or practice. For example, a physician who authorizes the withdrawal of a ventilator for a patient is morally accountable to a greater degree than the nurse who carries out the order. This is not to suggest that a nurse has *no* moral responsibility for what he or she does; or that in following an order the nurse does not *feel* as if he or she is directly responsible for what was done; or even that it is not justifiable for a nurse to refuse to acquiesce to such an order. The point is that it does not follow from the physician's right to refuse to perform a procedure that other members of the health care team have the right as well, if there is a morally relevant difference between their professional roles. Because nurses and pharmacists do not have decision-making authority to the same degree that physicians do, and this difference is morally relevant, there must be a reason *independent* of the physician's right to refuse that would morally justify a nurse's or pharmacist's right of refusal. (Our description of the formal differences among the health care providers is not an endorsement of those differences.)

Justifying the Refusal to Dispense

How, then, could a pharmacist justify a refusal to fill a prescription for an abortifacient drug? Pharmacists who hold the guild model of professionalism might appeal to the positive consequences of conscientious objection policies (i.e., professions that allow their members to follow the dictates of their religious tradition encourage scrupulousness, and this will enrich the profession and serve the best interests of the public in the long run). Besides, one could argue, women are always free to find a pharmacist who *is* willing to fill a prescription for mifepristone, and it is quite likely that such pharmacists are available. However, it is not clear that the interests of everyone concerned are best served by granting pharmacists the right to refuse to fill a prescription. The women whose prescriptions go unfilled by pharmacists claiming a right to conscientious objection certainly will not believe that their interests are being served by such a policy, and it is unclear why their interests should be outweighed by others'. Furthermore, pregnant women in rural settings might *not* have anyone else to turn to, should their pharmacists refuse to honor a prescription for an abortifacient drug.

The strongest argument supporting the right to refuse appeals to the principles of *nonmaleficence* and *respect for autonomy*. These principles would clearly be the cornerstones of the libertarian model of the pharmacist-patient relationship, but also may be found in the guild or societal models. The duty to avoid harming others is not a role-specific duty but one applicable to all moral agents, and thus is binding on pharmacists as persons. One might also justify pharmacists' right of refusal by appealing to their autonomy rights as members of the moral community rather than the profession of pharmacy. If one construes the principle of respect for autonomy broadly, the right to refuse to fill a prescription may be derived from the right to exercise control over one's life that is accorded to all persons.

In response to this argument, one might claim that becoming a member of a professional group involves forfeiting certain rights and accepting certain responsibilities. For example, the duty to rescue is not strong enough to require laypersons to enter a burning building to save someone's life. However, firefighters *do* have such an obligation, and we would say that a firefighter who refused to perform such an action was acting unethically because he or she has made a promise to society to assume a greater degree of risk than laypersons must assume.[12] By analogy, one might argue that although pharmacists should not be expected to relinquish their personal autonomy, their career choice *does* require sacrificing (or at least relegating to a less important position) some of their entitlements. Thus, it would be an open question whether the pharmacist's right to follow personal convictions must give way to the patient's request to receive a prescribed drug.

Paradoxically, grounding the right to refuse in a secular right to autonomy means that a pharmacist can claim to have moral reasons for refusing to fill a prescription without necessarily having professional ones as well. If the profession does not make provisions for conscientious objection, a pharmacist who chooses not to fill a prescription for an abortifacient on moral grounds (e.g., religious reasons) would be acting at once morally but unprofessionally. The concept of professional ethics, according to which professional behavior is shaped by moral precepts, then becomes incoherent. Thus, it is more convincing to argue for a pharmacist's *professional* right to self-determination in an attempt to secure a right of refusal.

A professional right to autonomy is the right to make decisions based on values, standards, and preferences established by the profession itself. Like other professional rights and responsibilities, this right is *prima facie*, in that it may give way to countervailing claims made upon the pharmacist. The libertarian, guild, and societal models of professionalism all secure a place for professional autonomy, even if they differ on its relative importance or the moral authority of the profession itself. One of the values that the profession of pharmacy could hold is that pharmacists who believe that abortion is morally wrong ought to be free to absent themselves from being involved in a patient's abortion.[13] One might argue that although pharmacists are not causally responsible for an abortion in the same way that physicians are, because pharmacists are only supplying the means for the procedure to take place rather than performing the procedure themselves, they do occupy a place in the causal chain of events leading to abortion, and to this extent bear some of the moral responsibility for this event, much in the way that nurses who participate in abortions do. Note that, because there are morally relevant differences between what pharmacists and physicians do, the pharmacist's right of refusal is *formally similar to* but not *justified by* the physician's right of refusal.

If the professional right to autonomy is not absolute, what kinds of situations, and which moral considerations, circumscribe it? Veatch has suggested that it is difficult to argue that a pharmacist who believes that homosexuality is immoral has the right to refuse to fill a prescription for AZT.[14] Even if one knew that a person who presents such a prescription is gay (and it is questionable that a pharmacist could know this), there is no causal relationship between filling a prescription for AZT and "participating" in a homosexual act. It is thus incorrect to hold that dispensing AZT implicates oneself in a practice one considers immoral. A pharmacist who refuses to fill a prescription for AZT is more likely acting out of prejudice than sincere moral conviction. There is no professional right to self-determination for choices based on sexism, racism, aesthetic preferences, or personal whims or idiosyncrasies.

Another situation that may limit the pharmacist's right to refuse to fill a prescription arises when a person is unable to have a prescription filled by anyone else, as would be the case in an isolated town with only one pharmacy. There, the person's right of access to health care may supersede the pharmacist's right of refusal, because as members of a health care profession, pharmacists have committed themselves to respecting the rights and promoting the welfare of patients.[15] Unless the profession changes its moral mandate, the guild model of professionalism would hold that a pharmacist's right to refuse cannot trump a patient's right to safe and effective treatment. It is likely that the societal model would similarly limit the pharmacist's right to refuse.

At opposite ends of the continuum are the libertarian and technician models of professionalism. Because libertarians reject the notion of even a basic right to health care,[16] a woman in the above situation would not have a right to the abortifacient drug, so a pharmacist has no duty to dispense it, unless he or she already has contracted to provide such a service. According to the technician model of professionalism, the pharmacist's personal values do not play a role in determining what the pharmacist ought to do, so a pharmacist has a duty to provide the service. It would be up to a defender of the technician model of professionalism in pharmacy to show why the pharmacist's values should play no role in determining what a pharmacist ought to do, for no other currently accepted model of professionalism in any area of health care adopts such a radical position.

CONCLUSION

From both legal and moral perspectives, the answer to the question posed in this chapter is, "It depends." Legally, a pharmacist may claim that refusal to fill such a prescription is sufficient to obviate the requirements of a State Board of Pharmacy's rules of professional conduct. If he or she can so convince a State Board (or court who may be reviewing the decisions of a State Board) then the pharmacist may continue to act in the knowledge that the profession will not take action against him or her.

If the pharmacist is an employee, then he or she will look to general employment law and to individual state and federal abortion and anti-discrimination laws to attempt to find a specific legal right on which to ground a refusal. We have seen that an individual employee might find it difficult to base a wrongful discharge action on the basis of a clear mandate of public policy where the refusal to act in line with an employer's wishes is based on individual, not collective, beliefs.

It may be possible to extend the current legal rights affecting those who participate in abortion procedures or who appeal to religious beliefs to pharmacists dispensing abortifacient drugs; however, such an extension would depend on a liberal and perhaps tenuous interpretation of the existing rights. We have seen that this might prove to be a difficult task with the employee having to find their way through an interpretive and definitional maze and rely on novel explications of existing laws. Many of those laws are framed in general terms or have a restricted scope. Fitting the particular requirements of the pharmacy profession into a system of general legal rights may not be easy.

An employee pharmacist who acts in the absence of a specific legal right to refuse to fill a prescription may find that he or she will be subject to certain disciplinary measures for such a refusal. These measures may range from simple warnings as to future conduct to lawful dismissal where the employer can show a pattern of disruptive behavior. This may not worry the renegade pharmacist. Indeed the deprivation of personal employment rights might be considered a cheap price for the statement of personal beliefs and convictions on the issue.

Where the pharmacist is self-employed the refusal to dispense may have little legal significance although it may have other implications such as loss of business or lack of patient confidence. Again that may not cause much consternation or anxiety. However, it would appear to be the case that the refusal to fill prescriptions for abortifacient drugs in the absence of a legal right to do so may have greater legal significance for an employee pharmacist than for an employer or self-employed pharmacist.

From a moral perspective, the answer to the question posed by this chapter depends upon the model of the professional-patient relationship one holds.

Discussion Questions

1. In Chapter 3: The Relationship between Ethics and the Law, Kenneth Mullan and James Brown discuss the distinction between ethics and the law. Imagine a situation in the future in which it were legal to dispense abortifacient drugs. Further suppose that political changes lead to the banning of these drugs, even though you have an ample supply of them left in your pharmacy. Should you continue to dispense them? Why or why not?

2. Much of the abortion debate has pitted the rights of one party (the right of women to choose what to do with their bodies) against the rights of another (the right of fetuses to life). What limitations are there in using rights language to frame discussions about the ethics of abortion? Are there other moral concepts we can use that would take us beyond an irreconcilable battle of rights? How would these concepts apply to the issue presented in this chapter?

3. Even if a pharmacist has a legal or ethical right to refuse to dispense an abortifacient drug, does that mean it is necessarily right to do so? Why or why not? How would the virtuous pharmacist rise to the challenge?

4. Revisit the case presented at the beginning of the chapter. What values are at stake? Can you think of an option open to Dr. S.S. that would enable her to promote *all* of these values? If not, may pharmacists reasonably disagree about what an ethically appropriate response would be?

5. What kinds of broad social changes might pharmacists work for so that the ethical questions raised by the case arise less frequently?

REFERENCES

1. West Virginia Code Title 15-1 (1993), 17.3.
2. Brushwood DB. Pharmacy Law. New York: McGraw-Hill; 1986:41.
3. Brushwood DB. Conscientious objection and abortifacient drugs. Clin Ther. 1993;15(1):206.
4. *Kalman vs. Grand Union Company* 443 A2d 728 (NJ Super 1982).
5. Title VII of the Civil Rights Act 42 U.S.C. 2000e-17 (1976).
6. *Trans World Airlines Inc. vs. Harding* 432 U.S. 63 (1977).
7. Engelhardt HT. The Foundations of Bioethics. New York: Oxford University Press; 1986.
8. Ozar DT. Three models of professionalism and professional obligation in dentistry. J Am Dent Assoc. 1985;110:173–77.
9. Veatch RM. Models for ethical medicine in a revolutionary age. Hastings Cent Rep. 1972;2:5–7.
10. American Dental Association. Principles of ethics and code of professional conduct. J Am Dent Assoc. 1990;120:585–92.
11. Beauchamp TL, Childress JF. Principles of Biomedical Ethics. 4th ed. New York: Oxford University Press; 1994.
12. Emanuel EJ. Do physicians have an obligation to treat patients with AIDS? N Engl J Med. 1988;318:1686–690.
13. Lee P et al. Pharmacist's refusal to dispense diethylstilbestrol for contraceptive use. Am J Hosp Pharm. 1989;46:1413–416.
14. Veatch RM. Pharmacist's refusal to serve patient with AIDS: analysis and commentary. Am J Hosp Pharm. 1990;47:153.
15. Weinstein BD. Ethical issues in pharmacy. In: Abood RR, Brushwood DB, eds. Pharmacy Law. Gaithersburg: Aspen; 1994:310–23.
16. Weinstein BD. Do pharmacists have a right to refuse to fill prescriptions for abortifacient drugs? Law Med Health Care. 1992;20(3):336–74.

Chapter 10

Professional Responsibilities Toward Incompetent or Chemically Dependent Colleagues

Lisa S. Parker
Michael L. Manolakis

In this chapter we explore the circumstances and ethical values that justify, indeed require, that pharmacists take action with respect to colleagues' misconduct. We discuss intraprofessional and external mechanisms for reporting, investigating, and disciplining professional misconduct and consider the role played by professional loyalty and other ethical values in decisions to use these mechanisms.

To place in context the importance of peer review of pharmaceutical care and the important role played by the individual pharmacist in ensuring the effectiveness of peer review mechanisms, we first consider the nature of pharmacy as a profession, the nature of the relationships among pharmacy colleagues, their relationships with other health care providers, and the responsibilities of pharmacists to ensure the quality of their colleagues' professional conduct. We then articulate three basic options that pharmacists have available to them when confronted with what they believe to be a case of a colleague's provision of poor quality care or of being chemically dependent. These options include: 1) doing nothing, 2) initiating some form of personal dialogue with the colleague involved, and 3) contacting a third party within the profession.

In the balance of the chapter we explore these three options in relation to both patient care cases and the profession's code of ethics. While no one is likely to argue that the first option, to do nothing, is acceptable behavior, looking the other way may seem an attractive alternative, especially with respect to early signs of chemical dependency or patient care that is debatably (rather than clearly) substandard. On the other hand, understanding the relationship among pharmacists as a collegial one seems to support the second option of personal intervention. While the personal intervention approach sometimes is successful, we argue that the third option (i.e., responsible intraprofessional reporting, investigation, and disciplinary mechanisms) offers the greatest promise of achieving the goals of professional self-regulation.

In the second section of this chapter, we consider two cases of substandard care in light of the provisions of the American Pharmaceutical Association's 1994 Code of Ethics for Pharmacists. We stress the importance of establishing standards of conduct and consider the relative merits of engaging in personal intervention or intraprofessional discipline when one discovers substandard care. In our third section, we discuss the ethical grounds for reporting, to both patients and peers, misconduct and inferior care.

In our fourth and fifth sections of this chapter, we consider the profession's response to chemically dependent pharmacists and the obligation of pharmacists to report their substance-abusing colleagues. We suggest that the profession might model its peer review mechanisms concerning poor quality care after the mechanisms that it has developed to address the problems of chemically impaired pharmacists.

PHARMACY'S PRIVILEGE AND RESPONSIBILITY OF SELF-REGULATION

Pharmacists practice in a wide variety of settings, each of which presents its own set of ethical dilemmas. Independent pharmacists can own the pharmacies in which they work, leaving the owner/pharmacist directly accountable to no one. They interact directly with the public, who often rely upon them for advice. Alternatively, hospital pharmacists are part of a health care team. They provide advice to physicians about the appropriate drug to be administered. They also make purchasing decisions about the hospital pharmacy's drug supplies and often decide which drugs to include on a hospital's formulary. Finally, pharmacists who choose to work within the pharmaceutical industry may eschew direct patient care and instead market and sell products to pharmacies and hospitals. In this competitive climate, these pharmacists may walk a line between using legitimate persuasive techniques to convince a client of a product's superiority and blatant bribery or misrepresentation. The diverse roles played by pharmacists complicate the self-regulatory task of pharmacy as a profession.

A profession, after all, is identified with and by the group of individuals who engage in particular professional practices. So it is the individual members of the pharmacy profession, acting individually and collectively, who establish, preserve, and inculcate in new members, professional standards of conduct. Pharmacy may appear to have an especially difficult time in establishing standards of conduct when the conduct of pharmacists varies so widely depending upon their work environment and role in health care. Entrepreneurial business activity may constitute a large portion of some pharmacists' jobs, while biomedical research may occupy others' attention. Nevertheless, as professionals with specialized knowledge, pharmacists are responsible not only for adhering to a prescribed standard of conduct, but also for setting that standard for themselves as a group.

Possession of specialized knowledge and skills is one reason that professions traditionally have been granted a large measure of self-regulatory authority. Those outside the profession of pharmacy, for example, may lack the knowledge necessary to establish and apply, in particular cases, a standard of care. Although nonpharmacists certainly could appreciate the importance of honesty and the obligation of truth-telling, they might, for example, have difficulty determining when, in fact, the truth about a pharmaceutical product had actually been told. Another reason that professions have been self-regulating reflects the economic, social, and political power typically wielded by members; as people in powerful and prestigious social positions, professionals traditionally have demanded and have been allowed substantial latitude in establishing the standards of their professional conduct.

Professionals themselves control the dissemination of their specialized knowledge and the perpetuation of their prestigious professional social role. Pharmacists go to professional schools, receive professional licenses, and typically belong to professional associations. These aspects of professionalism help to establish, preserve, and instill in new members the professional mores and standards of conduct characteristic of pharmacy. If these standards of conduct are set sufficiently high (e.g., a demand that pharmacists behave ethically and apply state of the art knowledge), then these self-regulatory mechanisms can operate to benefit both the profession and the public which it serves. If, on the other hand, the standards are not sufficiently high or are not stringently enforced, then self-regulation may establish and perpetuate a professional conspiracy of silence, shoddy professional practices, and poor service to the public and patients.

The relationship among professionals is traditionally highly collegial rather than hierarchical. Colleagues deem themselves to be equals in sharing the rights and responsibilities bestowed by virtue of their membership in the group and their pursuit of the group's common goals. Thus, even in settings where individual pharmacists are not self-employed (e.g., hospitals, large pharmacies or clinics, or corporations), they are still the equal colleagues of pharmacists in and outside of that setting, and policing of an individual pharmacist's conduct to assure that it is ethical and competent is left not only to the pharmacist's own conscience, but also to that of his colleagues.

At the same time, however, their collegial relationship and the requirement that pharmacists regulate their own professional conduct may come into conflict. Membership in a profession usually entails a sense of belonging and a sense of loyalty both to the profession as a whole and to the other individuals who comprise the whole. Establishing standards of conduct contributes to the unity of the profession. On the other hand, enforcing them, identifying departures from them, and applying sanctions to those who transgress against them may emphasize value differences, generate conflict, create disunity, and undermine professionals' senses of identity with the whole. Some of those who rightfully fulfill their responsibility to enforce the standards of professional conduct nevertheless feel that they are disloyal in doing so. Intervening to seek discipline of a colleague effectively creates a hypothetical hierarchy wherein one professional, who both represents and enforces the professional standards, stands above the alleged wrongdoer. In the context of collegial, nonhierarchical professional relationships, this stance is not easily adopted by the reporting colleague, nor has it been easily accepted by many who witness the professional's action. Those who fulfill their professional responsibilities to police their profession have sometimes been considered as professional dissenters or deviants.[1] (This sense of violating collegiality may be exacerbated when a junior colleague or subordinate exposes his or her senior colleague or supervisor.)

An unwillingness to extend themselves for the good of their colleague, their profession, and the public they serve (sometimes rationalized by a misguided sense of loyalty or supported by fear of reprisals) might lead some pharmacists to shirk their professional responsibility and to do nothing when confronted with another pharmacist's provision of substandard care. Of the three basic courses of action open to those confronting substandard care [i.e., 1) doing nothing, 2) personal intervention, and 3) intraprofessional mechanisms], doing nothing is clearly the least justifiable. The choice to *do nothing* traditionally has been rationalized by arguing, for example, that the involved party is nearing retirement, is under temporary domestic stress, or is overworked. In such cases, or so the rationalization goes, to raise questions about the practitioner's impairment either is unnecessary (because the concerns are obvious) or might exacerbate the problems (e.g., by increasing stress). The option of doing nothing, however, leaves the public, the profession, and the individual professional at risk. Doing nothing, thus, is almost never the correct choice.

Understanding the relationship among pharmacists as a collegial one seems to support pursuing the second option of *personal intervention*. This collegial approach of learning more about the circumstances leading to an apparent lack of quality care and offering personal assistance now probably is the prevailing practice in the profession and is a practice which, like other collegial aspects of the profession, is inculcated in new members by pharmaceutical education and literature.[2] While this approach sometimes is successful in persuading a practitioner to seek help with chemical dependency or stress, or to improve his practice standards, personal intervention may lead to: denial behaviors; a list of "excuses;" unfulfilled self promises to retrain or rehabilitate; attempts to talk the colleague out of reporting the misconduct or dependency; or a failure of genuine communication and the severing of personal and professional relationships which become strained beyond repair by the confrontation. We therefore argue that the path of personal intervention not only is the most personally demanding, but also presents the greatest risk of personal damage and professional disintegration. Sometimes it works to protect the public and rescue the impaired or incompetent professional and a stronger collegial bond results, but more often than not this approach achieves none of these goals effectively.

The third option, pursuing *intraprofessional mechanisms* for assuring professional conduct and high quality care, offers the greatest promise of achieving the goals of professional self-regulation. It clearly is the best choice in cases of chemical dependency wherein interpersonal skill and the ability both to fend off the dependent person's usual defensive responses and to monitor his or her progress in rehabilitation have been recognized not merely as desirable, but as necessary. The profession has recognized that by establishing intraprofessional channels for reporting, counseling, and monitoring chemically impaired pharmacists, everyone wins. The identity of the professional who reports an impaired colleague is reasonably protected, the impaired professional is offered a temporary "safe haven" in which his or her problems can be addressed away from the public's eye, and the public is protected from the risks of treatment by an impaired practitioner. The counselor, as a supportive third party, can help the dependent professional while keeping in mind the public's and the profession's interest in the provision of quality pharmaceutical care.

It is not clear, however, that reporting misconduct has had the same positive effect in situations where poor quality care is the issue. While the process of rehabilitation has documented success, there are no established programs of retraining for professionals who provide substandard care. Although it shares with dependency intervention programs the goals of protecting the public and preserving the standards of the profession, the peer review process often functions punitively, rather than supportively, with respect to the individual pharmacist whose patient care is deficient. Consideration of the following cases in light of the profession's guidelines for handling misconduct highlights the need to revise the existing peer review process. Nevertheless, when confronted with professional misconduct, using intraprofessional disciplinary mechanisms is superior to either doing nothing or accepting the risks to both oneself and the public of pursuing personal intervention alone.

COLLEAGUES, COMPETENCE, AND THE APhA CODE

To guide pharmacists' conduct in pursuit of their professional goals, indeed to shape those goals, the American Pharmaceutical Association formulated a "Code of Ethics for Pharmacists," hereinafter referred to as the APhA Code, that codifies the principles of conduct and shared goals to which those practicing in the profession historically have subscribed.[3] The version of the Code referred to here was adopted in 1994.

Although rules and principles do not tell the whole story about the ethics of a profession, examining the basic ethical principles adopted by any culture provides clues about that culture's values and about how members of that culture resolve ethical problems and regard members who act unethically. Just as basic principles of pharmacy allow for alternative treatment plans (e.g., inclusion of different and competing products on the formulary), the basic rules and principles of ethical conduct provide a framework for ethical decision making. In ethics, as in treatment planning, guidelines suggest which facts must be ascertained, what of value is at stake, and which of several possible courses of action should be ruled out from the outset as being unacceptable. Consider the following case and the guidance offered by the APhA Code.

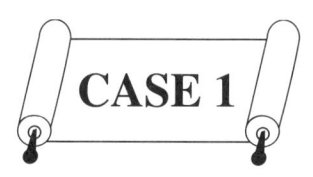

CASE 1

A.D., Pharm.D., has worked as a staff pharmacist at Metropolitan General Hospital for seven years. Her recent completion of a residency training program in oncology led to her promotion to the oncology satellite pharmacy, where she has worked for eight months. The director of the satellite, J.M., has been at Metropolitan for 15 years and maintains an excellent reputation among the pharmacy staff. Recently, on her morning rounds, A.D. was pulled aside by one of the staff nurses, who then expressed his relief that finally the nurses could all relax when it came to checking IVs. A.D., clearly caught off-guard by the comment, pushed the nurse for more information. The nurse reported that with increasing regularity, J.M. had sent the wrong IV antibiotic bag to patients; however, every error had been detected, and the nursing staff had become accustomed to triple-checking J.M.'s work. He also asked if A.D. was now going to be in charge, and if not, what should the nursing staff do about J.M.? A.D., hearing her name called by the rounding team, thanked the nurse, and indicated she would respond to his question soon.

A.D. had noticed that J.M. seemed rather uninterested in his work but attributed it to her own exaggerated level of enthusiasm. A.D. also knew that J.M.'s recent pharmacy review had been excellent, and that the pharmacy staff was unaware of any problems on the oncology satellite. What should A.D. do? How should she respond to the nurse?

Case Discussion

Suppose that A.D. turned to the APhA Code for guidance. The current Code's second principle states, "A pharmacist places concern for the well-being of the patient at the center of professional practice."[4] The task of applying general rules and principles in a particular case is not easy, because they do not always require the same conduct in each case. Often rules are too general to yield, by themselves, a correct course of action in a particular case. Indeed in this case, in order to fulfill their primary professional obligation, pharmacists must determine the standard of care owed to members of the public. A.D., for example, must be able to determine whether the well-being of these patients has been compromised by J.M.'s exercise of alleged suboptimal ability as a health practitioner.

Moreover, another principle offers what could be interpreted as conflicting guidance with respect to this particular case. This principle in the current Code states that "a pharmacist avoids…work conditions that impair professional judgment, and actions that compromise dedication to the best interests of patients."[4] Assuming that A.D. can determine that the nurse is correct in saying that J.M. is placing patients at risk of harm, A.D. may interpret this principle to require her to take action to protect patients from her colleague. A.D. might recall that the 1981 version of the Code required pharmacists to "expose, without fear or favor, illegal or unethical conduct in the profession."[5] She then apparently faces the difficult choice of acting to expose J.M.'s misconduct without herself bringing discredit to the profession. Although reporting and addressing a colleague's misconduct is ultimately to the credit of the professional who reports the misconduct and the profession that investigates it, interim publicity concerning the misconduct may appear to discredit the profession. Professionals should work to alter their colleagues' and the public's perceptions of reports of wrongdoing because, although the misconduct is wrong, any *publicity* concerning investigation of misconduct should be hailed as evidence that the self-regulatory function of the profession is working. The shame or discredit brought to a profession when one of its members acts negligently is only compounded by a lack of responsible action on the part of the profession. So long as the profession, acting through its members, responds in a timely manner to correct the mistakes and implement measures to ensure that they will not be repeated, the profession may take pride in the discharge of its professional responsibility. In contrast, it would be shameful for a profession to overlook mistake-making or, perhaps out of hubris or careless disregard, to fail to provide mechanisms for identifying, investigating, and redressing negligence or other wrongdoing. A.D., therefore, would be acting in an honorable and responsible manner to act on the nurse's allegations and her own concerns.

A.D. still faces various difficulties. First, neither the 1981 APhA Code which required pharmacists to "expose, without fear or favor, illegal or unethical conduct in the profession" nor the 1994 APhA Code tells her precisely to whom she should report her concerns about J.M.'s work. Second, especially in light of J.M.'s recent stellar pharmacy review, A.D. might risk her promotion by making unsubstantiated accusations. Nevertheless, the 1994 APhA Code grounds A.D.'s duty to take action in pharmacy's covenantal relationship with society. Its first principle defines

> the patient-pharmacist relationship as a covenant [which] means that each pharmacist has moral obligations in response to the gift of trust received from society. In return for this gift, the pharmacist promises to help individuals achieve optimum benefit from their medications, to be committed to their welfare, and to maintain their trust.[4]

Pharmacists are indeed the most trusted professionals.[6] A.D. would violate this "gift of trust" by failing to investigate the nurse's allegations. Investigation is justified and required by her commitment to patients' welfare. Finally, this societal gift of trust might be interpreted to ground the pharmacist's relationship with the nursing staff. Were she to ignore the nurse, A.D. could be perceived as implicitly condoning J.M.'s mistakes, and a health care team approach to providing optimum patient care would be jeopardized.

Engaging in a conspiratorial silence about substandard pharmaceutical care would surely lower the esteem of the profession by justifying the public's and other professionals' mistrust. If one of the reasons that pharmacy is self-regulating is that pharmacists possess specialized knowledge that the public and other health care professionals cannot be expected to have, then pharmacy has a special trust or duty to use that knowledge for the public's benefit.

Clearly A.D. must address J.M.'s alleged substandard care. Before we investigate her options, let us examine another difficult situation in which a pharmacist might turn for guidance to the APhA Code.

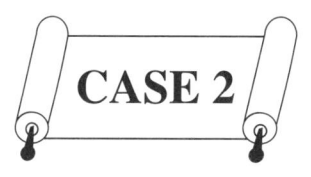

CASE 2

S.T., Pharm.D., has been operating a consultant pharmacy business for ten years as part of his community pharmacy practice. He currently serves most of the long-term care facilities in the surrounding counties. S.T. knows just about every physician and nurse on his side of the state, and he has earned the respect of the majority of his colleagues by keeping up to date with the changes in therapy and always trying to strike a fair deal.

On a recent visit to one of the nursing homes he serves, S.T. noticed that a number of the charts he was reviewing included orders for nonprescription medications that clearly interacted with the patient's prescription drugs. What was most surprising was that the physician who had made these errors, Dr. Z.K., was a respected physician in the area. Although Dr. Z.K. had limited his practice over the recent years due to his increasing age, he still appeared as vital as ever, and regularly attended the continuing education seminars that S.T. had coordinated.

Upon returning to his pharmacy, S.T. mentioned the mistakes he had caught to one of the staff pharmacists. The pharmacist responded with little surprise and noted that Dr. Z.K. recently had developed quite a reputation among the pharmacists for making errors on prescriptions. The pharmacist also remarked that even some of Dr. Z.K.'s patients had begun to express concern over the quality of his care, and then asked S.T. what he thought should be done about Dr. Z.K. How should S.T. respond?

Case Discussion

To fulfill their professional responsibilities, pharmacists must do more than just count and pour medications. Pharmacists occupying an entrusted role in society and on the health care team face the possibility of conflict within the pharmacist-physician relationship and indeed within the relationship between the pharmacist and a variety of other health care providers. Although pharmacists increasingly are playing a more active role in patient care management, it often still is true that the physician "has a desire to manage the patient's problems without interference, without usurpation of the management role by other health care professionals and with the understanding that the 'bottom line' rests with the physician in charge of the case."[7] The newly expanded responsibilities of pharmacists, particularly in the institutional setting, clash with traditional views of the physician as a unilateral decision maker and the pharmacist as one who should simply follow the physician's orders and fill prescriptions. Indeed, the fact that Dr. Z.K. had developed this reputation (i.e., making errors on prescriptions) among the pharmacists indicates that they were adhering to these traditional roles. The 1994 APhA Code, however, recognizes that pharmacists' primary loyalty must be to patients; above all, pharmacists, like other health care providers, have an obligation to avoid or prevent harm to patients. Just as S.T. acts as a conscientious pharmacist in keeping up to date on the latest therapies, he should act conscientiously in this area of professional responsibility. Both actions promote the welfare of patients and prevent harm to them.

Another principle in the 1994 APhA Code, however, might confuse S.T. It states that "a pharmacist respects the values and abilities of colleagues and other health care professionals" and that "a pharmacist recognizes that colleagues and other health care professionals may differ in the beliefs and values they apply to the care of the patient." Dr. Z.K.'s care could fall into this gray area involving justifiable differences of opinion. It is possible that Dr. Z.K. does not believe that the drug interactions seriously jeopardize the health of his patients. He may believe that these are actually the most effective drugs for particular patients' conditions and that the risk of the drug interaction is outweighed by the benefits of the treatment, or at the very least, he may weigh the risks and benefits of the possible treatments differently. The existence of a gray area where rules do not offer clear guidance does not suggest that this is an opportunity to ignore the demands of ethics. When the "letter of the law" does not clearly address the issue at hand, one looks to the "spirit of the law" for guidance in specific cases or in drafting more specific guidelines. In the absence of more specific guidelines, pharmacists must use their discretion and rely upon the fundamental ethical values which inform their practice and their professional code.

A gray area does not justify the option of doing nothing about alleged misconduct. S.T., for example, might want to know whether Dr. Z.K. had, in fact, weighed the risks of drug interactions against the likely benefits of the prescribed treatments, or whether he instead had been unaware of the likelihood of drug interactions. It may be difficult, however, for S.T. to ascertain this information himself. Thus, instead of intervening and investigating the matter himself, S.T. might refer Dr. Z.K.'s possible substandard care to an institutional, local, or state peer review body for further investigation.

All criticism of colleagues' work should be offered constructively with the intermediate goal of finding avenues for remedying deficiencies and for avoiding future instances of misconduct. In this spirit, A.D. (see Case 1) and S.T. (see Case 2) may choose to inform their respective colleagues of their findings of substandard care and of the steps that each will take (or has taken) to inform professional authorities. By informing J.M., A.D. would evidence her respect for him as a colleague who, she may presume, would want to know of his mistakes in order to correct them. The same would hold true for S.T. discussing his concerns with Dr. Z.K. According to the prevailing practice in pharmacy, except in unusual circumstances, A.D. and S.T. would discuss the mistakes that had come to their attention with J.M. and Dr. Z.K. before taking any other steps, such as reporting their concerns to local authorities. (If, for example, illegal actions were involved, or there were reason to think that J.M. or Dr. Z.K. might take steps to cover up evidence of negligence, A.D. or S.T. would be justified in not telling the respective parties of the discoveries or actions in reporting them.) According to the rationale underlying this prevailing practice, if J.M. and Dr. Z.K. did not respond to these personal efforts to remedy the professional deficiencies and the substandard pharmaceutical practices continued, then and only then should A.D. and S.T. carry their concerns, together with any substantiating evidence to the State Board of Pharmacy or Medicine (or some internal institutional review mechanism) for investigation.

In addition to imposing the difficult burden of personally assessing that the alleged misconduct or substandard care has, in fact, occurred, this personal intervention approach unfortunately assumes that both A.D. and S.T. will be in a position to monitor their colleagues' future professional conduct. It, thus, places a great practical and ethical burden on them; they must not only assess the sincerity of J.M. and Dr. Z.K. in desiring to correct their conduct, but also monitor J.M. and Dr. Z.K.'s success in doing so. Therefore, we argue that it is far more appropriate and efficacious for A.D. and S.T. to leave this responsibility to those bodies charged with this function.

While speaking to their respective colleagues first does respect their colleagues' autonomy (by allowing them to correct their conduct themselves) and maintain ties of collegial loyalty, it alone may not best serve either the patients' welfare or the profession's interest in its efficacious and autonomous regulation. We suggest that A.D. should report J.M.'s substandard treatment of the patients either to an institutional oversight body (e.g., the director of pharmacy or the quality assurance committee of the hospital) or to the State Board of Pharmacy for peer review and should monitor this process to ascertain that an investigation was indeed implemented and, if appropriate, that disciplinary action was taken. Similarly, S.T. should locate the appropriate body to initiate a review of Dr. Z.K.'s questionable treatment. Disciplinary action can range from a reprimand to the suspension or loss of one's license to practice. While it may seem harsh not to allow more latitude, it appears in both situations that patients habitually had been subjected to substandard treatment. Pharmacists in the positions of A.D. and S.T. should inform their colleagues of their intention to report the misconduct only if they can be certain that they will not allow themselves to be talked out of their acts of professional responsibility and that their colleagues will not destroy evidence; establish cover stories (including the possibility of blaming others for their own wrongdoing); or attempt to leave, escape investigation, or even blackmail their accusers. Few individual pharmacists are in a position to assure that these negative consequences will not occur upon confronting their colleagues; therefore, we recommend not informing one's colleagues of one's intention to report misconduct.

Moreover, because no one person can know whether a single case of wrongdoing, misconduct, negligence, or substandard treatment is actually a single isolated case, or whether it is part of a pattern of such incidents, we argue that all cases of misconduct or substandard treatment should be reported to a local peer review board so that a centralized database of reported infractions could be maintained. Maintenance of a centralized record of misconduct would enable regulatory authorities to identify those practitioners who show evidence of continued or seriously substandard provision of care. Ideally, local peer review groups, charged with a supportive and constructively corrective role, not a punitive one, should be established and should be the body to which pharmacists could turn first. If implicated practitioners did not respond to retraining or other efforts to protect their patients' welfare, or if their substandard practices persisted, then they could be reported to state review boards for additional intervention efforts and possible disciplinary action. Because of difficulties with the personal intervention approach, even in the absence of this ideal two-tiered (first supportive, then potentially punitive) system, pharmacists have an obligation to report substandard care to existing professional bodies.

SELF-POLICING AS A PROFESSIONAL RESPONSIBILITY

The obligation to report, investigate, and discipline professional misconduct is thus a very stringent one grounded in the ethical values of nonmaleficence, which requires that pharmacists avoid harming patients, and of beneficence, which requires that pharmacists promote the public's health and prevent harm to others. It also is grounded in concern for the autonomy of both patients who need medication and the pharmacy profession. Patients have a right to control and consent to what happens to their bodies. Their right to know if something adverse has been perpetrated upon them and their moral and legal right to seek redress in such cases is based upon recognition of their autonomy. The profession's right to autonomy is not a natural and absolute right, but a socially granted one which may be overridden by other rights and important interests. The profession's attempt at self-rule must be in accordance with its overriding goal of fulfilling the public's interest in receiving quality pharmaceutical care; therefore, the profession must give precedence to the interests of the public's health.

Throughout the chapter we refer to "professional responsibility," rather than "whistleblowing," a term that often is used in literature on the responsibilities of professionals. The former term has consistently positive connotations, while the latter has various interpretations and, accordingly, has met with varying degrees of approbation. Some accounts of handling professional misconduct distinguish, for example, between legitimate and illegitimate whistleblowing.[1] The so-called illegitimate whistleblower raises allegations of misconduct in order to further his own interests, perhaps vindictively, or acts irresponsibly by raising the allegations without having sufficient evidence to support his charges. Indeed, the 1994 APhA Code states that

> a pharmacist acts with honesty and integrity in all professional relationships. Patients, colleagues, and other health care professionals have a right to expect pharmacists to tell the truth. Pharmacists have a duty not to lie or to deceive others and to act with conviction of conscience.[4]

Of course, pharmacists need not be *certain* that their allegations of misconduct are true, but their suspicions must be sufficiently well-founded that further investigation clearly is warranted. A.D. must have a firmer basis than her feeling that J.M. is uninterested in his work to act on the nurse's allegations. Moreover, pharmacists should blow the whistle on alleged misconduct to protect public health and to preserve patient and professional autonomy, not to gain publicity or a competitive advantage, damage a colleague's reputation, or settle a difference of opinion. Legitimate whistleblowing thus is an act of professional responsibility. "Illegitimate whistleblowing," whether intentional or negligent, is not a response to misconduct; it itself is a type of professional misconduct. In referring to "whistleblowing," this chapter, therefore, consistently uses the term "professional responsibility."

Further complicating the notion of "whistleblowing" is the fact that some use it to refer to attempts to circumvent the profession's prescribed channels of self-regulatory authority by "going public" (e.g., talking to the press) or "going outside" (e.g., by reporting to a governmental agency).[8] One might appropriately go public or outside the profession with one's concerns if indeed one already had pursued internal means of addressing misconduct to no avail, or if one had good reason to believe that pursuing such channels would be both unproductive and seriously detrimental to one's professional standing. Whistleblowing in the sense of going outside of the profession is, thus, an ethically appropriate response to the inadequacies of internal self-regulatory mechanisms. Interestingly, research suggests that an organization's threat to retaliate against those who "go public" results in more, not less, external whistleblowing.[9] Perhaps the existence of internal threats of retaliation suggest to responsible professionals that internal channels of investigating alleged misconduct are unlikely to operate ethically.

We urge that promotion of patient welfare, and thus professional responsibility, demands that there are adequate internal channels of responsibility and authority to investigate, correct, and discipline alleged misconduct. These channels typically are established through professional organizations, but also should be established within clinical practices and other institutional settings (e.g., hospitals and companies) where pharmacists carry out their professional activities. Where these internal mechanisms do not exist or fail, pharmacists are justified in seeking extraprofessional mechanisms to address misconduct and protect patient welfare.

Because A.D. and J.M. (see Case 1) work within a single institution, A.D. has channels of oversight and peer review that probably are not available to S.T. in Case 2. A.D. may choose to take her concerns about J.M.'s mistakes in practice to the hospital director of pharmacy or to an institutional body charged with investigating charges of professional staff negligence and misconduct. Indeed, were she to report J.M. directly to the State Board of Pharmacy, her hospital colleagues and supervisors might consider her to be "going public," albeit *within* her profession. They might appreciate the opportunity to investigate J.M.'s conduct "in house." If, on the other hand, A.D. reported J.M. to hospital bodies and no investigation ensued, or if she felt that she could jeopardize her employment by reporting to internal bodies, then she would be justified in turning to the state review board immediately. Indeed, if J.M. sits on the internal review board or is the only supervisor to whom A.D. may appropriately turn within the institution, she would be justified in reporting J.M. directly to the state board to avoid the possibility (or even appearance) of an internal cover up, as well as the possibility of reprisals against her being made with impunity. A.D.'s appropriate course of action requires her judgment and permits her some latitude in determining how best to protect both patients' welfare and the profession's esteem in the eyes of the public and colleagues.

For cases involving chemically impaired pharmacists, a network of supportive, nonpunitive, intraprofessional channels already has been established. These bodies may serve as models for establishing similar mechanisms for dealing with poor quality pharmaceutical care not involving chemical dependency. Indeed, institutions, like A.D.'s hospital, may find this model instructive. All institutions should have mechanisms for investigating and resolving allegations of negligence, misconduct, and chemical impairment. Pharmacists who find themselves working in institutions that do not yet have such mechanisms in place should work to establish them *before* the identification of any concerns about inappropriate conduct.

PROFESSIONAL RESPONSIBILITY AND THE CHEMICALLY DEPENDENT PRACTITIONER

Practicing pharmacy while impaired through chemical dependency constitutes a clear case of unacceptable professional conduct. In 1982, the APhA House of Delegates adopted a policy stating that

> the APhA believes that pharmacists should not practice while subject to physical or mental impairment due to the influence of drugs—including alcohol—or other causes that might adversely affect their abilities to function properly in their professional capacities.[10]

In addition, court decisions have been recorded that hold pharmacists to high standards of care due to the dangerous properties of the drugs they distribute.[11] These policy and regulatory statements, when combined with ethical duties grounded in beneficence and nonmaleficence, obligate those having reasonable knowledge that a pharmacist is a substance abuser to take some type of action.

Currently, alcohol and drug dependency are viewed as having a biologic, as well as an environmental, basis. Instead of being accused of moral weakness, those afflicted should be offered therapeutic alternatives. Perhaps for this reason, the second part of the policy adopted by APhA in 1982 states,

> APhA supports establishment of counseling, treatment, prevention and rehabilitation programs for pharmacists and pharmacy students who are subject to physical or mental impairment due to the influence of drugs—including alcohol—or other causes, when such impairment has potential for adversely affecting their abilities to function properly in their professional capacities.[10]

In one 1985 examination, no state laws mandating that pharmacists report their impaired colleagues were discovered; although such laws do exist for some health professionals, "health professionals prefer to rely on a voluntary reporting system, because they believe that such reporting is an ethical duty that should not be replaced by law."[11] In addition, increasing the threat of impaired colleagues losing their licenses deters reporting and contravenes current theories of nonpunitive rehabilitation.

Since the adoption of these rehabilitative policies, APhA has worked to provide programs and other support to effectively address the problem of impaired pharmacists. APhA sponsors the Pharmacists Section of the University of Utah School on Alcoholism and Other Drug Dependencies, an intensive training program for those working with impaired pharmacists.[12] APhA published a manual, "Helping the Impaired Pharmacist—A Handbook For Planning and Implementing State Programs," to assist state and local pharmaceutical associations in implementing or strengthening their own impaired pharmacist programs. In a 1988 survey, respondents from 40 states reported having chemical dependency assistance programs. Twenty-five of these are administered by state pharmacy associations. Such programs most commonly are "recovery oriented, multidisciplinary treatment" programs "consisting of identification, verification, intervention, evaluation, treatment, and after-care."[12] Typically they are confidential, nonpunitive, and therapeutically oriented.[12]

Chemical dependency among pharmacists is a documented problem. A survey of pharmacists and pharmacy students in one New England state revealed that 18% of the pharmacists and 35% of the students who had ever used a drug either became dependent or were at risk of drug abuse. The drugs most often abused were marijuana, stimulants, tranquilizers, and opiates.[13] In addition, 43% of 1370 pharmacists in North Carolina who responded to a 1984 survey knew at least one pharmacist whom they considered impaired, and 24% said they had worked with someone who was abusing or addicted to drugs.[14] Although estimates of impairment vary, about 10% to 15% of all pharmacists could be impaired by alcohol alone at some point during their careers.[14] This percentage is based upon a national estimate of alcoholism of 10% in the general population and the finding of an incidence of alcoholism at one and one half times the national average for health care providers. It is not unreasonable, however, to assume that this figure actually should be projected as being greater for pharmacists, who not only are at higher risk for stress and burnout, but also have easy access to drugs.[10] A nationwide survey of recovering chemically dependent pharmacists shows that men are more at risk than women (83% respondents were male), and 60% (of the 87% who provided this information) graduated in the upper third of their class. Finally, 54 of the 86 respondents identified one or both parents as alcoholic.[15]

Moreover, many pharmacists, like many dentists, work alone or with limited supervision,[16] and independent pharmacists, like anesthesiologists, have virtually unlimited access to drugs with minimal risk of detection by colleagues. Their isolation may indeed result in pharmacists' reliance upon alcohol or drugs to relieve stress resulting from inadequate opportunity to share frustrations with coworkers. Indeed, by the time the pharmacist's problem has progressed to the point that he comes to work obviously under the influence of drugs, this is at a late stage in the disease and his life already is falling apart.[17]

Persons with a chemical dependency often delude themselves into believing that they are in control of their addiction. For pharmacists this denial is bolstered by social expectations (e.g., the view that pharmacists, of all people, should know how to handle drugs) and surveys that identify pharmacy as the most trusted profession.[6] Therefore, until some catastrophic event shakes them into the reality of their problem, pharmacists often believe they can cease their substance abuse at any time. Even then, there is a reluctance to admit to their addiction and to seek treatment for fear that this will mean the automatic loss of their pharmacy license.

Because chemically dependent pharmacists, in most instances, are not capable of acknowledging and stopping their addictions alone, a special burden to intervene falls on those with whom they have direct contact in the work environment. Unfortunately, the previously mentioned study of 86 recovering pharmacists found that close friends or family generally were the first to approach the impaired pharmacist and only rarely was this step initiated by a colleague or employer.[15] Pharmacy schools need to rectify this situation by educating students about chemical dependency and treatment. They then will be more confident and able to identify and assist their impaired colleagues at an earlier stage.[15]

Colleagues initially may intervene personally by discussing the impairment with the chemically dependent pharmacist. Although this gives him an opportunity to seek treatment and shows respect for his autonomy, this approach rarely is successful and could indeed lead to retaliatory action against the concerned colleague. Moreover, unless the individual colleague takes the burden upon herself, direct personal intervention also does not afford the opportunity to monitor the impaired professional's success in recovering from his dependency problem. Respect for the profession's autonomy and the concomitant privilege to self-regulate, as well as the overriding concern for the efficacious prevention of harm to patients, should instead prompt the concerned colleague to seek intervention assistance through institutional or intraprofessional channels specifically established to assist and monitor impaired pharmacists.

For those who know of, or strongly suspect, a pharmacist with a substance abuse problem, advice hotlines commonly are available to facilitate contact with state or local peer assistance programs involving direct intervention and referral.[12] Those using hotlines to seek assistance for impaired pharmacists are guaranteed confidentiality. This promise of confidentiality is offered to decrease the likelihood of any retaliatory action being taken against those who contact the pharmaceutical society on behalf of a chemically dependent pharmacist. The guarantee of confidentiality, however, increases the opportunity for injustice to be done to innocent practitioners, particularly in a constrained economic climate where competition may motivate malicious tactics. Unfortunately, it is not inconceivable that an unscrupulous professional would wrongly point an accusing finger toward a professional peer for personal gain or retaliatory purposes. The moral responsibility for the accuracy of reports must lie with those who report an addicted associate. Thus, some mechanism of accountability should be instituted to deter and discipline those who would bring frivolous or malicious accusations.

Once the peer assistance program is contacted, typically a small group of specially trained intervention team members conduct an investigation to determine if a problem exists. In the event that there is a problem, they meet with the impaired pharmacist and discuss treatment options and encourage him to pursue this plan before he runs the risk of losing his license to practice.[12] Pharmacists enter a treatment program with the ultimate goal of returning to practice. They typically are monitored closely by the recovery program and sometimes even by the original intervenors.[17,18] (This process should serve as a model for the supportive peer review mechanism, described earlier as a means of addressing poor quality pharmacy practice not related to chemical impairment.)

The pharmaceutical profession's creation of these intraorganizational, self-regulating mechanisms discourages pharmacists from "blowing the whistle" to journalists or to others external to the profession. To do so before first taking steps to address the impaired colleague's problem within the professional arena, would be contrary to the essence of self-regulation, embarrassing to the profession and the individual impaired colleague, and possibly alarming to members of the public. If, however, after having informed the appropriate parties, there is no discernible progress towards the pharmacist's recovery, one may be obligated to take a more public action (e.g., informing state licensing agencies or patients).

In all cases of reporting a suspected impaired pharmacist—publicly or intraprofessionally—one must be guided by clear conscience, an absence of malice in motive, and accurate evidence justifying a reasonable belief that a dependency problem exists. Such evidence permits one to feel especially confident in seeking assistance for a pharmacist whose dependency is currently and obviously impairing his ability to provide quality pharmaceutical care. Suppose, however, that the pharmacist's chemical dependency has not yet caused any obvious impairment to his ability to practice and there is only a perceived potential for harm. How then does one justify intervening? Consider the following case.

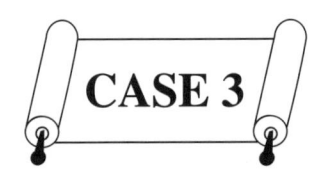

CASE 3

Pharmacist E.V. owns Proper Care Pharmacy where he has practiced for nearly 30 years. H.P., a graduate of the local college of pharmacy, recently became a partner with E.V. She purchased 40% of the business through an agreement with E.V. in which she put a percentage of the money down and would provide state of the art clinical services for the balance of the deposit. The agreement further stated that after five years, H.P. would have the option to buy the remaining 60% of the business.

H.P. had noticed over the past few months that E.V.'s mood seemed to shift radically during the latter stages of the afternoon. He also had been arriving later than usual in the morning, and he had asked her to work for him on several Saturday mornings when she was scheduled for a day off. On one of these mornings, H.P. was confronted by a patient who demanded that she receive all the pills she was due. She told H.P. that she had been short-changed before with her tranquilizers and that a few of her friends were having the same problem. H.P. suspected that E.V. may have become dependent upon a prescription drug.

Recalling the lessons she learned about dependence when she was in school, H.P. decided that she should speak with E.V. and offer her support, as well as identify the intervention program offered by the state pharmacy association. One day, during a quiet moment, she gently approached the matter by describing the incident with the patient, as well as her personal observations. She encouraged E.V. to seek help with the state association and told him the story of a classmate who had completely recovered from a chemical dependency through the program.

E.V. thanked her for her concern but insisted that there was no problem. He told her that he probably had miscounted the prescription and attributed it to an increasing amount of pressure he had come under lately. In addition, the anniversary of the loss of his son was taking its toll. He promised that he would pay more attention to the work schedule, as well as his performance behind the counter.

Less than two weeks later, H.P. noticed E.V. replacing a prescription bottle on the shelf. Her suspicion was raised since inventory was not being counted and there were no prescription orders being filled at that moment. Resuming her activity in the diabetic center, she watched as a long line developed at the prescription counter. Realizing that her help was needed, she went back to assist her partner. Arriving behind the counter she quickly noticed that there was no order to the unfilled prescriptions, the prescriptions were in disarray, and E.V. was nowhere in sight. After she called his name, E.V. stumbled out from around a corner. Realizing that he was under the influence, H.P. stepped in and dispensed the remaining prescriptions. When the pharmacy was empty, she restated her concern that he seek help. H.P. told E.V. that she felt bad having to cover for him and was thankful that no mistakes occurred. He angrily responded that she had exaggerated the whole problem and that he just needed some time. Besides, he argued, it would be worth her time to be patient since she had already invested her life savings in the store, and if he went, so would all of those who trusted him to dispense their prescriptions.

Three months have passed, and E.V. still has not sought any help. Although there have been no more complaints of miscounted prescriptions, he has been arriving at work later and later. What are H.P.'s options? What should she do?

Case Discussion

H.P. could approach E.V. again and insist that he get help this time; however, since she has done this twice already with little effect other than raising his ire, it is unlikely that a third attempt would produce a successful outcome. H.P. could report E.V.'s substance abuse to the State Board of Pharmacy, which could initiate an investigation. Some type of disciplinary action, including the suspension or loss of his license to practice, could result if E.V. were found to be practicing "while subject to physical or mental impairment due to the influence of drugs—including alcohol."[10] The investigation of the complaint would likely include the examination of prescription records, as well as the authorities' interviews of the accused pharmacist, his staff, his acquaintances, and perhaps his patients. Such an investigation would result in public exposure of his problem, perhaps without really dealing with the dependency problem itself. Again, it is not unreasonable to anticipate E.V.'s resentment and retaliation toward his previously trusted colleague and partner, H.P., as well as a deterioration of his health if he continues using alcohol and drugs in response to this additional stress.

At this point, at least from the perspective of H.P., the situation remains in a largely preventive stage since she has no evidence that any patient has yet suffered more than inconvenience because of E.V.'s addiction. Therefore, taking such a drastic step as reporting E.V. to the State Board of Pharmacy, while offering protection to the patient community, would be a no-win situation for him, H.P., and other staff of Proper Care Pharmacy and their families who depend upon the income generated by E.V.'s practice.

At this stage a reasonable option for H.P. would be to contact a pharmacy association intervention program and seek help for E.V. This action would seem to offer the best ethical balance among: 1) her obligation to prevent harm to patients, to E.V., to his staff, and to the profession (through an erosion of the public's trust); 2) her responsibility and desire to preserve her investment and to support herself (and perhaps her own family); and 3) her responsibility and desire to respect the autonomy of all those affected by E.V.'s chemical dependency, specifically, E.V., and his patients.

Having been previously unsuccessful in motivating E.V. to seek help, by now contacting an intervention program, H.P. addresses the chemical dependency problem directly while still offering him maximal confidentiality and a chance to rehabilitate. Unlike state regulatory agencies, chemical dependency assistance programs take no punitive action against the pharmacist. By limiting the negative consequences for E.V. as much as possible, while affording him the greatest opportunity for a positive outcome, H.P. also best protects her future and E.V.'s collegial relationship with her.

If H.P. were not aware of a local peer assistance program, she could contact the Pharmacists' Recovery Network through the APhA and without identifying anyone, describe her situation and ask for guidance concerning the most ethically appropriate action. H.P.'s situation as the concerned subordinate or junior partner of the impaired practitioner has many parallels within the profession (e.g., the pharmaceutical student who observes the impairment or inappropriate practices of an instructor; or the junior colleague who has concerns about a more senior or more prestigious member of the field). Turning to the APhA is an appropriate course of action for anyone seeking guidance about an impaired practitioner or someone whose professional practices appear substandard.

In reviewing possible courses of action for A.D., S.T., and H.P., it should be clear that the "do nothing" alternative mentioned early in this chapter is unacceptable. In these three cases, this chapter argues for third-party intervention, not for direct, personal intervention. While there is no question regarding the acceptance of the third-party intervention strategy as the prevailing practice in cases involving chemical dependency, there has not been the same level of professional acceptance for similar third-party approaches in cases of substandard practice not related to chemical dependency. To bring the profession's responses to these three cases in line with each other, a greater effort should be made at the state level to ensure the availability of a well-publicized, nonpunitive third-party support system addressing cases of negligent misconduct or substandard practice, similar to those support systems now in place for cases of chemical dependency. Although it is unlikely that the profession will be able to move quickly toward this objective, in light of the deficiencies of the personal intervention approach in identifying and monitoring the retraining of professionals providing poor care, we nevertheless advocate reporting poor quality care to the State Board of Pharmacy.

CONCLUSION

If pharmacists are to serve the public, and deserve and maintain the public's trust and esteem, they must learn to be effective self-regulators.

In the course of their pharmacy school education and through continuing education programs and publications, pharmacists must learn to act autonomously, taking upon themselves the responsibility to promote and prevent harm to the public health. Educational, regulatory, and professional policies, structures, and mechanisms should seek to create an open and collegial environment in which pharmacists are expected to identify and seek help in correcting their mistakes and faults (e.g., a chemical dependency problem or a lack of preparation or skill), as well as those of their colleagues. A supportive and corrective professional response to mistake making, rather than a punitive one, may encourage pharmacists to assume this self-regulatory responsibility.

High-quality care is the primary goal of pharmacy and, therefore, when poor care has occurred or is likely to occur, pharmacists have a responsibility to correct or prevent it. In doing so, they promote good and prevent or correct harm, which are the goals of the ethical duties to act beneficently and nonmaleficently. By assuming this responsibility, by identifying and correcting their own faulty work and that of their colleagues, and by informing patients of such faulty work when it occurs, pharmacists act as responsible, autonomous individuals and also promote the autonomy and health of their patients.

Professional Responsibilities... 217

Discussion Questions

1. Loyalty is a virtue invoked both in favor of and against reporting colleagues' substandard practices. To whom might a pharmacist, who has knowledge of a colleague's misconduct, feel a duty of loyalty? Why? How should he weigh these conflicting loyalties? Why?

2. What is the relationship between competent practice and ethical practice in pharmacy?

3. Evaluate the strengths and weaknesses of various responses to a colleague's poor quality patient care. If the colleague's substandard treatment resulted from his chemical dependency, would your response be different? Should it be?

4. How does the diversity of institutional and workplace settings in which pharmacists practice complicate the task of determining how they should respond to suspected misconduct on the part of their colleagues? Should pharmacists respond differently when they observe a fellow pharmacist offering substandard pharmaceutical care than when they observe a physician, nurse, or other health care provider offering substandard health care?

5. Suppose that while on rounds in the medical intensive care unit of your local hospital, you observe the attending physician make two errors concerning dosage when writing his orders and also ignore a possible negative drug interaction. What would you do? When?

    Suppose that the physician explains why he believes he made the errors; knowledge of another's reasons for mistake (or motives for action) often affects how one feels about the mistake (or bad outcome) and what one deems an appropriate response. Suppose that he explains that he probably made the errors because he had been up all night, before coming in for rounds, with his colicky baby and therefore was tired. Suppose instead that he says that he had been out too late the night before with friends, had a bit too much to drink, and therefore was tired. Do these different explanations affect how you feel about his error or the course of action that you choose? Should they make a difference? How? Why?

    Next, suppose that you learn from other colleagues that these are not isolated errors that the physician has made, but that errors of this sort are a common occurrence. Does knowing this information lead you to a different course of action? If so, what and why? If not, why not?

6. What are your school's policies concerning chemically impaired pharmacy students and faculty? Do the grading practices of your school encourage students to be responsible professionals?

(Continued)

Discussion Questions continued

If the dean of your school asked you to make recommendations concerning the curriculum and policies of your school so that they better reflected the school's commitment to training responsible professionals, what recommendations would you propose? Why do you think that it is important to establish mechanisms to investigate allegations of negligence or chemical impairment before any allegations are made?

REFERENCES

1. Swazey JP, Scher SR. The whistleblower as a deviant professional: professional norms and responses to fraud in clinical research. In: Whistleblowing in Biomedical Research. President's Commission for the Study of Ethical Problems in Medicine and Biomedical and Behavioral Research. 1981.
2. Lowenthal W. Ethical dilemmas in pharmacy. J Med Ethics. 1988;14(1):31–4.
3. Manolakis ML. Why APhA should reject its code of ethics. Am Pharm. 1991;NS31(11):46–8.
4. American Pharmaceutical Association. Code of Ethics for Pharmacists. 1994.
5. American Pharmaceutical Association. Code of Ethics. 1981.
6. Bruner CT. Pharmacists should not borrow prescription drug products for personal use. Am J Hosp Pharm. 1989;46:703.
7. Shea M. When pharmacist and physician disagree. In: Difficult Decisions in Medical Ethics: Proceedings of the Eighth and Ninth Conferences on Ethics, Humanism, and Medicine Held in 1981 and 1982 at the University of Michigan, Ann Arbor. New York: A.R. Liss; 1983:203–9.
8. Elliston F et al. Whistleblowing Research: Methodological and Moral Issues. New York: Praeger Publications; 1985:8.
9. Near JP and Miceli MP. Retaliation against whistleblowers: predictors and effects. J Appl Psychol. 1986;71:137–43.
10. The impaired pharmacist. Am Pharm. 1985;NS25(6):37.
11. Simonsmeier LM, Fox LA. The law and the impaired pharmacist. Am Pharm. 1985;NS25(6):63–8.
12. McNees GE, Godwin HN. Programs for pharmacists impaired by substance abuse: a report. Am Pharm. 1990;NS30(5):33–7.
13. McAuliffe WE et al. Use and abuse of controlled substances by pharmacists and pharmacy students. Am J Hosp Pharm. 1987;44:311–17.
14. Normark JW et al. Impairment risk in North Carolina pharmacy students. Am Pharm. 1985;NS25(6):60–2.
15. Bissell L et al. Pharmacists recovering from alcohol and other drug addictions: an interview study. Am Pharm. 1989;NS29(6):19–30.

16. Metge CJ, Brown PA. Setting up a program: how one group went about it. Am Pharm. 1985;NS25(6):49–51.

17. Bunting GA, Talbott GD. One road to recovery: the Georgia program. Am Pharm. 1985;NS25(6):52–4.

18. Sheffield JW. Establishing a rehabilitation program for impaired pharmacists. Am J Hosp Pharm. 1988;45:2092–98.

ACKNOWLEDGMENT

The authors gratefully acknowledge the contributions of Lissa Wettick, Research Assistant, University of Pittsburgh.

Chapter 11

Power and Professional Responsibility: The Social Context of Pharmacy

Andrew Jameton
Amy M. Haddad

The topic of this chapter is the power of pharmacists in relationship to their professional responsibilities. Pharmacists' sense of empowerment depends partly on their sense of effectiveness in their job roles. Since pharmacists depend on the cooperation of others for their success, the ability of pharmacists to communicate and to mediate is essential to their power. Social factors such as income, class, race, gender, educational level, and professional standing affect communication processes and the ability of pharmacists to mediate among patients, physicians, and other health care providers. Thus, social factors play a role in determining the power of pharmacists to meet their responsibilities.

Pharmacists also maintain their sense of empowerment in relationship to their ideals and values in practice. Their ideals of practice may conform with or conflict with the expectations of others and their role responsibilities. When their ideals and roles harmonize, pharmacists are more likely to feel empowered. Social factors also affect pharmacists' values and ideals, and thus affect their sense of empowerment.

The pharmacy profession is becoming increasingly diverse in the social backgrounds of its members. This contributes a wider range of values that can be expressed in pharmacy practice. For example, more traditionally masculine values of technical proficiency, directness, and objectivity now combine with more traditionally feminine values of compassion and nurturance. Increasing diversity provides opportunities for pharmacists to become more effective and flexible as mediators and in expressing their ideals; at the same time, it increases the potential for uncertainty about values in practice. The level of educational achievement of pharmacists has been widely discussed in the pharmacy literature. This social factor is likely to have diverse effects on both the relationships of pharmacists with each other and with other health professionals.

One important area of concern is the pharmacist-patient relationship. We will present a case study and analysis of this relationship. Social factors can affect the pharmacist's ability to work with the patient in powerful and subtle ways. Social factors affect: 1) the ability of the pharmacist to trust the patient, 2) the range of choices available to the pharmacist in serving the patient, 3) the potential to benefit the patient, and 4) fairness in handling uncertainties with regard to the patient's wishes and needs.

Another important area of concern is the pharmacist-physician relationship. A case study and analysis of a disagreement between a pharmacist and a physician will be presented. Social factors similarly affect the pharmacist's power and objectives in resolving this disagreement. The nature of the institution in which both pharmacist and physician serve may affect the resolution of this disagreement.

The chapter concludes with some proposals to strengthen the pharmacy profession by strengthening its ideals and its ability to mediate among others in the context of expected long-term global changes.

PHARMACY AS MEDIATION

The growth of medical technology and the increasing public interest in ethical issues in health care has given rise to the field of *bioethics*. Philosophers, theologians, and health care providers who contribute to this field are sometimes known as *bioethicists*. A major theme in bioethics in the last twenty years has been the balance of power between patients and health professionals. Although the views of bioethicists are better represented as conflicting than consensual, bioethicists have generally tended to support empowering the patient and to criticize excessive professional power expressed by paternalism and restricted information flow to patients. Ethicists have generally defended equalization of power between professionals and patients largely through improved communication, informed consent, and more patient involvement in making decisions.

Despite these recommendations, health professionals retain considerable power as compared to the patient through various forms of influence: in particular, the authority to dispense and prescribe medications is a key element of the professional powers of pharmacists and physicians. If patients could generally buy, on the open market, pharmaceuticals that are now legally available only by prescription, many patients would likely medicate themselves, however unwisely, without benefit of professional consultation. Furthermore, if correct and understandable information about drug use were readily available from the media, on television and in newspapers, and from friends and neighbors, the power of, and need for, physicians and pharmacists to counsel and inform patients would diminish.

Bioethicists, to the best of our knowledge, have not seriously defended elimination of the prescription system, nor have they argued for vast changes in the nature of what the media communicate. Instead, bioethicists have generally considered it beneficial for patients to be subject to the expert judgment of physicians and pharmacists with regard to access to a wide range of therapies. Health professionals also should play a key role in educating and informing patients about use of the therapies. Some might regard these powers as essentially paternalistic (or parentalistic), but there is general agreement that the market in pharmaceuticals should be controlled in part by professional expertise. Understanding the hazards of pharmaceuticals requires specialized knowledge in pharmacology and therapeutics. Patients may show poor judgment for a variety of reasons including the influence of advertising, poor public education, inability to assess risk rationally, or powerful feelings induced by illness. Marketers, wittingly or not, have taken advantage of this vulnerable clientele, as demonstrated by the history of the marketing of many nonprescription (OTC) and prescription pharmaceuticals.[1]

Thus physicians, pharmacists, and other health professionals might be thought of as mediators, who obtain their professional power and authority through several kinds of mediation. As information sources, pharmacists mediate among the patient's needs, scientific knowledge, and pharmaceutical company claims. As professionals among other professionals, they mediate and cooperate with these professionals to resolve disagreements among themselves as to how to best serve the patient's needs. Furthermore, as prescribers and retailers of pharmaceuticals, they mediate between the interests of patients and the interests of providers and marketers.

Social Factors in Effective Mediation

Influenced by a variety of internal and external factors, the patterns of power and professional responsibility in the pharmacy profession continue to shift. External factors affecting these patterns include changes in reimbursement for services, the general structure of health care services, U.S. demographics, and U.S. health problems. Internal factors include changes in the demographic composition of pharmacy, the ethical conceptions of the professional responsibilities of pharmacists, and the basic paradigm of pharmacy practice. The last is changing from a more business-oriented model to the patient-centered pharmaceutical care model proposed by Hepler and Strand.[2] Simply put, this model proposes that pharmacists can best fulfill their goals by emphasizing their advising and consulting functions among health care team members rather than their physical function as hands-on suppliers of pharmaceutical materials.

There is no clear consensus on the social functions of pharmacy. As pharmacy struggles to determine which paradigm best suits contemporary and future pharmacy practice, the profession also searches for clarity of purpose and identity, combined with recognition of its authority and legitimacy. The profession of pharmacy has steadily gained responsibility for patient counseling and education; yet clinical knowledge and expertise often remain unrecognized by health care colleagues and the public. If we understand professional power as the ability to exercise professional judgment and to influence others accordingly, pharmacy professionals must depend heavily on the cooperation of others with their professional goals in order to exercise their power. If pharmacy professionals have goals that integrate poorly with the work and aims of others, they are more likely to feel powerless; however, if their aims are consistent with those of others and facilitate the pharmacy mediating role, then they are more likely to feel empowered. The pharmacist must, therefore, work in tension between his or her individual sense of purpose or service in working with patients and with his or her actual situational, role-dependent ability to fulfill that sense of purpose. Moreover, since pharmacists work in hierarchically organized and stratified institutions in which some occupational groups and positions possess more power than others, pharmacists are likely to feel more influential than those lower in the hierarchy and less influential than those higher in standing. Thus, pharmacists' personal sense of empowerment will depend in part on whom they perceive as an appropriate group with which to compare themselves.

The struggle for recognition and power is further modulated by various social differences (e.g., gender, race, class) of the members of the profession individually and collectively. Each individual professional pharmacist brings a social background that, together with her professional image and position, tends to affect how the pharmacist views her authority in relationship to others, and how she is perceived as an authority. As the social characteristics of the profession change, we can expect changes in the attitudes of those both inside and outside of pharmacy toward the power and authority of pharmacists.

For example, the traditional status of the community pharmacist as merchant tended to impose obstacles upon women and minorities wishing to enter the profession, since one could not become a pharmacist without also establishing a business. Traditional business and employment practices have long made it more difficult for minorities and the poor to obtain credit, own property, and gain customers. This business barrier also was present for women. In 1988, 23.3% of actively practicing male pharmacists were pharmacy owners or partners as compared to only 4.5% of their female colleagues.[3] A corollary study in the same year observed that women pharmacy owners believed that they were at a disadvantage when compared to men. Respondents stated that they were not accepted as owners, had additional home and family responsibilities, and had difficulty obtaining financial support.[4]

Pharmacists also tend to be members of the middle to upper-middle class with average incomes over $50,000 annually. The income level of pharmacists tends to create opportunities and barriers for socializing with potential business partners and colleagues outside of the work setting. These informal networks provide opportunities to establish cooperation and to exchange information.

Physicians are key to most mediation that pharmacists engage in to improve patient care. Because pharmacists have different incomes and education from physicians and work in locations distant from physicians, social differences can hinder building the full cooperative relationships needed for effective mediation. Similar differences may affect communication between pharmacists and drug company representatives or pharmacists and their employers. As pharmacies become increasingly owned by large corporations, face-to-face opportunities for mediation and negotiation with those most in control of the business aspects of pharmacy are diminishing. Differences among races and nationalities also may affect informal networks of power and authority with financial impacts via referrals, institutional contracts, and discounts. Most importantly, pharmacists and patients are often of different social class—this may hinder patients from asking important questions, hinder pharmacists from empathizing with patients, and limit pharmacists' knowledge of practical everyday obstacles hindering or facilitating the ability of patients to pursue medication regimens.[5]

Since communication styles, access to personal contact, estimates of authority, and the ability to empathize are affected by such factors as hierarchical position, social status, gender, race, and income, these social variations may impact the outcome of moral deliberations in pharmacy practice and the ability of pharmacists to implement their moral judgments. Despite the importance of these cultural variables to decision and communication processes, the tradition in ethical theory has been to abstract as much as possible from particular social circumstances and to attempt to articulate moral considerations as generally as possible without considering particular differences among people. As a result, these phenomena are often unexamined in the traditional principle-based approach to ethics emphasizing impartiality and abstraction.[6]

Yet, even though social factors often enter illegitimately into decisions, it is important to consider their actual patterns of impact. Moreover, it may even be legitimate to take such factors into account when attempting to estimate the consequences for patients of health care decisions. For example, an anthropological study of confidentiality and AIDS in the hospital showed that the social class of patients tended to influence how professionals handled information. Indeed, a patient in need of help from Medicaid and other social welfare institutions would often be in such a state of dependency on these institutions that the good of the patient could arguably require the easy flow of information, unhindered by confidentiality, among institutions.[7] Similarly, pharmacists may feel torn between equality and the need to take special circumstances into account in their assessments of patients' needs.

This chapter will reflect on the various forms of power and authority that pharmacists engage in when acting as mediators among these parties. It will do so by calling attention to the subtle but persistent influence social variables exert on ethical understanding and decisions in pharmacy practice. The next section of this chapter will describe current trends. The second and third sections will each treat a case illustrating the potential ethical implications of these trends.

CURRENT SOCIAL TRENDS IN PHARMACY

The face of pharmacy is changing. The number of women pharmacists has greatly increased. In 1950, only 4% of active pharmacists were women. By 1988, that proportion had risen to over 26%, an upward trend expected to continue. In 1963 to 1964, 13% of students enrolled in the final three years in colleges of pharmacy were women. By 1990 to 1991, pharmacy programs awarded almost 63% of entry level degrees, whether baccalaureate or doctorate, to women.[8]

Although well represented in the workforce, disparities exist at management levels, with only 36% of the women reporting management positions compared with 68% of the men.[9] Additional studies show women underrepresented in managerial positions and overrepresented in staff positions.[10,11] However, this percentage should improve since one in five women entering the profession over the last five years has gained a managerial position, a ratio comparable to men over the same time period.[12] Nevertheless, women pharmacy students appear unconvinced that these opportunities exist, as indicated by a study regarding gender differences and management aspirations of pharmacy students. Woodward and colleagues, in a study of 604 pharmacy students, found that more men (88.6%) than women (56.7%) aspired to management positions, the major difference being accounted for in the different interest in pharmacy ownership.[13]

Women account for 40% of hospital pharmacists, but the majority of women pharmacists work in community settings with 34% in chain and 19% in independent pharmacies.[9] Three out of 10 women pharmacists took time off from their careers to be mothers. Women over 40 were more likely to have taken time off for family rearing. Generally, the women returned to the work force within a year. Women worked on average 9% fewer hours per week (42 hours) than men (46 hours). Salaries were not statistically different between men and women.[9] Growth in the number of women pharmacists is expected to account for all growth in the active supply of pharmacists in the next decades.

The minority composition of pharmacy practice has been changing during the last two decades, although much less dramatically. The authors found it difficult to find good historical numbers on minority presence in pharmacy, an indicator in itself of a historical inattention to minority membership. It is estimated that in 1988 there were 16,500 minority pharmacists in active practice, 10.5% of the total of active pharmacists, as compared to 4.2% in 1974 and 8.9% in 1980. The number in 1988 included 4800 African-Americans, 3400 Hispanic-Americans, 7700 Asian-Americans, 300 Native Americans, and 300 other minority individuals.[9] Over 11% of pharmacy students were identified as minority in 1990 to 1991 (7.9% African-American, 3.5% Hispanic-American, and less than 1% Native American).[8] Although the percentage of minorities represented in pharmacy is less than the percentage in the overall population, pharmacy fares better in minority representation than nursing (8.5%), dentistry (2.6%) and medicine (7%).

The three-phase transition from 1) a male-dominated profession to 2) one of a large number of novice female and some multicultural practitioners with a large number of experienced white male practitioners in positions of authority (management, independent owners, and supervisors), and then 3) to one of an equitable distribution among gender and cultural identifications will certainly mean a change for pharmacy. What these changes will mean in regard to practice and ethics specifically cannot be accurately predicted. Yet, we can expect that many of the issues women and minorities in medicine have faced will appear in pharmacy as well. Such concerns as rate of promotion, balancing personal and professional life, management and communication styles, identification with social groups, reconciling individual values with standard professional values, and setting priorities in patient care can be expected to arise.

Since pharmacists are of a different standing than physicians, and since a majority of pharmacists are expected to be women, there are likely to be differences as well. If women in medicine have been associated with a humanizing trend in medicine, can we expect similar trends in pharmacy to be even more strongly expressed? Or, as women are achieving greater equality in society generally, will such differences be less marked than in the past, when men and women tended to express sharply differentiated role expectations? Will multiple cultures entering pharmacy increase the varieties of conceptions of service within pharmacy? Will it extend the potential range of the profession to inform and influence patients? Will pharmacy evolve into a more patient-centered, less technical profession?

Diversifying Values and Empowerment

These possible changes, should they occur, have desirable features. A stronger expression of values (e.g., community, service, nurture, and caring), more closely associated with women's roles than men's, can be expected to foster equality of patients and to strengthen the power of those in roles where mediation is key. Furthermore, a greater presence of pharmacy practitioners with varying cultural backgrounds can provide greater flexibility within the profession to set goals and to communicate among various cultures present in the United States.

These developments also pose hazards for pharmacists. First, for women, those with a dedication to service have often been exploited by concepts of service requiring great self-sacrifice, as in the claim that, "...the needs, demands, and difficulties of other people should be woman's major, if not exclusive, concern and that meeting these must take precedence over all other claims."[14] Similarly, minorities have faced obstacles and messages of shame from the majority culture making it challenging for some to assert fair compensation for service and their knowledge of human needs and relations.[15] Second, the broad pharmacy mandate of communication and mediation has not been clearly defined for, or especially visible to, the public. Since the functions of a pharmacist are already unclear to outsiders, the move to a more care-centered practice might further obscure the actual contributions of the pharmacist to patient care.

Although the long tradition of combining pharmacy with owning a small business has been a unique feature of pharmacy practice, the tradition of graduating from pharmacy school and opening one's own "store" is rapidly going the way of the corner bakery. Most pharmacists who now enter community pharmacy do not go into business for themselves, but seek employment from independent and corporate-owned pharmacies. Thus, women and minorities entering pharmacy as a business are now entering in a position of less power than on the older model. As employees, pharmacy professionals have less control over their hours, prices, policies, and the other business conducted in conjunction with pharmacy services. For instance, pharmacists who own their own businesses can decide without consultation, although not without financial pressures, whether to carry cigarettes or alcoholic beverages; but, pharmacists working for a franchise of a large corporation must rely for control over cigarette and alcohol sales on the cooperation of a vast array of managers and stockholders. Moreover, the employed pharmacist has little role in choosing the location of a corporate-owned pharmacy and, thus, little choice in the community it serves most immediately.

On one hand, pharmacists may feel disempowered by these changes because they find that their context lacks support for their ideals. On the other hand, pharmacists may still feel adequately empowered in either of two ways. One way to feel empowered is to narrow goals. For example, a pharmacist may focus on tertiary care and pay less attention to opportunities to affect public health (e.g., smoking and drinking habits). Similarly, a pharmacist may maintain a sense of objectivity toward, or distance from, clients, or cultivate general and equal feelings of support and affection for them; and may, thereby, limit concern about the choice of clientele. Another way to feel empowered is to speak up consistently for one's ideals of service—vocal pharmacists may find a supportive response among management also interested in the goals of service to the public.

As the values guiding pharmacy practice become more diverse, pharmacists may feel more ambiguity about their roles. For instance, pharmacy practice combines both technical and emotional skills. Women pharmacists may seek rewards for such traditional feminine behavior as compassion, nurturance, gentleness, and attentiveness, and yet also be rewarded for types of masculine behavior, such as technical proficiency, directness, objectivity, and strength. Initial uncertainty of the student over the choice of working environment (i.e., between the more traditionally masculine model of independent businessman, in contrast to the service employee model) may give the student the opportunity to project both "masculine" and "feminine" versions of future work. Furthermore, once at work, pharmacists may suffer from conflicting pictures of their roles, since the ideal pharmacist may be expected to embody both "feminine" and "masculine" behaviors in order to meet the demands of the profession.

These ambiguities apply increasingly to expectations of men as well as women. Men also are subject in many cultures to conflicting messages regarding roles: they are to be cooperative as well as independent, dominant as well as submissive, expressive as well as objective, and nurturing as well as aggressive. As men and women enter pharmacy with these conflicting self-images, they both nuance the neutral institutional definitions of the pharmacist's role and struggle to maintain their own sense of identity in the face of corporate and organizational pressures. Moreover, the images of gender and culture can be expected to affect the patient's perception of how pharmacists express their professional role.

Multiplying the cultures of those practicing pharmacy is likely to diversify even more widely the potential self-perceptions of pharmacists' roles. Any cursory glance at health values held by various cultures indicates widely varying assessments of the importance of health, the methods for maintaining health, and the explanations of health and disease, even though there is much overlap among cultures and much variation within them. Although this process of diversification is likely to increase the level of controversy among students and professionals, we believe that such discussions will prove healthy to the profession, enhance pharmacy's potential to serve a wide variety of populations, and deepen its understanding of its goals.

Social Factors in Pharmacist-Patient Relations

In order to explore the themes of mediation, gender, culture, power, and professionalism, we find it helpful to consider cases. We will present two cases in this chapter, each illustrating different aspects of pharmacist-patient relations.

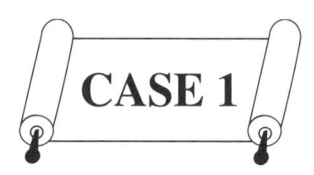

CASE 1

This was the third month in a row that pharmacist J.J., R.Ph. received a one-month prescription for oxycodone hydrochloride and acetaminophen (Percocet) from M.S., a 37-year-old housewife. M.S. had injured her lower back and her physician prescribed Percocet for the pain. The prescriptions were appropriate regarding dosage and indication. Yet three months was, in J.J.'s judgment, too long a course of therapy for a drug with such a high abuse potential. He was concerned that M.S. was abusing the drug and, further, that he was contributing to her addiction.

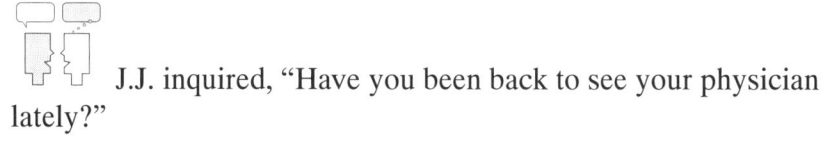

J.J. inquired, "Have you been back to see your physician lately?"

"Why, yes," M.S. replied. "Just today. I guess I'll have to take this medication longer since my back just hasn't gotten better." Pharmacist J.J. is left with what looks like a legitimate prescription and a problem.

Case Discussion

If we were to approach this case, as bioethicists have, with a focus on general ethical principles, we would become involved in such socially neutral and abstract concerns as conflicts in professional judgment regarding medication use and abuse, respect for M.S.'s autonomy in managing her regimen; the balance of risks and benefits to her of addiction on one hand and pain relief on the other; and conflicting loyalties for J.J. among responsibility to the patient, the physician, and the community. Yet, we know that the American public holds seriously conflicting views regarding appropriate use of addicting and pain-relieving medications. We also know that the diagnosis of back pain is itself heavily laden with multiple interpretations. Although no consideration of gender or culture is likely to be involved in stating the abstract ethical concerns here, when we reflect on the pharmacist's ethical concerns in full, we recognize that many different stories could be told about what is happening with M.S. Furthermore, these more complete stories, these "thicker narratives," inevitably involve expectations that are likely to vary in J.J.'s mind, irrespective of whether they actually vary in real life, depending on gender, race, class, age, religion, and other variables.

J.J. has a range of options open: he can fill the prescription in silence; refuse to fill the prescription without explanation; talk with M.S. about his concerns; talk with the physician about his concerns; talk with both patient and physician; work with an informal social network; or refer the matter to another authority. What pharmacist J.J. decides to do, and should decide to do, depends on what he knows and projects about the situation and the people involved. What he actually knows about the physician and patient and his actual history of relations with them may involve whether he has worked with them professionally for years and gotten on well, knows them both to be of impeccable credentials, knows them both personally and professionally, has or lacks informal social networks through which he can learn more or communicate information, knows them both to sell drugs at parties and cooperate in insurance fraud, or whatever. And, how much J.J. must guess about these crucial matters depends on to what degree he is a stranger to them or shares community with them. What J.J. guesses M.S.'s situation to be, and with what assurance he is able to guess, will very likely depend to some degree on his own cultural background and that of the physician and patient. J.J. also needs to care enough about M.S. to take the trouble needed to help resolve the problem, and his ability to care about M.S. may likewise depend on some of these factors.

Modifying Cases

Some ethicists find it helpful in composing and analyzing ethics case studies, to vary the group identifications of all of the characters involved as a crude sensitivity test for our abstract intuitions. If we find that we have the same gut reaction and the same sense of the story for a variety of backgrounds, we feel that we are less likely to have erred morally. Yet, in this case and many like it, how J.J. is likely to handle the case, and perhaps should handle the case, may vary depending on what he believes his relations to be with the cultures and communities involved.

For instance, what if we change the gender of the pharmacist and the patient? The pharmacist now becomes female and the patient a male. Changing the gender of the participants in the case study may change the way J.J. is likely to perceive pain and to legitimize medicating it. If J.J. believes the pain to be "honest," "legitimate" pain, J.J. is more likely to hazard continued medication before confronting the problem of addiction. Numerous studies of the influence of gender on decisions regarding drug therapy in pain management have shown gender effects on decisions. Descriptive ethics studies in nursing have demonstrated that women nurses view pain differently in their men and women patients. One study found that nurses selected less medication for female patients than male patients in two vignettes which varied only for the gender of the patient.[16] However, another study found that female cancer patients receiving radiation were more likely to receive, and likely to receive stronger, narcotic analgesics upon staff initiative than were corresponding male patients.[17] Other researchers have reported that concern about addiction is stronger in male medical students than females.[18] Do such gender variations exist in pharmacy? One study of the perceptions of pharmacy students indicated that the gender of the student affects judgments about cancer pain management. Holdsworth and Raisch found that male students were more likely than female students to judge that cancer patients were being adequately medicated, more worried that patients may be addicted, and less concerned about undermedication.[19]

If pharmacist J.J. were to call M.S.'s physician and share his concerns with the physician regarding the possibility of abuse, the gender of the physician might also make a difference to the discourse. We might imagine that a female pharmacist, more than a male, might be less likely to question the legitimacy of the pain complaint. However, a male pharmacist might be more willing to set aside concerns particular to this patient and to settle the issue with a simple rule concerning authority: fill the physician's *prima facie* legitimate order unless presented with obvious evidence of a problem. The way the conversation proceeds between pharmacist and physician also may depend on styles of communication characteristic of differing genders; this may affect the ability of physician and pharmacist to reach an agreement on how to handle this delicate matter.[20]

Four Key Considerations

Turning our attention to race and culture, we have a broad range of possible combinations to choose among pharmacist, physician, and patient. Rather than try to specify cases from what is an essentially endless list, let us consider four key factors in handling this case that are likely to be affected, and may legitimately be affected, by these cultural variables: trust, mediation, patient benefit, and fairness.

First, the pharmacist must decide whether to trust the physician, the patient, or both; this will affect whether the pharmacist fills the prescription without question and whether and how he or she speaks with one or both of them. The decision to trust depends on the pharmacist's actual knowledge of the physician and patient and the sense of community membership he or she has with them. We can't predict for sure whether similarity or difference in background will increase or decrease trust, but it will affect the level of knowledge involved in making the judgment and the reliability and extent of community relations on which the pharmacist can depend. For example, a suburban white male pharmacist who abused alcohol and drugs in his youth before entering pharmacy school may see a kindred spirit in the similar young white male standing before him with back pain and a prescription for Percocet, and immediate mistrust may be the first reaction. Alternatively, the pharmacist may not feel entirely comfortable and may still feel new to the community after several months. The pharmacist may feel that it is not appropriate to raise these concerns until acquiring better acquaintance with the community and individuals involved.

Second, the actual choices available to the pharmacist may depend on the community. The pharmacist is, as we suggested, a mediator, and in that role, his or her actual ability to have an impact depends on the quality of his or her relations with others. Is the patient or the physician likely to trust him or her? Is his or her judgment respected? Moreover, the actual alternatives open to the patient may be determined by the concrete resources available to the patient, which varies according to a range of cultural variables. Suppose, for instance, that upon investigation the pharmacist recognizes that a program of drug rehabilitation treatment is needed for M.S. Is there a good program available; does M.S. have appropriate insurance; and is M.S. of such a culture and situation that she can actually get treatment? Is M.S. the sort of person who could understand and handle the problem readily or with great difficulty? Although these are problems of big cities housing diverse cultures and scarce resources, these also are problems of small towns and intimate, uniform communities.

Third, what is actually beneficial to M.S. may well depend on these cultural and communitarian concerns discussed above. What can be done effectively for the patient depends on what resources are available. Moreover, what needs to be done depends on whether the pharmacist has an addicted patient with a legitimate pain problem who is otherwise managing well, an addicted patient with no pain problem and otherwise good health, an addicted patient with deteriorating health and a pattern of self-abuse, or a patient who is giving or selling Percocet to others. Whether the pharmacist is able to find out what is going on or whether the pharmacist must make a guess, rightly or wrongly, about what is going on, depends in part on the perception of the patient, with all of that person's details of culture, class, and background expressed, or hidden, (e.g., in clothing, manner). For example, if a prediction of the likelihood that the patient will adhere to a new regimen is required to make a recommendation on a therapy, the pharmacist inevitably enters into a realm in which concrete predictors are rare and in which perceptions of social factors tend to play a distressingly large role in the minds of practitioners.

Fourth, in making such guesses, the pharmacist faces the ethical problem of fairness: on one hand, the pharmacist may stereotype the patient (e.g., by race, class) and, thereby, unfairly trust or mistrust the patient; on the other, the pharmacist may fail to take into account indications of a possible problem suggested by the total presentation of the person standing before him or her. Making a responsible choice about the patient's benefit, and ability to manage the situation, depends to some degree on the patient's actual situation as well as to uncertainties concerning the patient which may be affected, in part, by class, gender, and cultural factors.

EDUCATION AND INTER- AND INTRAPROFESSIONAL RELATIONS

The health care system is an essentially hierarchical, stratified, and increasingly bureaucratic one. In this system, physicians as a group have more power and authority than do pharmacists. The role of the pharmacist has evolved from a "handmaiden" role (a stereotype found in the pharmacy literature of the last century even though at the time the majority of pharmacists were male) to a more collegial one. The move to the single entry-level degree for pharmacy, the Doctor of Pharmacy degree, may help to place pharmacists in a more equitable position on the health care team, especially since other professions are setting similar entry level requirements. Lengthier education and the provision of pharmaceutical care also will engender a stronger distinction between the service and the product the pharmacist offers patients. Although it appears that the brass ring of "fee-for-service" is becoming less and less likely a model for reimbursement for physicians, other health professionals such as nurses and pharmacists still pursue it. It is difficult to predict how pharmacists will be reimbursed in the future, but if they are reimbursed more for their services and less for the products they sell, then they will be more in keeping with the medical profession.

The proposal to separate the pharmacist's advice from the act of providing the product brings up deeper questions about what it means to be a pharmacist. As recently as 20 years ago, dispensing was considered the *sine qua non* of pharmacy. However, dispensing in isolation from the patient and other health professionals has left many pharmacists dissatisfied:

> At the same time, a new breed of clinical pharmacists argued persuasively that professional redemption lay in a radical shift from a product-oriented to a patient-oriented practice, a practice that emphasized expanded patient counseling and, in a sense, a return to patient-care functions reminiscent of an earlier generation of pharmacy practitioners.[21]

If the dispensing function is removed from pharmacy practice, we are left with what has become known as clinical pharmacy practice, composed largely of doctoral-prepared pharmacists practicing in hospital settings. Thus, an unintended split has formed between those generally with bachelors degrees who practice in a community setting and those with doctoral degrees who practice in the hospital setting. Differing levels of education have led to different types of professional organizations appealing to the particular focus of each group, such as the National Association of Retail Pharmacists and the American College of Clinical Pharmacists. This split unfortunately fosters elitism and division within the profession. The shift to a single entry level of the Doctor of Pharmacy degree may help to relieve some of this conflict, but it will reopen the debate over the legitimate and unique functions of pharmacy, since pharmacists with different levels of education continue to practice in all types of settings.

Like other health professions considering higher entry-level degrees, not all of pharmacy is in agreement with the professional doctorate. The academic community, although not unanimous, has tended to support strongly the move to the doctoral degree. National pharmacy organizations have moved slowly to support the doctoral entry level, although some, such as the National Association of Chain Drug Stores, have maintained strong reservations. It is clear that if all entry-level pharmacy practitioners have more education, there will be a need for higher starting salaries. It is not as clear whether increased academic preparation will make appreciable differences in performance in non-hospital settings. Thus, for example, corporate-owned pharmacies may well prefer to employ an even less well-prepared person, such as a pharmacy technician, although state laws regarding pharmacy practice may prevent such strategies.

Graduates of Doctor of Pharmacy degree programs are still in the minority. Of the first professional degree graduates in 1991 to 1992, 82.9% received baccalaureates and 17.1% received Pharm.D. degrees.[8] Many practicing pharmacists and educators voice concerns about the need for the professional doctorate and question if there is any concrete difference between a baccalaureate pharmacy graduate and a Pharm.D. beyond the title "Doctor." Yet, title alone often confers status—colleagues with the title "Doctor" are on equal footing at least regarding how they address one another, and from this point can move more comfortably to addressing each other by given names.

Pharmacist-Physician Relations

In the past, pharmacists have been called upon to protect the physician's reputation as outlined in the 1852 Code of Ethics:

> [I]t is his [the apothecary's] duty, when possible, to accomplish the interview without compromising the reputation of the physician. On the other hand, when apothecaries commit errors involving ill consequences, the physician, knowing the constant liability to error, should feel bound to screen them from undue censure, unless the result of a culpable negligence.[22]

The duty to protect professional reputation was considered to be reciprocal in this version of the Code of Ethics. The 1922 Code of Ethics contains a similar tenet admonishing the pharmacist to protect the reputation of the physician, but the section asking the same discretion and protection from the physician is missing.[23] Although protecting the physician disappeared from the Code after 1922, the obligation of mutual protection continues to exist as an unwritten principle.

Pharmacists and physicians disagree about the status of the pharmacy profession and which functions are most appropriately performed by pharmacists. In a 1983 study, over 60% of pharmacist respondents stated that they were professional equals of physicians compared to 45% of physicians. Both groups in the same study agreed that patients did not regard pharmacists and physicians as professional equals.[24] A 1989 study showed improvement: Ninety percent of pharmacists stated that they were truly health care professionals while only 54% of the physician respondents would grant pharmacists this status.[25] Pharmacists stated that their most important function was advising patients on general health matters (57%) followed by filling prescriptions (46%). Physicians did not see pharmacy function in the same manner and stated that the most important function was filling prescriptions (64%) followed by counseling patients on prescriptions (37%). Physicians stated that advising patients on general health matters was the most important function only 6% of the time. Perhaps physicians are uneasy about pharmacists taking over the physician's role in the area of advising patients.

Expertise and Empowerment

Given this schism between medicine and pharmacy, it is interesting to note that the pharmacy profession is proposing even greater involvement with the patient, which may further threaten the physician's relationship with the patient. The following case study highlights some of these conflicts in decisions regarding life-sustaining treatment.

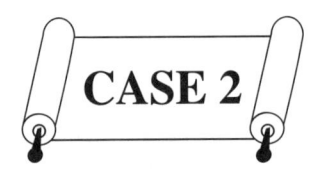

CASE 2

It appeared to everyone on the health care team who was working with C.H. that treatment had shifted from helpful to harmful. All team members, that is, except Dr. H.A., C.H.'s attending physician and oncologist. To team members, Dr. H.A. seemed unaware that C.H. was not responding to the experimental chemotherapy and was, in fact, doing worse. C.H. remained alert and aware of her deteriorating condition. She often spoke of discontinuing treatment with the nurses and other members of the team. Yet, she never mentioned this when Dr. H.A. made rounds.

D.J., a Pharm.D., specialized in nutritional support and had worked with C.H. since one of her earlier admissions over a year ago. Dr. D.J. was responsible for managing the total parenteral nutrition (TPN) that sustained C.H. at this point, as she was too weak and anorectic to take any food by mouth. Dr. D.J. did not feel that she could rightfully say anything about discontinuing the chemotherapy, even though she felt that this was the compassionate thing to do. After all, she reasoned, Dr. H.A. is an oncologist. However, Dr. D.J. was less certain about what her stance should be regarding the TPN. Not only was she the expert on the team regarding TPN, she also knew that nutritional support can be a physiological burden to patients in the end stage of terminal disease by causing fluid overload. Dr. D.J. believed clinically and ethically that the right thing to do was to discontinue the TPN, but how could she convince Dr. H.A.? Dr. D.J. reflected on just what her responsibilities were to C.H. as the pharmacist on the team and how she could best fulfill them.

Case Discussion

This case study outlines the ethical issue of power and authority within the health care system, and it indicates the differing relationships that members of the health care team hold with the patient. "The degree of power one has over another is dependent on the extent of imbalance in the relationship."[26] In the preceding case, C.H. has the least amount of power in relationship to her position in the hospital hierarchy. Dr. D.J. has more power than C.H., but still finds herself in a position of relative helplessness as she cannot necessarily affect the goal she is seeking (i.e., to discontinue the TPN).

Dr. D.J. clearly has expertise in the realm of nutritional support. Yet Dr. D.J. lacks full control over the issue on which she has, perhaps, the most expertise on the team. The legitimate power to make the decision, to sign the order on the record, is held by Dr. H.A. Thus, Dr. D.J.'s power and influence on the health care team is somewhat ambiguous. Of three sources of the power to control others' decisions—expertise, institutional legitimacy, and coercion[27]—Dr. D.J. has the influence of her expertise and the power of coercion available, since the institution does not legitimize her expertise with a parallel level of discretion. She might, although perhaps not ethically, attempt to coerce Dr. H.A. through the complex accumulation of debts and exchanges that grow up among members of health care teams as they work together over the years. Alternatively, she might be able to convince Dr. H.A. with her clinical expertise. If she is unable to use any of the types of power mentioned, she may be unable to do what is best for C.H.

Dr. D.J.'s power in relation to Dr. H.A., thus, becomes a crucial concern, and how Dr. D.J. communicates, perhaps with the assistance of other team members, with Dr. H.A., has considerable potential impact on C.H. There are a number of ways in which the conversation with Dr. H.A., which at its best would be a straightforward mutual analysis of various courses of therapy, could go wrong. For instance, 1) Dr. H.A. might feel inappropriately interrupted by someone of lesser standing in the hierarchy when he is thinking primarily about his communications with other physicians and those above him to whom he must answer; 2) he may fail to engage in the discussion because he does not immediately appreciate the depth of Dr. D.J.'s concern; 3) he may perceive the question or expression of concern as an effort to challenge his position in the hierarchy, which indeed it also may be, or as an expression of a lack of confidence in his expertise, which it also might be; 4) he may estimate Dr. D.J.'s expertise incorrectly because he lacks acquaintance with her skills or misperceives them because of his perceptions of her social background or profession; or 5) he may see the conversation as part of the series of debts and exchanges ("We did it your way last time; let's do it my way this time") between him and Dr. D.J. or the pharmacy department. Culture, class, race, and gender affect all of these possibilities. Insofar as they affect the likelihood of success in improving C.H.'s welfare, they need to be considered by Dr. D.J. in choosing whether to pursue the question and with what nuances of communication and approach. Dr. D.J. thus faces a complex dilemma about the ethics of communication. She can simply regard Dr. H.A. as an obstacle to her patient's welfare, in which case the aim of the conversation is the manipulation of Dr. H.A. on behalf of her patient, an entirely morally respectable role considering that Dr. D.J.'s professional responsibility is to mediate on behalf of C.H.'s welfare. Alternatively, she also can maintain respect for Dr. H.A. as well, and, in her efforts to maintain the quality of professional relationship, perhaps undervalue her responsibility to C.H. Dr. D.J., overly conscious of hierarchical and other social differences, also might undervalue her own standing and expertise, and thus, fail to exercise the full degree of influence open to her. Dr. H.A. is capable of a complementary and parallel set of dilemmas, and the patient C.H. also faces a similar set of considerations as she struggles among the poles of respect for team members, efforts to manipulate them, and the potential to doubt her own judgment.

INSTITUTIONAL FACTORS

Class, culture, race, and gender also may enter into the background structure of the institution in which this conversation takes place. A well-funded institution likely will provide more private spaces for conversation, more personnel and, thus, more time for conversation, and perhaps a broader range of therapeutic options.[28,29] On the other hand, an institution with financial constraints may have imposed protocols controlling the use in total parenteral nutrition (TPN) which may supersede the professional judgment of both Drs. D.J. and H.A. Furthermore, the patient's particular insurance or HMO plan may limit what can be done for her: perhaps TPN or a similar therapy is required for her to have her continuing hospital stay reimbursed.

Behind these multiple potentials stands an important debate in ethics about power and relationships in institutions. Most people seem to accept the hierarchical relations of bureaucracies as natural and inevitable, and indeed, desirable and rational. The question of fairness among cultures or genders becomes, first, one of equal opportunity across social factors to obtain access to the positions of power in organizations; and second, of appropriate regard for individuals working within the hierarchy depending on their expertise and their institutionally defined responsibilities for supervision, delegation, obedience, and discretion. Some ethicists, however, have increasingly attacked the hierarchical construction of health care itself. They believe that the neutrality and beneficence of this form of organization is an illusory ideal. They believe that much greater equality of standing, power, and rewards is called for. They believe, moreover, that since scientific objectivity and neutrality in medicine are illusions, given the diversity of our actual communications and relations among one another, that we should strive for more individualized and face-to-face methods of communicating and making professional judgments.[30] For this latter group of ethicists, the potential impact of social factors require careful attention in deciding ethically how to resolve disagreements among experts.

IDEALISM, VALUES, AND EMPOWERMENT

Our intention here has been to suggest some connections among ethical concerns and the changing demographics of pharmacy and its context. We have focused on the individual pharmacist as a mediator among other health professionals, patients, providers of pharmaceuticals, and scientific understanding of drug effects. We have suggested that complex interactions of ethics and social factors tend to have an effect, and sometimes should have an effect, on pharmacists' moral decision-making. Justice is being served by the increasing cultural and gender diversity of pharmacists; we hope that social conditions in the United States will increase, rather than hinder, the pace of increasing equal opportunity and diversity of health occupations. At the same time, we note the tension involved in maintaining both equality and diversity, since one supports similarities and the other differences. Likewise, professional consensus over goals and ideals should embrace a wider range of visions of pharmacy practice as coalitions grow within the profession expressing diverse culturally based conceptions of pharmacy practice. And again, sameness and difference within the profession will require balance between these polarities. Since the profession's power is essentially a mediating one, the enhancement or diminishment of its power, and more exactly, its contours of influence, will depend to a large degree on the relationship of pharmacists to the other parties in the myriad of negotiations over pharmaceutical use. These groups—patients, physicians, health professionals, businesspeople— are also becoming more diversified, and so pharmacists in their ethical decision-making will need to pay increasing attention to communication styles and diverse expressions of values as they maintain cooperation with others in improving health care.

To conclude, we would like to make some recommendations for expanding the concept of pharmacy practice beyond the traditional limits of personal service, which we believe will help to enhance the authority and reputation of pharmacy practice; and, thereby, assist pharmacists in expressing their ideals of service effectively in their mediation role. Our suggestions are based on two uncertain predictions: we expect that the historical and international sweep of the next 50 years is likely to be distinguished by two major themes: 1) an increasing international dominance of large corporations in the control of human and physical resources through the growth of international trade (pharmaceutical companies being major examples of this dominance),[31] and 2) increasing inequality among rich and poor combined with an overall decline of human health and increasing scarcity of natural materials available for health care (e.g., through diminishment of forests, arable land), and greatly increased population.[32]

As mediators, pharmacists stand at a symbolically important and potentially influential point between increasingly hierarchical control of human relations through expansion of international business practices, and responsible and humane stewardship of substances promoting human health. We, thus, make several suggestions to enhance pharmacy's role and its beneficial impact in the next century.

- Since all health care employees, including pharmacists, are likely to face a diminishment of their influence in the workplace hierarchy, the pharmacy professional organizations should become more active in advocating public policy, business practices, and education regarding the healthy use of pharmaceuticals.

- As the population grows and mass media become even more essential to public education, pharmacy organizations should become more active in educating the public about appropriate use of pharmaceuticals through the media.

- Pharmacy organizations should become more active in defending the environment and promoting equality internationally, since without progress in these areas, burgeoning poverty and public health problems, combined with destruction of the natural resource base for pharmaceuticals, are likely to hinder the ability of pharmacists to be of service.

- Pharmacy organizations should be aggressive in promoting equal access to the profession for all genders, classes, races, cultures and should increase support of primary and secondary public education to distribute the prerequisites of entry into pharmacy education as widely as possible.

- The pharmacy profession should extend its range of concern to include not only the appropriate use of pharmaceutical substances, but also the appropriate avoidance of toxic and harmful substances.

- As mediators, pharmacists should join as individuals and groups with others in public health prevention efforts concerned with toxic wastes, hazardous substances, and environmental pollution.

We think pharmacy's broadening of its agenda, its assertion of humane values, its efforts to humanize the workplace, and its efforts to work with other groups in ameliorating the global problems of the next century will do much to enhance the power, reputation, and standing of pharmacy.

DISCUSSION QUESTIONS

1. What are your ideals of pharmacy practice? What would you like ideally to do as a pharmacist?

2. How comfortable are you working with physicians, nurses, other pharmacists, patients, or people of differing cultures?

3. You are concerned that a patient is receiving a prescription for no valid medical reason. How would you think about responding ethically to this problem?

4. To what extent would you like to act as a health advisor to patients?

5. What is the responsibility of pharmacists to such public health concerns as drug abuse, toxic chemicals in the environment, or public health problems in general?

6. To what extent are your ideals and values the same ones you grew up with? How closely are they linked to your own cultural background?

REFERENCES

1. Silverman M, Lee PR. Pills, Profits, and Politics. Berkeley: University of California Press; 1974.

2. Hepler CD, Strand LM. Opportunities and responsibilities in pharmaceutical care. Am J Pharm Educ. 1989;53(Winter Suppl.):7S–15S.

3. Schondelmeyer SW et al. Pharmacists' compensation and work patterns: overview of 1988 National Survey. Am Pharm. 1989;NS29:697.

4. Shepherd MD, Proctor KA. Women and pharmacy ownership. Am Pharm. 1988;NS28:28–33.

5. Waitzkin H. The Politics of Medical Encounters: How Patients and Doctors Deal with Social Problems. New Haven: Yale University Press; 1991.

6. Benhabib S. Situating the Self: Gender, Community and Postmodernism in Contemporary Ethics. New York: Routledge; 1992.

7. Brown KH. Descriptive and normative ethics: class, context and confidentiality for mothers with HIV. Soc Sci Med. 1993;36(3):195–202.

8. American Association of Colleges of Pharmacy. Profile of Pharmacy Students. Alexandria, VA; 1993.

9. U.S. Department of Health and Human Services, Public Health Service. Seventh Report to the President and Congress on the Status of Health Personnel in the United States. Washington, DC; 1990.

10. ASHP Report on the status of women in hospital pharmacy. Am J Hosp Pharm. 1986;43:1766.

11. Lurvey PL. Career longevity of men and women pharmacists. Pharm Bus. 1991;2:14.

12. Pharmacy Affairs Department. Schering Report X: A Profession in Transition: The Changing Face of Pharmacy. Kenilworth, NJ: Schering Corporation; 1988.

13. Woodward JB et al. Management aspirations and gender differences in pharmacy students. J Pharm Mark Manage. 1993;7(3):3–24.

14. Adams M. The compassion trap. In: Gornick V, Moran BK, eds. Woman in Sexist Society. New York: New American Press; 1971:555–75.

15. Collins PH. Black Feminist Thought: Knowledge, Consciousness, and the Politics of Empowerment. New York: Routledge; 1990.

16. Cohen FL. Postsurgical pain relief: patients' status and nurses' medication choices. Pain. 1980;9:265–74.
17. Pilowsky I, Bond MR. Pain and its management in malignant disease. Elucidation of staff-patient transactions. Psychosom Med. 1969;31(5):400–4.
18. Weissman DE, Dahl JL. Attitudes about cancer pain: a survey of Wisconsin's first-year medical students. J Pain Symptom Manage. 1990;5:345–49.
19. Holdsworth MT, Raisch DW. Perceptions of pharmacy students concerning cancer pain and its treatment. Am J Pharm Educ. 1993;57(Spring):29–34.
20. Tannen D. You Just Don't Understand: Women and Men in Conversation. New York: Ballentine Books; 1990.
21. Buerki RA, Vottero LD. Ethical Responsibility in Pharmacy Practice. Madison: American Institute of the History of Pharmacy; 1994:20.
22. Code of Ethics. J Am Pharm Assoc. 1921;10:900–01.
23. Code of Ethics. J Am Pharm Assoc. 1922;11:728–29.
24. Pharmacy Affairs Department. The Schering Report V: Pharmacists and Physicians: Attitudes and Perceptions of Two Professions. Kenilworth, NJ: Schering Corporation; 1983.
25. Pharmacy Affairs Department. The Schering Report XI: Pharmacists and Physicians: Professional Allies or Professional Adversaries? Kenilworth, NJ: Schering/Key Laboratories; 1989.
26. Erlen JA, Frost B. Nurses' perceptions of powerlessness in influencing ethical decisions. West J Nurs Res. 1991;13(3):397–407.
27. French JP, Raven B. The bases of social power. In: Cartwright D ed. Studies in Social Power. Ann Arbor: University of Michigan Press. 1959:150–67.
28. Duff RS, Hollingshead AB. Sickness and Society. New York: Harper & Row Publishers, Inc.; 1968.
29. Guillemin JH, Holmstrom LL. Mixed Blessings: Intensive Care for Newborns. New York: Oxford University Press; 1986.
30. Harding S. Whose Science? Whose Knowledge? Thinking from Women's Lives. Ithaca: Cornell University Press; 1991.

31. Barnet RJ, Cavanagh J. Global Dreams: Imperial Corporations and the New World Order. New York: Simon & Schuster; 1994.
32. Postel S. Carrying capacity: earth's bottom line. In: Brown LR et al., eds. State of the World 1994: A Worldwatch Institute Report on Progress Toward a Sustainable Society. New York: W. W. Norton & Company; 1994.

Chapter 12

Medicating by Media

Pamela L. Redden
Mary Ellen Waithe

Mass media coverage of pharmaceuticals has expanded from news reports on research in progress, and stories about recently released medications that will benefit large sections of the population, to coverage about undesirable side effects of widely used pharmaceuticals and medical devices. In the 1960s there was protracted mass media coverage of the deformities caused by thalidomide. In the 1970s the media covered reports of adverse consequences to adult women whose mothers had taken DES (diethylstilbestrol) before conception. During the 1980s coverage of the Dalkon Shield class action suit seemed to alternate with coverage of the defects in the Jarvik 7 artificial heart. In every case, the public interest was served by bringing information to the attention of patients and the health care community about risks of adverse side effects that had not been widely known to health professionals or to pharmacists.

In recent years, two very different consequences have been the result of mass media coverage of prescription drugs. First, has been the effect of news reports of increased morbidity and mortality among patients who were prescribed benzodiazepines. As a consequence of this coverage, many authorized prescribers ceased prescribing a variety of benzodiazepines for fear that patients would suffer unwanted side effects (and, perhaps consequently commence litigation against the health professional). Second, has been the effect of both news coverage and mass media advertising to patients and to health professionals promoting the use of a variety of preparations designed to prevent conception or to treat conditions like baldness. Although there has been media attention to the undesirable effects of Prozac as well as to the advertising of Procardia XL,

N.E.E. 1/35 female contraceptive pills, and other preparations, the effects of media exposure on these preparations will not be analyzed because of space limitations. What we wish to accomplish in this chapter, can be achieved by focusing on three preparations: Dalmane (a benzodiazepine), Rogaine (minoxidil), and Norplant (subdermal levonorgestrel implants).

Both organized pharmacy and individual pharmacists have a role to play in the dissemination of accurate, scientifically valid information to patients and to health professionals. We will argue that this role extends substantially beyond that of consulting with inquiring patients who receive, and physicians who prescribe, (or, in the case of the benzodiazepines, cease to prescribe) medications and devices that have been the subject of news reports and advertising. In ways discussed in the following pages, health professionals and patients regularly receive biased information generated by the media. The authors will argue that individual pharmacists sometimes have duties to verify that when health professionals write prescriptions they do so based on scientific knowledge about the efficacy, side effects and contraindications of the prescribed pharmaceutical. We also will argue that organized pharmacy must flex its muscle and require pharmaceutical merchandising and marketing practices to meet standards of pharmaceutical ethics that reflect the moral norms of the pharmacy profession.

ETHICAL ISSUES

Are marketing objectives ethically defensible when they stress maximizing health professional and patient perception of the benefits of a pharmaceutical while minimizing perception of its risks of harms and other costs? To answer this question, we must determine 1) what conditions must be met for a pharmaceutical to be licensed at all, and 2) whether particular methods of marketing pharmaceuticals to health professionals and to patients are ethical.

Licensing Pharmaceuticals

In order for a pharmaceutical preparation (i.e., drug) to be licensed at all, the scientific efficacy of the preparation for the treatment of specific conditions must be demonstrated. The pharmaceutical must be able to achieve the results which it is intended to achieve. It must be demonstrated to behave biochemically in a way that is consistent with the current state of knowledge regarding the expected behavior of the components that constitute the pharmaceutical preparation. If it does not behave in the expected manner, then some scientifically valid, verifiable explanation for its atypical biochemical behavior must be available. Second, there must be adequate animal research, followed by adequate human clinical trials to determine clinical indicators for the preparation, effective and toxic dosage levels (if any), contraindications for use including interactions with other preparations, and adverse reactions. On balance, for the treatment of specific disorders, the pharmaceutical preparation should do more good than harm.

However, the avoidance of harm in itself is insufficient to determine the pharmaceutical's ethical acceptability. It must also be *comparatively* efficacious: the benefit of treatment with the pharmaceutical preparation should equal or exceed the benefit in most cases of alternative treatments (including, but not limited to alternative pharmaceutical treatments) as well as the benefit of no treatment at all. The weighing of benefits and harms should, of course, include a financial cost-benefit analysis. There may be other treatments available which offer greater medical benefit, but only the patient, in consultation with a physician, can determine whether a more expensive, less effective preparation is more desirable than one that may, for example, be less costly and more effective, but that tends to have highly unacceptable side effects.

Public's Right to Know: Role of Journalism in Health Care

Investigative journalism can be credited with generating many positive changes in the delivery of health care. For example, *Life* magazine's photoessays of thalidomide-disfigured toddlers generated global public outrage about the side effects of medications prescribed for women of childbearing years. Investigative journalism adopted for itself the role of "public watchdog" over the side effects of routinely prescribed medications. The careers of well-known journalists were sometimes made when they created public outcry about medical and pharmaceutical practices. For example, Geraldo Rivera was a young, little-known New York City television reporter when his investigation of the conditions at Willowbrook Hospital for the mentally retarded catapulted him to national fame.

On the theory that an informed public can and should hold the health professions and pharmaceutical industries accountable, a "patient's rights" movement developed during the 1960s. The movement spurred a fundamental departure from the public's conception of the traditional doctor-patient relationship. Slowly but surely, major aspects of that relationship changed, generally in the direction of requiring health professionals to fully inform patients of the benefits and risks of medical procedures as well as of medications. Patient insert leaflets soon became standard components of prescribed medications, and informed consent quickly became a precondition to medical treatment of any type. In general, investigative journalism could be credited with providing the impetus to public demand for what are now perceived to be minimal ethical standards for the practice of every health profession.

Unfortunately, two insidious factors are at play regarding the consequences of such well-intentioned investigative journalism. First, there is the public's tendency to believe that what is true of one member of a class of medications, such as benzodiazepines, is true of all members of that class. An untutored public may well draw the unwarranted conclusion that if Halcion is unsafe or ineffective, so are all benzodiazepines. Second, individuals tend to hope that a medication, like Rogaine, reported to be somewhat effective in a minority of cases for which it is prescribed, will be extremely effective in their own case. Everyone hopes to be the exception, everyone hopes for a "miracle." There is a third, and ultimately more dangerous, consequence of journalistic reports. According to a Report of the American Psychiatric Association,[1] many physicians practicing outside of a teaching and research environment have ceased prescribing *all benzodiazepines* presumably in response to mass media reports about triazolam (Halcion), diazepam (Valium), and excessive use of hypnotic sedatives for the elderly. That is to say, mass media reports sometimes took the place of the scientific literature that *should* have governed physicians' decisions whether or not to prescribe other benzodiazepine medications.[1]

Truth in Advertising

Media advertising of the availability of new preparations has generated patient demand for specific, named pharmaceuticals. At the time that this chapter was in preparation, a number of prescription pharmaceuticals were being directly advertised to consumers in print and television media. Among them are Habitrol, ProStep, Nicoderm, Cardizem, Rogaine, and Seldane. The advertisements generally urge patients to consult with their health professional to determine whether a particular pharmaceutical "is right for" them. Often they offer a toll-free number that can be called to obtain additional information about, and possible referrals to, physicians who prescribe that pharmaceutical. The advertisements are usually carefully produced to appeal to prospective consumers who want to be informed about treatment for unnamed medical conditions. The advertisements are careful not to suggest that consumers self-diagnose or self-treat. The advertisements do not mention symptoms, nor do they claim specific efficacy of the preparation for the unnamed medical condition, nor contraindications, nor side effects. Rather, the implication is that the condition has already been diagnosed because the prospective consumer knows full well the nature of the problem (e.g., male-pattern baldness), or that the consumer is already under the care of a health professional for an undisclosed medical condition, but the physician may not have thought about changing the patient's medication to a more effective, less costly formulation.

Consent and Refusal: Informed or Induced?

We will assume for the sake of argument in this chapter that all who are treated with pharmaceutical preparations are rational, competent adults who give consent free of coercion or undue influence. For the sake of argument, we will also assume that advertising, media hype, and sales pitches from pharmaceutical representatives do not vitiate genuine, competent, voluntary consent. The mere fact that there has been mass media exposure given to a pharmaceutical does *not* imply that a physician's decision to prescribe (or to cease prescribing) and a patient's decision to seek a prescription (or to refuse to continue using a medication) are less than freely given. What we wish to explore in this section is whether such consent is *adequately informed*. In order to render appropriate advice to a patient, the health professional must first be adequately informed. Ideally, to be so informed, health professionals rely on two types of information. First, they rely on up-to-date reports of the latest research and treatment experiences of other health care professionals and regulatory agencies regarding the preparation. Second, health professionals also rely on consultation with knowledgeable members of the pharmacy profession. The ideal world, however, is not the real world of medicine. Realistically, health professionals are subjected to a variety of advertising techniques, as well as to media-driven patient demands for particular medications. In addition, they are often held accountable by more informed patients for continuing to prescribe medications that have recently been the subject of headline-grabbing press reports. Understandable constraints on taking time away from treating patients to instead keep up with the professional literature may well mean that authorized prescribers in private practice who are not active in research and teaching are susceptible to bias when it comes to deciding which medications will meet their patients' needs.

In what way may the prescribing physician be biased? It is arguable that physicians generally are less competent than pharmacists in evaluating pharmaceuticals. Physicians in private practice often are more exposed to pharmaceutical sales representatives and to anecdotal reports as well as media hype than they are to the expert pharmaceutical literature. If the American Psychiatric Association Report reveals anything, it reveals that general practitioners and psychiatrists are among those health professionals who often do not go the "extra mile" needed to be well-informed about either positive or negative claims made about pharmaceuticals.

Positive claims are relayed to the health professional by pharmaceutical sales representatives who adopt the role of advocate for the medication and the pharmaceutical house manufacturing it. The sales representative usually is not a pharmacist, but a salesperson with limited technical competence. Though the Food and Drug Administration requires pharmaceutical manufacturers to provide balanced information about medications (i.e., both positive and negative effects), the disadvantage of relying on the sales representative for unbiased information is obvious.

The pharmacist should have the role of providing balanced information to physicians; however, the physician and pharmacist generally have little or no interaction, and when they do interact professionally, usually it is because the physician (or other authorized prescriber) perceives a need to be better informed. Generally, pharmacists do not routinely supervise or monitor physician prescription practices except in rare circumstances (e.g., when the situation warrants an ethics complaint for substandard practice, or when a pharmacist is routinely consulted as a member in a team practice). The health professional who does not perceive the need for a more objective source of information is exposed primarily to the biased positive claims about a pharmaceutical preparation's properties. The health professional who "thinks he understands" all he needs to know about the pharmaceutical preparation, and uncritically accepts information given by the sales representative may well be biased when assessing the appropriateness of a particular medication for a particular patient.

In the ideal physician-patient relationship, the physician has a commanding knowledge of the current state of research regarding each medication that is prescribed. In such a relationship, the physician (or other authorized prescriber) is not only capable of making well-informed recommendations, but actually does make well-informed recommendations to a patient. Conversely, the patient always is free to do two things: succumb to fears created by media coverage of the dangers of a prescribed medication and, consequently, to refuse to use this prescribed medication; or believe the advertising claims made about a medication and request a prescription for the advertised preparation. The physician, however, is *never* morally free to do likewise. The physician always has the moral responsibility to make medication recommendations to the patient consistent with the highest standards of the medical profession. Therefore, the physician, in making every medication recommendation, *is always limited morally by the constraints logically invoked by expert knowledge of the medication* as interpreted in light of, and applied to, each patient's particular case. The constraints are the conclusions logically entailed by reasonable interpretations of relevant scientific knowledge. This important point warrants deeper analysis and explanation.

In formal, mathematical logic, the premises of a formal argument entail the argument's conclusion. In pharmacy, indeed in any science, arguments are complex and their premises are often themselves the consequences of a series of other arguments (e.g., theories about biochemical transformation and interaction). It is not necessary for physicians (or other authorized prescribers) to understand complex theories of pharmacokinetics: it is sufficient for the protection of patients from unethical prescription practices that their physicians defer to the scientific consensus regarding the pharmacokinetic properties of a pharmaceutical preparation when making medication recommendations. Note that we say "consensus." We recognize that science is not static: new data regularly are reported and interpreted in the professional literature. Proof of the suitability of a medication requires only a very low level of proof. It does not require proof "beyond a shadow of a doubt," as required in cases of capital crimes. Such a high level of proof is unrealistic for the science of medicine or of pharmacy. Rather, a lower standard, akin to the "clear and convincing" evidentiary standard, probably satisfies the ethical requirement that physicians prescribe medications within the logical constraints of the science of pharmacy. If there are clear and convincing data reported in rigorously refereed professional journals that a particular medication is efficacious for treatment of specific disorders with patients who fit a particular medical profile (but *not* otherwise), a physician (or other authorized prescriber) is constrained by the science of pharmacy to prescribe that medication in a manner consistent with scientific consensus. When it comes to prescribing pharmaceuticals (or discontinuing the prescription of pharmaceuticals) the authorized prescriber always must make recommendations that are consistent with the current state of knowledge of pharmaceutical science, broadly construed. The prescriber must be knowledgeable of the current cumulative wisdom regarding a preparation's efficacy, long- and short-term side effects, contraindications, therapeutic dosage, toxicity, and the clinical indications for the use of that drug. In addition, the prescriber must be knowledgeable of comparable alternative preparations and must determine *with respect to each patient that the recommendation is an appropriate one.*

In 1990, the American Psychiatric Association (APA) concluded that media reports of excessive prescribing of benzodiazepines and concerns for the safety of benzodiazepines have contributed to a

> ...discrepancy between past research survey data and current clinical impressions regarding estimates of benzodiazepine use and dose escalation. This lack of correspondence is between survey data from the past decade when long half-life [and low therapeutic potency] drugs [such as Dalmane] were most commonly prescribed and current clinical perceptions now that short half-life, more potent benzodiazepines [like Halcion] are widely prescribed.[1]

The Report indicated that in many cases, with patients who present with specific symptoms (e.g., anxiety, insomnia, panic disorders), long-term benzodiazepine use, particularly of long half-life, low-therapeutic potency benzodiazepines (e.g., chlordiazepoxide, diazepam, halazepam, prazepam, clorazepate, flurazepam), is clinically effective in reduction of symptoms.

Although long half-life, low-therapeutic potency benzodiazepines produce patient dependence upon the medication, *they do not cause addiction* (i.e., they do not create the kind of dependence that is marked by the need to escalate the dosage). In identifiable cases, prescription of these benzodiazepines is clinically warranted. Unfortunately, prescribers apparently have generalized to the long half-life, low-therapeutic dosage benzodiazepines what may have been clinically observed (or garnered from the media) about the short half-life, high-therapeutic potency benzodiazepines such as triazolam (Halcion). The clinical psychologist who is not knowledgeable of such basic, crucially relevant information as the distinction between long and short half-life and high and low therapeutic potency of a medication cannot knowledgeably recommend either the use or discontinuance of that medication. It is our judgment that in such a situation, the prescriber cannot competently inform the patient. Therefore, patient consent (or refusal) *fails to be informed*. Because the patient relies primarily upon the authorized prescriber, rather than upon the dispensing pharmacist, to analyze current pharmaceutical knowledge about the prescribed medication, the patient is unaware that the consent he or she has given is uninformed and, therefore, ethically invalid. Unfortunately, in our experience, some dispensing pharmacists, as well as some pharmacists consulting in a medical group practice, have been no better informed than were the physicians whose benzodiazepine prescription practices prompted the American Psychiatric Association study. When we understand how such bias has developed, we can understand why it is morally imperative for the profession of pharmacy to protect its patients' health and moral rights to make informed medication decisions.

MEDICATING BY MEDIA
Regulation of Advertising Media

The Food and Drug Administration (FDA) in the United States regulates all direct marketing to prospective patients of prescription medications. Until recently, the FDA refused to approve advertising of drugs by brand name on television, unless the advertisements included full disclosure of side effects and contraindications. In essence, the pharmaceutical company was required to present in television advertising, all information customarily found on the patient information insert provided with the medication. Since the cost of such advertising is usually prohibitive, direct television marketing of prescription medications has been virtually nil. The FDA has made exceptions to the full disclosure rule for "reminder advertising" (i.e., advertising to announce a new formulation of a pharmaceutical preparation, or pricing information). Reminder advertising may not contain information about conditions the preparation is used to treat, nor about dosage, or contraindications.[2] According to a 1989 article in *Advertising Age*:

> Lexis Pharmaceuticals was the first company to advertise a brand name prescription drug without FDA objection.
>
> Going one step further, Lexis in 1989 tested the same TV spot in the Kansas City area with the addition of a rebate offer. It offered a $40 rebate on the cost of a gynecological examination for women who buy a six-month supply of the Lexis pill.
>
> 'Lexis definitely increased the comfort margin for how prescription drugs can be advertised,' said Bill Purvis, assistant to the director of the FDA's drug advertising and labeling division. 'They're keeping it within the bounds of pricing information and that is acceptable,' he said, 'but what it's done is open the door for companies like Upjohn who are asking how they can do similar advertising for their prescription drugs.'[2]

Cynicism about the FDA's requirements for direct mass media advertising is revealed in a statement made by William McDaniel Jr., the President of Consumer Health Marketing. Consumer Health Marketing specializes in developing media campaigns to promote consumer use of prescription drugs. According to *Advertising Age*, Mr. McDaniel, referring to FDA approval of direct television marketing other than "reminder advertising," said that:

> ...I don't think it's an easing of restrictions...I think it's going to be judged on a case-by-case basis, and the FDA is going to reserve the right to review and reject ads *based on criteria that only they fully understand*.[2]

While the FDA can establish criteria for advertising pharmaceuticals, only the First Amendment regulates media news coverage of prescription medications.

Media and the Marketing of Medications to Health Professionals

In an ideal world, ideal pharmaceuticals (i.e., perfect pharmaceuticals) are preferable to those that are less than 100% reliable and to those that have any undesirable side effects. Failing the ability of the pharmaceutical industry to develop ideal products, it seems best to accept the fact that medications will not always do exactly what we want them to do, and will sometimes create in individual patients undesirable side effects. From the perspective of those who must market non-ideal medications, it would appear to be desirable to promote these medications in such a way as to maximize the authorized prescribers' and patients' reasons for accepting the medication while minimizing their reasons for deciding against its use. In essence, successful pharmaceutical marketing must maximize health professional and patient perception of the product's beneficial effects, and minimize the perception of the product's harmful effects.

Pharmaceutical manufacturers use a wide variety of advertising techniques. First, direct advertising in prestigious journals confers on newly approved pharmaceutical preparations an aura of respectability (and may well affect editorial staff decisions regarding the publication of scientific reports critical of that preparation). Second, sales representatives are employed by the pharmaceutical manufacturer to provide health professionals with information packets that are intended to favorably influence the prescription decisions. Third, much indirect advertising in the form of note pads, pens, calendars, and other office supplies are given to subliminally influence favorably a prescriber's decisions. Fourth, supplies of free samples of drugs are routinely distributed to health professionals, hospitals and clinics. Fifth, food, beverages, and speakers are donated to assist health care institutions in their educational programs or these costs are reimbursed by pharmaceutical manufacturers.

Benzodiazepines: Scaring Health Professionals

Media reports of several different events led to a scare among health professionals regarding the use of benzodiazepines (e.g., chlordiazepoxide, halazepam, prazepam, clorazepate, diazepam, flurazepam, triazolam, temazepam, alprazolam). In one particular instance, a patient, after much trial and error, and after considerable medical and psychological evaluations, was able to regulate her sleep cycle only when treated with flurazepam (Dalmane). The flurazepam facilitated the patient's ability to own and operate a small business. Without regulation of her sleep cycle, the patient, who had chronic insomnia secondary to chronic anxiety, was unable to hold a job or to engage in other activities for which regular sleep is a prerequisite. When the patient relocated her business, it was necessary to change health care providers. Her new physician refused to continue prescribing flurazepam. When the patient requested a joint consultation with a pharmacist and her physician, both health professionals insisted that the patient was a "drug addict" and that they allegedly would be held responsible if the patient committed suicide by overdose. The physician and pharmacist, citing their own professional expertise, refused to consider any professional literature regarding the safety, effectiveness, and low abuse potential of that benzodiazepine.

The scientific literature on flurazepam from 1980 through 1992 encompasses more than 400 articles. Of particular interest is the literature on the safety and effectiveness of flurazepam, and its low potential for abuse. Two anecdotal cases of suicide associated with flurazepam use were described in the literature during this time period. In one case[3] the patient ingested household bleach which, together with the flurazepam, produced hypernatremia and death. In the second case, an elderly woman, initially thought to have suffered a cardiovascular accident, was discovered at autopsy to have taken an overdose of flurazepam.[4] Attribution of cause of death to flurazepam on the basis of serum samples extracted from the pulmonary arteries or veins (which are the usual sites for post-mortem blood testing) has been questioned because flurazepam concentration is highest in solid organs and pulmonary vessels secondary to post-mortem redistribution of this drug into these sites.[5]

In recent decades, prescriptions for benzodiazepines have substantively replaced those for barbiturates because benzodiazepines:

- are more effective for relief of anxiety and stress;
- have fewer and less severe side effects;
- are less likely than barbiturates to produce toxic and lethal overdose;
- tend not to interact with other medications; and
- produce fewer and less severe withdrawal symptoms than barbiturates.

Tolerance to benzodiazepines can develop with doses that are less than therapeutic; and dependence can develop with therapeutic doses without the development of further tolerance. *Benzodiazepines, therefore, have a very low potential for abuse.* According to the Report of the American Psychiatric Association, the abuse of benzodiazepines is rare and appears to be limited to patients who have histories of alcohol or other substance abuse. Due to the strong inverse relationship between drug half-life in serum and the severity of withdrawal symptoms, benzodiazepines should only be used long term in patients who present with anxiety serious enough to create substantial discomfort or disability. Therefore, the long-term prescription of benzodiazepines is appropriate when other therapies have been ineffective for the treatment of chronic anxiety, and is especially appropriate for patients with chronic insomnia secondary to chronic anxiety which impairs normal social function. When anxiety is chronic and produces profound sleep disorders that prevent patients from undertaking usual activities (e.g., maintaining employment), therapeutic doses of benzodiazepines are indicated, especially when psychotherapy had failed to relieve chronic anxiety. Benzodiazepines should, of course, be used cautiously in patients who have a history of drug or alcohol abuse because these patients also are likely to abuse benzodiazepines.

Popularizing Triazolam (Halcion)

Triazolam (Halcion) was tested in the early 1970s in clinical trials involving more than 9000 patients (primarily prison inmates). In 1977 triazolam was approved in Belgium and the Netherlands for use in doses up to 1 mg. Two years later, reports of amnesia, hallucinations, paranoia, depression, and aggression in patients who received triazolam resulted in a 6-month suspension of sales of this drug within the Netherlands while the scientific data on triazolam was evaluated. Early in 1980, triazolam sales were reinstituted in the Netherlands, albeit at a maximum dose of 0.25 mg. In 1982, the U.S. Food and Drug Administration approved triazolam for use at a maximum dose that was twice that which was permitted in the Netherlands (i.e., 0.5 mg).

Triazolam was preferred by patients to the alternative sedative-hypnotics, temazepam (Restoril) and flurazepam (Dalmane), then both widely prescribed. Unlike its competitors, triazolam (Halcion) tended not to cause morning-after sedation. It was, therefore, perceived by the public and physicians alike to be safer: patients could safely operate machinery, drive cars, and resume normal activities the next morning without pharmaceutically induced "hangover" or impairment. Within five years after Halcion appeared on the U.S. market, its manufacturer, Upjohn, reduced its recommended dosage to 0.25 mg in response to reports of adverse side-effects (e.g., aggression, episodic amnesia, hallucinations).

Diazepam (Valium), Gender, and Sex

In 1979, following constituent demands for a federal investigation of diazepam-dependence alleged by many women who had been taking the preparation for several years, the U.S. Senate Subcommittee on Health and Scientific Research under the chairmanship of Senator Edward M. Kennedy convened hearings on the safety of diazepam. Those hearings were followed by "…a flood of testimonials in the media about adverse reactions and dependence, and congressional inquiries to various agencies."[6]

One investigator noted that the British General Dental Council guidelines required that sedative administration in dental practice be witnessed.[7] Failure to do so resulted in later accusations and a lawsuit for sexual assault.[8] Allegations against a dentist were made by seven women who claimed to have been victims of sexual assault while under treatment by the dentist. The complainants had been prescribed and administered diazepam preparatory to dental procedures. Experts testified that benzodiazepines in general, and diazepam in particular, sometimes cause the experience of erotic sexual fantasies, particularly in women patients.[9]

Institutional Abuse of Benzodiazepines

Accounts in the popular press about the use of benzodiazepines as a behavior control mechanism in nursing homes made reference to anecdotal reports of falls in geriatric patients for whom benzodiazepines were prescribed. Subsequently, the (U.S.) National Institutes of Health Development Conference on the Treatment of Sleep Disorders of Older People recommended against the use of hypnotics for treatment of insomnia in the elderly because hypnotics have the potential to be habit-forming and too high a dose tends to be prescribed for the elderly.[10] Still other studies compared the use of neuroleptics, benzodiazepines, and non-benzodiazepine sedative-hypnotics on nursing home geriatric patients' levels of agitation and other adverse side effects.[11,12] Investigation of the risk of accidental injuries (primarily due to falls) revealed that accidental injuries increased during months in which benzodiazepines were prescribed for treatment of insomnia in nursing home populations.[11]

Overprescription of Diazepam (Valium)

The National Institute of Drug Abuse (NIDA) review of benzodiazepines concluded that significant additional study was needed for a fuller understanding of the pharmacokinetics of benzodiazepines, in particular, mapping of receptor locations, the identification of endogenous ligands, the production of benzodiazepine antibodies and the relationship between benzodiazepine receptor occupancy in the brain to the reinforcing effects of specific benzodiazepines. Of greater political interest perhaps were the NIDA's findings that:

1. Excessive doses of benzodiazepines over prolonged periods are needed to produce physical dependence upon benzodiazepines in persons with unstable personalities.
2. Dependence upon benzodiazepines is less than for alternative sedatives and hypnotics.
3. Risk of dependence can be minimized by discontinuing the pharmacotherapy as soon as the underlying cause that produces the need for the therapy can be eliminated.
4. Most importantly, risk factor of dependence and the dangers to society are of such a low order that no extension of control on the prescription of benzodiazepines is needed.[6]

Despite the conclusions of NIDA, the public perception of the widespread abuse of diazepam led New York State to require in 1989 that prescriptions for all benzodiazepines be written on triplicate special forms to enable the state to monitor patient *and* practitioner abuse of the substance. The result was a reported drastic drop in the number of prescriptions for benzodiazepines[11] accompanied by a substantial increase in prescribing of medications that were viewed by the profession to be far more hazardous.[13] According to *Medical World News*[14] physicians who did not wish to risk the possibility that they would be called upon to explain their prescription practices simply substituted more toxic, less effective preparations such as meprobamate (for which there was a 125% increase in New York while nationally there was a decrease of 9%) and chloral hydrate (for which there was a 136% increase in New York while nationally there was a decrease of 0.4%).

The British Ban on Triazolam (Halcion)

In May 1988, Great Britain's Committee on the Safety of Medicines ordered a review of triazolam (Halcion), and in the fall of 1991, banned triazolam from the market in the United Kingdom. The ban was controversial, especially in light of many letters by British physicians to the medical journal *Lancet* attesting to the efficacy and safety of triazolam. Although the British government had been investigating the safety of triazolam, it was not until information about systematic errors and falsifications in Upjohn's original clinical trials came to light during a much-publicized murder trial in the United States (a discussion of this case appears later in this chapter) that the government had the data it needed legally to justify a ban. The reason for the ban was that Upjohn had falsified its application to market the preparation in the U.K.[15]

To summarize: from 1989 to 1991 separate, but highly negative factors contributed to physicians' reluctance to prescribe benzodiazepines:

- the abuse of diazepam, its reported contribution to sexual fantasies in females;
- the New York State triplicate script requirement;
- the causal linking of triazolam to a violent murder;
- the British Government's ban on triazolam;
- reports of nursing home abuse of benzodiazepines as a nocturnal patient control method in an at-risk population; and
- the NIH study on contraindications of benzodiazepine use in the elderly.

These highly publicized events undoubtedly heightened physicians' concerns regarding benzodiazepine safety and perhaps regarding their own potential liability for malpractice. The conclusion that benzodiazepines were not routinely to be prescribed was a legitimate conclusion for practitioners to draw from the popular media reports on the scientific information then available. But the mass media did not report on *all* of the relevant scientific information. In particular, it ignored the task force Report of the American Psychiatric Association. Whether the conclusions that practitioners drew from the mass media reports warranted what became a general unwillingness among health professionals to prescribe any benzodiazepines for *any* patient, is not clear. What is clear from that Report, however, is that during the late 1980s large numbers of health professionals, without making any distinctions among very different drugs of the class benzodiazepine, refused to continue prescribing other benzodiazepines even where continued prescription was warranted.

Marketing Contraceptive Implants to Health Professionals

Levonorgestrel implants (Norplant), used for many years in other countries, has been approved by the FDA in the United States. Norplant consists of five fan-like tubes impregnated with progestin that when implanted subdermally release the hormone in measured amounts over a five-year period.[16] By preventing ovulation and by changing the character of the female endometrium 50% of the time, as well as by altering the consistency of cervical mucous to prevent sperm entry, levonorgestrel reliably prevents pregnancy despite a high rate of menstrual irregularities (e.g., vaginal spotting, amenorrhea). Low-dose levonorgestrel subdermal implants have been marketed to health professionals in traditional and now-familiar ways. There have been full and multi-page advertisements in medical journals and feature articles in journals such as *Medical World News*[17] and *American Health*.[18] Journals that specialize in reproductive technologies, such as *Family Planning Perspectives*, have run feature articles on the results of clinical trials of Norplant.[19]

There has been the usual provision of office supplies to health professionals and clinics: notepads, pens and other articles bearing the "Norplant" name. Patient information booklets also have been created for distribution to women seeking family planning and contraceptive services at specialized clinics. Interestingly, although birth control products are generally marketed to primary care physicians in private practice, Norplant marketing seems to be directed to particular clinics. This strategy, when combined with the generally accepted idea that Norplant is suitable for those least likely to use oral contraceptives or spermicides correctly, raises the question whether Norplant is selectively advertised to a specific audience via health professionals who are themselves selectively targeted. Patient demand for Norplant also has contributed to health professional interest in the preparation and the device through which it is administered. Medicaid totally covered the cost of Norplant in the District of Columbia and in all 50 states, making it widely accessible and desirable to poor women. In addition, there has been indirect marketing to health professionals through news coverage of punitive uses of Norplant as a condition for probation of a woman convicted of child abuse.[20]

Marketing Minoxidil to Health Professionals

Minoxidil, long used to treat hypertension as an oral agent, was coincidentally noted to cause excessive facial and body hair growth. Subsequent studies designed to determine whether a topical application of minoxidil could intentionally produce hair growth on denuded scalp secondary to male pattern baldness, were positive.[21] Topical minoxidil (i.e., Rogaine) acts by normalizing hair follicles in the area of alopecia. Of note are the American Medical Association's conclusions that the most severe baldness and baldness of more than five years' duration are not responsive to treatment, and that patient satisfaction with the degree of hair regrowth approximated only 30% in most trials.

Marketing followed the proven route of combining large space advertising in respectable medical journals, especially in conjunction with publication of scientific reports in those journals. This was supplemented with the usual advertising by sales representatives (e.g., personal visits, free office supplies). The promotion of Rogaine, a product of limited efficacy, but designed for a cosmetic purpose (i.e., baldness) proved challenging for the industry. Two novel approaches appeared to be particularly useful in marketing Rogaine to health professionals. One was the emphasis on the product's safety and absence of side effects excepting local allergic reactions. Second was the use of gender-specific advertising aimed at establishing to health professionals that hair loss, although male pattern in type and largely hereditary, was a distinctly unnatural condition that required pharmacologic intervention. Additionally, the Rogaine campaign has subtly introduced the idea that any health professional capable of diagnosing male pattern baldness can now offer treatment. This was a distinct change that might provide both ego satisfaction and financial reward to health professionals because previously only specially trained physicians could administer definitive treatment for baldness. What may have been unique is the use by Upjohn of a referral list of physicians who treat male-pattern baldness. Since minoxidil is the only nonsurgical treatment available for that condition, it would be expected that only those surgeons who specialize in performing "hair implants" would be named on the list. That is not the case. Listed physicians include internists and general practitioners.

PATIENTS AND MEDIA APPEALS

In this section we will explore two types of media coverage that appeal to the public to take action regarding a prescription medication. First, we will explore the role of investigative journalism. Next, we will examine the nature of media advertising primarily in print and television. Depending on the pharmaceutical preparation, investigative journalism and media advertising have played different roles in informing the public about benzodiazepines, subdermal levonorgestrel contraceptive implants, and minoxidil.

Benzodiazepines: Scaring the Public

In 1988 a middle-aged woman with no prior history of assault murdered her 83-year-old mother. The expert testimony of court-appointed psychiatrists was to the effect that the deceased woman's daughter, 57-year-old Ilo Grundberg, was involuntarily intoxicated by triazolam (Halcion) and had acted involuntarily in killing her mother. As soon as the criminal proceedings against her were dropped, Ms. Grundberg filed a multimillion dollar civil suit for negligence against Upjohn. The litigants reached an out of court settlement for an undisclosed amount one day before the trial.[22] Thereafter, the side effects of triazolam were widely disseminated in the popular press noting that patients experienced memory loss, anxiety and hallucinations.[22,23] A substantial portion of the popular press coverage on triazolam focused on the then-recent British government ban on the sale of this drug. Upjohn, the pharmaceutical manufacturer of triazolam, had provided incomplete and unverifiable data in its 1972 application to market this drug in the United Kingdom. The information came to light as a result of the publication of the allegations against Upjohn by Ilo Grundberg.[15] Before the British ban on the sale of triazolam, the *New York Times Magazine* in February 1989 cited reports of deaths and injuries caused by falls attributed to benzodiazepine use by geriatric patients.[24]

Norplant: Marketing Low Dose Levonorgestrel Subdermal Implants

In the late 1980s news about the anticipated approval by the FDA of subdermal contraceptives began to appear in magazines, including those with a predominantly female readership. When low-dose levonorgestrel subdermal implants received FDA approval, news coverage of its release further stirred patient interest. In December 1990, both *Time*[25] and *Newsweek*[26] published articles on the Food and Drug Administration's approval of a "highly effective, totally reversible" birth control device that "could last up to five years." Women's magazines including *Ms.*[27] and *Self*[28] published articles with titles such as "Birth Control Goes Skin Deep," and sidebars on birth control updates in their "women's health" sections. In the first year of Norplant's manufacture, Wyeth-Ayerst Laboratories reported a backlog of thousands of orders of the implant.[29] The demand for Norplant was phenomenal, and mass media as well as word of mouth contributed to that demand. According to the *New York Times* in 1992, 500,000 women used Norplant—*a fivefold increase over the previous year*.[30] Planned Parenthood clinics nationwide began distributing Norplant as soon as it became available. One school district even announced plans to make the implantable contraceptive available to female students through clinics based in public schools.[29] During the first two years of its availability, 13 state legislatures considered statutes proposing mandatory use of Norplant by women who received government welfare benefits because of its potential economic benefit in decreasing the number of pregnancies among women who qualified for public assistance.[29]

Marketing Minoxidil

Rogaine (minoxidil) is the subject of what can only be described as a media blitz. The pharmaceutical manufacturer of Rogaine (i.e., Upjohn) advertised on television, with FDA approval, that Rogaine is intended to treat male-pattern baldness. One of the first television commercials opened with a head-and-shoulders view of a handsome, calm, reassured white male who appeared to be in his late thirties to early forties and who sported what can only be described as a "Kennedyesque" head of hair. This hirsute male calmly addressed viewers concerned about hair loss. Unquestionably, the unspoken message was that "men who suffer from male-pattern baldness can regain a full head of thick, healthy hair." (The original name chosen by Upjohn was "Regain," a name that the FDA objected to.) The advertisement provided no information about costs or usage, but listed a toll-free telephone number through which viewers could order a free videotape that further explained the product. That video came with a $10 coupon good toward the purchase of the preparation once a prescription has been obtained. To assist the prospective patient in locating a physician who might write such a prescription, the cover letter accompanying the videotape and coupon listed the name of half-a-dozen physicians in the caller's postal zip code. After responding to questions that constituted a "demographic survey" the caller was informed that the physicians on this list had been randomly selected from among those physicians who ordinarily treat male-pattern baldness.

In late 1993, a new, essentially similar commercial promised to send the viewer a certificate to cover the cost of the physician appointment; thereby, eliminating all financial cost to the prospective patient of seeking a prescription from a physician and commencing treatment. Around that same time, a similar television commercial appeared, but *directed at women concerned with their own hair loss*. While neither of these actions vitiate informed consent or violate a patient's right to exercise choice, they are, at the very minimum, unvirtuous for different reasons. After one physician visit and one month's trial use of Rogaine, the male patient will be unable to determine Rogaine's efficacy in his own case because it typically takes several months and a return visit for a follicle count to determine whether there has been any new growth. Female patients, even those who suffer from male-pattern baldness, may well react differently than males, but there have been no published clinical trials with female subjects; and, therefore, there is no reason to believe that they will experience comparable results.

EXPLORING A RANGE OF RESPONSES TO THE ISSUES

In this section we will explore several perspectives on responses by pharmacists to the issue whether patients have given informed consent to the prescription of Rogaine or Norplant. We shall also explore the question regarding what should a pharmacist do when a health professional discontinues prescribing a benzodiazepine. The perspectives from which we will explore these questions include several different models of the pharmacist's role. We will investigate in turn, the concepts that the pharmacist is the servant of the pharmaceutical company, that the pharmacist is the servant of the physician, and that the pharmacist is a patient advisor and/or advocate. Before turning to those perspectives, however, we should explain what is meant by "servant." Then we will explore the role of organized pharmacy in giving voice to each of these perspectives.

The Private Servant Analogy

A private servant is one who does the bidding of the person served: usually either the employer or the designee of the employer. The role and responsibilities of the servant are clear: to do what is asked within a given scope of agreed-upon duties. So if a housekeeper is asked to mop the kitchen floor both he and his employer reasonably can expect that he will do so. If a housekeeper is asked to pick up groceries, that task is likewise reasonably expected by him and by his employer to be performed because it is within the scope of the traditional duties of someone holding that position. Duties become increasingly less clear the further the assigned task departs from the scope of duties agreed upon by employer and employee. Likewise, the duty (e.g., of a secretary to fetch the employer's coffee) becomes increasingly less expected as social consensus about the nature of the position diverges from custom and tradition. Therefore, when the housekeeper is told to mow the lawn or to clear brush, neither he nor his employer can reasonably expect compliance because that task is not within the traditional scope of the servant's duties. The housekeeper or the secretary may acquiesce and complete the task as requested, however, it seems clear that he need not do so. Other accounts of the nature of a "servant" are possible of course, however, this account seems to capture contemporary American consensus about that role. Simply put, there are legitimate expectations one may have of a servant, and there are those tasks that the servant may agree to perform, but need not.

There is a second, normative source of constraint on the expectations that an employer may legitimately have of a servant. For example, the housekeeper may be expected to screen phone calls, but to disclose information about an overheard phone conversation would be unethical because custom and social norms make it clear that housekeepers have duties to preserve their employers' confidences and to respect their privacy. By accepting an offer of employment, an employee acquires certain moral duties towards the employer. Those duties are *prima facie* duties, rather than absolute duties. That is, there are situations when moral obligations are overridden by other, more compelling moral duties. For example, if the housekeeper is asked to "do away with" one of the children, or to cover up or participate in any other criminal activity, the moral duty to respect the employer's privacy and to treat the phone conversation as confidential is "trumped" by a higher moral duty, for example, the duty to obey just laws against killing. Therefore, if the overheard telephone conversation was material to the employer's plans to murder his offspring, the housekeeper would clearly have a duty to violate the principle of confidentiality and inform the authorities in order to protect innocent parties from harm. Both the defined scope of duties and the criminal and moral law pose constraints on servants' duties.

It is also a matter of broad social consensus that good servants possess certain "virtues." In many cases, the "good" servant will attempt to protect the employer from the employer's own vices. For example, the "good servant" might inform "Sir" that "perhaps he has had a few too many" and it might be time to call it an evening. Likewise, the "good" servant will sometimes be the messenger of apologies to those whom the employer has offended. That is to say, the virtuous servant helps the employer to avoid or to atone for the exercise of vice and to engage in virtuous actions.

Pharmacist as Servant of Pharmaceutical Companies

When a licensed professional pharmacist is employed by a pharmaceutical company to participate in the design, research, and development of pharmaceuticals, it would appear that the pharmacist has many primary duties to the employing company. For example, the pharmacist has a duty to accurately report results of research to the employer, to engage in those research projects assigned by or initiated by the employer, to preserve as confidential "trade secrets" related to research and development of medications, as well as other obligations. But when the employer requests or makes it clear that it expects a pharmacist to falsify data, or to publish clinical trials results that are not supported by the data, the pharmacist, even on the "private servant" model, has clear ethical duties to refuse. Depending upon what occurs subsequently, the pharmacist may have a duty to report the request to the authorities. The criminal and civil law, as well as the moral law, require noncompliance; and in cases where the employer cannot be persuaded to report findings of pharmacy research accurately, those laws may require the pharmacist to step outside the employment relationship and "blow the whistle" to the authorities. The virtuous pharmacist/servant will first attempt to convince the employer that the requested behavior is morally wrong, and will provide opportunities to "do the right thing" by submitting for publication only those conclusions that are logically entailed by an application of the relevant theories of pharmacy science to good data. The virtuous pharmacist/servant will remind the employer of the disastrous consequences to the company's public image as well as to its "bottom line" when lawsuits were brought by those who, in the past, were harmed by its preparations.

When the professional pharmacist is employed in or (as is becoming less common) owns a dispensing pharmacy, there is a *prima facie* duty not to misrepresent to health professionals or to patients opinions about a manufacturer of pharmaceuticals. For example, it would, on the face of it, be unethical for the pharmacist to say to a patient or to a prescribing health professional something along the following lines: "If I were you, I wouldn't use/prescribe a medication made by UpJohn. After all, if they misrepresented Halcion's safety, they might be misrepresenting the safety of this preparation." Such an attempt to cause another to draw broad generalizations about a manufacturer's entire line of products based on knowledge of unethical practice regarding one of its preparations would inject unnecessary bias into the decision-making process engaged in by the health professional and the patient because it represents *as a fact* what is, at best, a suspicion for which the pharmacist lacks sufficient evidence.

Pharmacist as Servant of Physicians

If we extend the analogy of "pharmacist as servant" to the relationship between pharmacists and physicians, we see that the pharmacist is likewise required to fill a prescription as written by the physician. But there is a disanalogy between pharmacist and servant: the pharmacist is the physician's peer in a related profession, while the housekeeper or secretary usually is not the peer of the employer. Pharmacist and physician both are licensed professionals, with publicly recognized comparable expertise in related areas of health care. The pharmacist has the duty to consult with and advise the physician. The physician has the duty to practice medicine within the constraints imposed by medical science and also the science of pharmacy. The function of the pharmacist in the physician-pharmacist relationship is to provide expertise *in an area in which the physician has the responsibility to exercise expertise but often lacks the knowledge and training to do so*. And it is the fact of this significant disanalogy between the "private servant" and the pharmacist that is the source of the pharmacist's moral duty to intervene when, in the pharmacist's professional judgment, physician-authorized pharmacotherapy poses risks to the patient or to public health.

The Pharmacist as Public Servant

The "private servant" model of the pharmacist as servant of the pharmaceutical company, the physician, or the patient lacks one important feature that characterizes professional pharmacists. Professional pharmacists also are "public servants" in that the concept of professional that is implicit in the accreditation and licensure of schools of pharmacy and of individual pharmacists respectively, entails that the practice of the profession be in the public interest. That interest is a broad one, and it is one that professional pharmacy traditionally has served well. When it became clear that generic versions of pharmaceuticals once manufactured only by brand name would make what would otherwise be expensive medications available to less affluent segments of the population, organized professional pharmacy lobbied for and received authorization to dispense generics. Pharmacy practice that is in the public interest ranges from serving the public's need for development of "orphan" pharmaceutical therapies to serving the public's interest in being knowledgeable consumers of pharmaceuticals. Indeed, many of the chapters in this book focus on particular public interests that pharmacy serves. Insofar as pharmacists' practice of their professions threaten a public interest, those practices become morally suspect and require moral justification. For example, the use of radioactive substances in chemotherapy poses grave risks to the health of patients, health care providers and, when contamination occurs, the public. When the practice of pharmacy poses a threat to the public interest, the pharmacist is morally obligated to take steps to safeguard that interest.

In particular, pharmacists should remain knowledgeable, not only of the professional literature regarding the safety and efficacy of medications they dispense, but also of the media coverage of pharmaceuticals. The bulk of this paper is devoted to a description of the various roles that mass media advertising and investigative journalism play in increasing public understanding and misunderstanding about widely-prescribed medications. Pharmacists who are aware of potentially misleading claims made in patient "information" booklets, as well as in advertising and news coverage of pharmaceuticals, are in a unique position to ascertain the extent to which their patients have been inappropriately influenced by information garnered from those sources. Likewise, they are in a unique position to provide the patient with readily understandable, unbiased, accurate information that will render the patient's consent truly informed. In this way, individual pharmacists can serve the public's interest in becoming knowledgeable consumers of pharmaceuticals. It seems clear that the vehicle of organized professional pharmacy is one through which individual pharmacists can act in unison in ways that demonstrably serve the public's interest in health. In the example given earlier where the pharmacist tried to dissuade a patient from accepting prescribed medications originating from a manufacturer who had concealed harmful side effects of a different medication, the pharmacist's comments may undermine public confidence in the pharmaceutical industry. As a public servant, the pharmacist is morally required to act in ways that neither compromises the health of individual patients, nor of the public, nor undermines confidence in the health professional, the medical community, the profession of pharmacy or pharmaceutical manufacturers.

Pharmacist as Patient Advisor/Advocate

If the role of the pharmacist is viewed as that of patient advisor, then clearly the pharmacist has duties to assure that the patient's consent to pharmacotherapy is informed. At a minimum, this means that the pharmacist should have reason to believe that the patient understands the nature and purpose of the medication, the method of its administration and its dosage, as well as contraindications to its use. Since it is not an uncommon practice for family members to pick up prescribed medications, direct contact with the patient is often impossible. Similarly, since it is not an uncommon practice for patients to have different prescriptions filled at different pharmacies, it is likely that the pharmacist will not have direct access to information about other medications that the patient may be using but which cannot be taken concurrently with the most recently prescribed medication. Likewise, it is not uncommon for patients to see more than one health professional, and the primary care physician may not always be aware of what the gynecology nurse-practitioner and clinical psychologist might have prescribed. In such circumstances, the role played by patient information inserts that accompany prescribed medications is extremely valuable. With many prescribed medications, the pharmacist might need to document that the patient did not disclose to the pharmacist that she was concurrently using any medications for which the dispensed medication was contraindicated.

The situation is somewhat different, however, if the pharmacist perceives herself to have the role of patient advocate. The nursing literature is replete with numerous articles describing that profession's adoption of the role of patient advocate, and students of pharmacy who perceive their profession developing a similar role would be well advised to review that literature. In this section we will limit our discussion to a brief synopsis of the role of patient advocate. Were the concept of the nurse as patient advocate to be adopted by the pharmacy profession, dispensing and hospital pharmacists (as well as other pharmacists with direct patient contact) would view themselves as physicians' peers and equals and would take the position that as professional pharmacists it is their responsibility to monitor pharmaceutical aspects of patient care and to intervene with other caregivers, including physicians, in certain circumstances. Those circumstances would include, at least, the following:

- when a pharmacist has reason to be concerned that the patient has not given informed consent to the medication;
- when the pharmacist's knowledge of pharmaceutical science reasonably supports a conclusion that the physician is uninformed of (or inappropriately weighs) the risks that *commencing or discontinuing* a particular medication or class of medication poses to the patient's health;
- when pharmacotherapies inappropriate for the treatment of the patient's condition are ordered by the physician; and
- when the prescribed medication is contraindicated for concurrent use with another medication.

The form that the pharmacist's intervention should take would vary with the circumstances. If the pharmacist is concerned that the patient has not given informed consent to the medication, an appropriate level of informing may be all that is required before dispensing the medication. However, if the consent is not "informed consent" because the patient has been misinformed by the health professional, it would appear to be within the scope of duties of the pharmacist to determine the nature of the misinformation. Is the authorized prescriber misinformed about the medication and for that reason misinformed the patient? If so, then there is room for the pharmacist to provide the physician with information sufficient to make knowledgeable treatment recommendations to the patient. If the authorized prescriber is well informed and has deliberately misled the patient, the pharmacist would appear to have a positive duty to delay dispensing the medication until the patient has been properly informed. Similarly, if the physician is simply not up to date on important developments regarding pharmacotherapy, and the risks to a patient's health may be greater or different than the physician may have supposed, it appears that the pharmacist would again have a duty to delay dispensing the preparation until the physician has had an opportunity to weigh the now-known risks to the patient. The pharmacist would have a moral obligation to draw to the authorized prescriber's attention a summary of the relevant new scientific developments. Conversely, when, as in the case of the benzodiazepines and other preparations, there is a risk of harm to the patient of suddenly discontinuing the medication, the pharmacist has a duty to so inform both the physician and patient of the likely consequences of abrupt discontinuation. This is a particularly difficult duty to fulfill unless both patient and physician have been informed of the dangers at the time that the prescription is filled. Monitoring abrupt discontinuance of a medication can be fraught with potentially insurmountable difficulties. There may be many reasons why a patient has not requested a refill of a prescription medication. The patient may have moved or may have filled the prescription at another pharmacy. Tracking patients who fail to present for a refill of a medication that should not abruptly be discontinued would certainly strain the personnel and financial resources of most dispensing pharmacies. For this reason, pharmacists should take care at the outset to confirm that both the patient and authorized prescriber are well informed of the risks of suddenly discontinuing certain medications.

In another situation, when pharmacotherapy inappropriate to treatment of the patient's condition has been ordered, the pharmacist must first verify that she is knowledgeable of the diagnosis. Pharmacists often are unaware of the diagnosis of the underlying condition for which therapy is ordered. In such a case, the pharmacist needs to consult with the physician and confirm the patient's report of the diagnosis. In most outpatient situations, the pharmacist will have no knowledge of the diagnosis and should not as a matter of course confirm each diagnosis with the physician. In some situations, and with certain kinds of pharmaceutical preparations, it may be desirable for the pharmacist to verify the condition with the nursing or medical staff. Pharmacists are sometimes, but not always, in a position to verify that a patient is not presently taking medication that will render a newly prescribed medication ineffective (or be rendered ineffective by it). Similarly, pharmacists are not always in a position to know what other medications the patient might be using that would be toxic when combined with a newly prescribed preparation. However, many pharmacists use automated patient record keeping systems that do enable the pharmacist to track patient use of multiple prescribed medications. Indeed, the pharmacist is often the only health care professional who is in a position to know that the psychiatrist, gynecologist, and internist have prescribed mutually inefficacious substances or substances that are toxic when taken in combination. Clearly, because there are potentially fatal consequences to the patient, whenever possible, the pharmacist should make every effort to determine what medications are being simultaneously used by a patient, and, if necessary, contact all prescribing health professionals with the goal of reaching mutually compatible medication decisions.

Organized Professional Pharmacy: The Voice of Ethics?

Organized pharmacy can support the efforts of individual pharmacists and serve the public interest in having access to safe, effective pharmacotherapies. It is through professional associations of pharmacists that codes of professional responsibility for pharmacists can address some of the issues we have addressed here. It is organized, professional pharmacists who jointly can insist that when health professionals prescribe medications, they do so based on adequate knowledge of developments in the science of pharmacy. It is organized, professional pharmacists who can support action by individual pharmacists who suspect that a health professional's reasons for prescribing or for discontinuing the prescription of a preparation may be founded on nonscientific grounds. Professional pharmacy organizations can affirm that it is the appropriate professional role of the pharmacist to confirm with the authorized prescriber, and sometimes with the patient, that the prescription decision is a well-founded one to which the patient has given informed consent. It is organized, professional pharmacy that can achieve outcomes of patient understanding that are as much in the patient interest as was obtaining the authority to dispense generics. It is organized, professional pharmacy that can insist that investigative journalism temper sensationalist and erroneous generalizations about classes of medications with accurate information that is presented in a way that the public can understand. It is organized professional pharmacy that can act in the public interest to thwart medicating by media.

Discussion Questions

1. A medication is widely reported in the popular press to cause kidney failure in an unacceptable number of patients but remains on the market with FDA approval. When the pharmacist is presented with a prescription for that medication, does the patient have a right to know about the press report? If so, by whom should the information be given?

2. A new, heavily advertised over-the-counter preparation receives heavy consumer demand in your pharmacy. Its usefulness is variable and it is costly. It is available by prescription at a concentration that although costly, is generally efficacious. A customer picks up the over-the-counter preparation and asks you, the pharmacist, "whether this stuff works or not." How should you reply?

3. Representatives of Cure-all Pharmaceuticals have recently begun to track the number of specific product prescriptions written by physicians to whom they have made specific "product pitches." These physicians practice in the Medical Arts Building where you are employed as a pharmacist. What ethical issues might be raised for you in this context? How should you resolve those issues?

4. Are there any situations where pharmacists are absolved of responsibility when they follow a physician's orders to omit the patient advisory information that accompanies a preparation?

5. What advertising constraints, if any, should be placed on the pharmaceutical industry? Explain how those constraints, or the lack of constraints would serve the public interest.

6. A patient for whom Halcion has been prescribed recalls a news report in which then-President George Bush vomited on the Prime Minister of Japan during a state dinner. The President's physician had stated that because of that incident the President was no longer prescribed triazolam (Halcion). The patient states that as the spokesperson for a large corporation, she cannot risk a similar incident. She asks you whether she should discontinue triazolam or switch to another medication. She asks if you could recommend an alternative.

7. A patient for whom you have filled scripts for fluoxetine (Prozac) asks numerous questions about the risk of psychotic episodes. He heard that several people committed murders while taking it. He wants you to reassure him that it will not make him violent. What should you say?

(Continued)

Discussion Questions continued

8. A young mother of two is picking up a prescription for Ventolin suspension for her six-year-old who has had repeated respiratory infections and has been hospitalized twice for pneumonia. Her younger child has chronic bronchitis. The mother has tried unsuccessfully to give up cigarettes. The family has difficulty making ends meet and do not qualify for public assistance. She asks about the success of various nicotine "patches" stating that she is sure her pediatrician will prescribe it because he has warned her that her smoking harms her children. How should you respond?

REFERENCES

1. Benzodiazepine Dependence, Toxicity, and Abuse: A Task Force Report of the American Psychiatric Association. Washington, D.C.: American Psychiatric Association; 1990:1, 12–13, 55.

2. Nicorette, Rogaine seek TV OK. Advert Age. 1989;60(51):31.

3. Ward MJ, Routledge PA. Hypernatraemia and hyperchloraemic acidosis after bleach ingestion. Hum Toxicol. 1988;7(1):37–8.

4. Svenson J. Obtundation in the elderly patient: presentation of a drug overdose. Am J Emerg Med. 1987;5(6):524–26.

5. Pounder DJ, Jones GR. Post-mortem drug redistribution—a toxicological nightmare. Forensic Sci Int. 1990;45(3):253–63.

6. Szara S, Ludford J, eds. Benzodiazepines: a review of research results. 1980 NIDA Res Monogr 33. Rockville, MD: Department of Health and Human Services National Institute on Drug Abuse; 1981.

7. Brahams D. Benzodiazepine sedation and allegations of sexual assault. Lancet. 1989;333(8650):1339.

8. Brahams D. Medicine and the law: benzodiazepines and sexual fantasies. Lancet. 1990;335(8682):157.

9. Brahams D. Medicine and the law: benzodiazepine sex fantasies—acquittal of dentist. Lancet. 1990;335(8686):403–4.

10. The treatment of sleep disorders of older people. NIH Consensus Statement. 1990;8(3):1–22.

11. Coccaro E et al. Pharmacologic treatment of noncognitive behavioral disturbances in elderly demented patients. Am J Psychiatry. 1990;147(12):1640–645.

12. Trimble M, ed. Benzodiazepines Divided: A Multidisciplinary Review. New York: John Wiley & Sons; 1982.

13. Weintraub M et al. Consequences of the 1989 New York state triplicate benzodiazepine prescription regulations. JAMA. 1991;266(17):2392–397.

14. Bankhead CD. Triplicates shift N.Y. scripting. Med World News. 1991;32(5):24–6.

15. Webb J. Sleeping pill ban puzzles doctors. New Scientist. 1991;132(1790):13.

16. Burkman RT. Modern trends in contraception. Obstet Gynecol Clin North Am. 1990;17(4):759.
17. Higgins LC. Users give four-star nod to a five-year implant. Med World News. 1990;31(11):24.
18. Podolsky DM. The five-year contraceptive. Am Health. 1989;8(7):16.
19. Turner R. Hormonal implants prove to be highly acceptable, although nearly all users experience side effects. Fam Plann Perspect. 1990;22(5):234–35.
20. New York Times. 1991 Jan 10:A20.
21. Olson et al. Topical minoxidil in early male pattern baldness. J Am Acad Dermatol. 1985;13:185–92.
22. Cowley G, Springen K. Sweet dreams or nightmare? Newsweek. 1991;118(9):44–51.
23. Cowley G. Hard times for Halcion. Newsweek. 1991;118(16):61.
24. Dobkin BH. Sleeping pills. New York Times Magazine. 1989 Feb 5:39–40.
25. Purvis A. A pill that gets under the skin. Time. 1990;136(27):66.
26. Cowley G. A birth-control breakthrough. Newsweek. 1990;116(26):68.
27. Carr D. Birth control goes skin deep. Ms. 1989;18(1-2):77.
28. Weinhouse B. Birth-control update. Self. 1990;12(9):88.
29. New York Times wire service. Dispute arises over poor using Norplant. Cleveland, Ohio: The Plain Dealer; 1992 Dec 19:E-1, 6.
30. New York Times wire service. Contraceptive use: facts and figures. Cleveland, Ohio: The Plain Dealer; 1992 Dec 19:E-6.

ACKNOWLEDGMENTS

Thanks to Ronald Mortus RPH, MBA, Director of Pharmacy, Meridia Huron Hospital, East Cleveland, Ohio for his wisdom. Terence Isakov, MD and Basil Waldbaum, Pharm.D., MD, Mayfield Heights, Ohio provided good examples of media influence on professional judgment. Jennifer Heyl, M.A. assisted with research and Cindy Kunsman, Cindy Bellinger, Doris Mathews, and Geneane Ford assisted with preparation of the manuscript.

Chapter 13

Drug Research with Human Subjects

Eric D. Kodish
Bruce D. White

Pharmacists are a vital link, with legal and moral standing, in the drug delivery chain and the American health care system. Pharmacists are independent practitioners who must exercise *independent judgment*; independent judgment that includes independent *ethical judgment*.[1] As independent practitioners, pharmacists must consider whether ethical principles are being violated when patients are participating in drug research activities.

One might ask: *What ethical dilemmas might pharmacists confront when involved in human drug research activities?* Enlightened practitioners would have no difficulty with an appropriate response to this question because they understand that pharmacists are "commonly faced with patient-specific and system-wide decisions concerning the use of specific products within a category, or in advising prescribers about the use of one category of drugs versus another" and that these decisions are influenced by ethical factors that are open to interpretation.[2] Following are just a few obvious examples:[3]

- Is the subject *freely consenting* to participate in the research study? Would it matter that the patient is dying of a "terminal illness" with no alternative therapy available?
- Is the subject truly *informed* about the risks, benefits, and adverse effects of participating in the research protocol? Would it matter that the drug has been used only in animal studies previously?

- Should investigators tell subjects about how the research study is *being financed?* Would it matter that the project is funded entirely by a pharmaceutical manufacturer interested in marketing a new product?
- Is the study *designed* properly? Would it matter that the literature fails to support the hypothesis?

Although these cases may not be problematic for pharmacists who have had the opportunity to explore options and contemplate solutions, there are other more subtle ethical dilemmas. Consider the following.

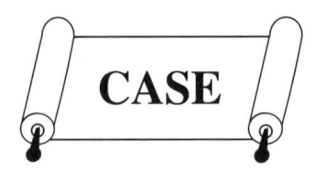

CASE

A pharmacy resident had her research protocol approved by the facility's institutional review board (IRB) for the protection of human subjects. The study is designed to evaluate the clearance of vancomycin in patients with renal failure who are being dialyzed twice weekly. In order to evaluate vancomycin levels properly, trough serum drug concentrations have to be monitored and blood samples taken daily until the next dose is due. The resident has had some difficulty in recruiting patients because few of the center's dialysis patients receive vancomycin.

When rounding in the dialysis unit one morning, the resident identifies a potential subject just before the next scheduled dose of vancomycin is to be given. However, the patient is stuporous and lacks the capacity to give an informed consent. The patient's next of kin and representative is his wife who is not present, but is en route to the hospital. However, the patient's son is present.

Case Discussion

In this case, the resident faces at least two immediate ethical dilemmas or questions:

- Is it ethically permissible to withhold the vancomycin dose for some limited time (e.g., one hour or so) in order to obtain consent from the patient's representative to include the patient in the study group?

- Who may give consent for the patient? Since the wife is not readily available, is it ethically permissible to ask the son to give consent to include the patient in the study group?

There may be "pressures" (e.g., those listed below) to obtain immediate consent from the son if the patient is to be included as a research candidate:

- The dose of vancomycin probably should not be withheld too long after the time it is due in order to maintain the serum concentration of the drug within its therapeutic range.
- It may be important to seek consent from every possible subject since the number of potential candidates is small.
- The resident may have little remaining time to complete the project within the residency period.
- The project may be of significance to other patients who must receive vancomycin—it is possible that the appropriate dose could be reduced in other similar patients; the study might provide very beneficial information.

However, countervailing arguments may be more important:

- Is the son a proper surrogate since the wife is in transit? Would the son really be the appropriate person to voice the patient's preferences?
- Should one even consider withholding the dose for any period of time—might that be too great a risk for the patient?

These are very practical concerns and issues that must be addressed and balanced by the pharmacy resident responsible for the research project. Similar questions must be asked with each research project.

If there is to be adequate and appropriate research, by implication, there also must be research *subjects*. And therein lies the rub because researchers and society must proactively encourage and permit human experimentation, an activity inherently dangerous to the few individuals who are the initial subjects of a research protocol. Thus, scientists and authorities must attempt to strike a legal and moral balance between the needs and rights of individuals (as a dying AIDS patient with often only a slight chance that a drug might work against the illness) and the needs and rights of the community to be safe from the dangers of untried and ineffective products and the experimentation to research these drugs.[4] As one might imagine, it has been difficult to develop a responsible system that meets everyone's needs without any inconvenience or difficulty. One must expect though that even with the most stringent of standards, "mistakes" or errors of judgment or errors of scientific calculation will likely occur somewhere in the process.[5]

Drug products are prescribed to benefit patients; yet practitioners know that all drugs have untoward effects that might harm the patient too. With every prescription order, physicians and pharmacists must try to balance two ethical principles: beneficence ("trying to do good") with nonmaleficence ("trying not to cause harm"). From the beginning, physicians are taught to practice *primum non nocere* "first, do no harm." Similarly, drug research requires that physicians and pharmacists balance the same two principles for equivalent reasons.[6] The pharmacist, and the physician, must weigh the risks against the benefits of drug use and pharmaceutical research. It often is not a matter of knowing which choice is "right" and "wrong," but often which is the best of two poor choices.[7]

Historical Framework

Efforts to regulate foods and drugs in the United States began, for all practical purposes, with the Pure Food & Drug Act of 1906. The impetus for passage of this law came with the publication of Upton Sinclair's *The Jungle*. This book exposed then current abuses in the food processing industry; Americans were so shocked that they demanded action in the form of this new regulatory statute. Enforcement rested with the Department of Agriculture's Bureau of Chemistry and its renowned chief, Dr. Harvey W. Wiley. However, by the 1920s, little change was noticeable in food and drug marketing practices. So long as the manufacturer and distributor did not "falsely misrepresent" the product (that is, out-and-out lie about ingredient components), most drugs could be sold without restriction.

As might be expected, the worst happened. In 1937, the Massengill Company, in an attempt to market a liquid form of sulfanilamide (the first of the sulfa antibiotics), found that the drug would dissolve in diethylene glycol and that the resulting solution had a reasonable appearance and taste. "Elixir Sulfanilamide" was not tested for toxicity; unfortunately, it was lethal! Over a hundred people, many of them children, for whom the product was originally developed, died a painful death from taking the antifreeze-laden preparation. The Food and Drug Administration (FDA), the successor agency to Dr. Wiley's Bureau, moved quickly to seize most of the product, but under the 1906 law could only act because the product was technically "mislabeled" (an *elixir* is a product with an *alcohol* base, not a glycol base). This incident led to enactment of the Food, Drug, & Cosmetic Act (FD&CA) in 1938 and the banning of harmful substances from interstate commerce; the new law allowed establishment of a new-drug approval "process." New drugs, to be marketed thereafter, had to be at least tested and proven "safe" (in animal and then limited human trials) before they could be sold to consumers.

Soon after World War II, a technological revolution occurred in the pharmaceutical industry. Within twenty years, the number of marketed drug products increased two-hundred-fold! Congress became concerned about the nature—or rather, the lack—of competition in the market for new, patented drugs. But, there was little interest in modifying current marketing practices, until the "thalidomide story" broke in 1962. Apparently an FDA examiner, Dr. Frances Kelsey, on her own initiative, and without overt evidence of danger, held up approval of the William S. Merrell Company's new drug application (NDA) to market thalidomide (a mild sedative) in the United States. Remarkably, this product proved to be the cause of an outbreak of phocomelia, grossly underdeveloped limbs in newborns, in Europe. With this near-miss, Congress was able to amend the FD&CA to require that claims of effectiveness in an NDA thereafter had to be supported by "substantial evidence." With this amended law, the need for research in American pharmaceutical manufacturing practice became firmly established.[8]

But then, mere product safety and effectiveness is no guarantee that the product will be used safely and effectively by practitioners. One only has to recall the abuses that were tolerated in the name of clinical research before the days of institutional review board (IRB) regulation. The classical description of these abuses appears in a 1966 *New England Journal of Medicine* article by Harvard anesthesiologist Henry K. Beecher.[9] Thus, "research" extends to individual daily use at the bedside; physicians and pharmacists must constantly reassess benefits to patients in light of current dangers.

THE STRUCTURE OF DRUG RESEARCH IN THE UNITED STATES

The regulatory system for the development of new drugs in this country is primarily intended to protect individuals from the potential for harm. Because of the history recounted above, the greatest danger in drug development has been the loss of life or serious morbidity resulting from the unregulated use of new agents. With the goal of preventing untoward toxicity as the major and explicit focus of the regulatory bureaucracy, the introduction of new and potentially important medications has been relatively restricted.

The system is now divided into four major phases of research. Phase I trials are defined as the first time a new agent is used in a human subject. These studies generally are evaluations of the toxicity and pharmacology of a new agent, and efficacy is not a scientific endpoint of the study. Phase I trials usually are performed with a small number of subjects, and drug doses gradually are escalated during the trial. Data are reported on how well a therapy is tolerated, questions of dosing, pharmacokinetic information, and what the observed side effects have been. The effectiveness of a drug for treating a particular condition may be reported, but these data are not the primary reason for the Phase I study. Phase I trials may raise several important ethical issues. These include the possibility of sacrificing the few for the good of others (the many), vulnerability of human subjects, and the potential need for special safeguards when doing research on patients who have end-stage conditions. Other issues that arise include the quality of informed consent, questions about patient/subject motivation, the nature of altruism, and the potential for coercion in these kind of studies.

Phase II trials are performed on medications that have been shown to be safe and well tolerated in Phase I. These trials address the question of efficacy of a particular drug for a particular condition in a fairly small cohort of patients. Patients/subjects are given the same dose, and response to the treatment is measured. The response data often are compared to historical control data to determine the relative value of the Phase II drug compared with more conventional standard treatment. The ethical issues raised by Phase II research involve the question of how to decide which patients one may enroll in this sort of trial, and what the potential advantages and disadvantages of "standard" treatment compared to the experimental treatment may be. Again, morally valid informed consent is of paramount importance in Phase II research.

Phase III research protocols are large-scale studies that often, but not always, use a randomized study design. These trials build on Phase I and II data by testing a drug determined to be safe in a Phase I study and potentially effective on a smaller scale in a Phase II study. Phase III trials can be viewed as the final hurdle to approval of the drug by the FDA. Ethical issues unique to Phase III trials relate to questions about the necessity of continuing a trial until a particular statistical end point is reached, and how a decision on the early stopping of a Phase III trial comes about. A host of other important ethical issues in Phase III research are discussed below in the section on randomized clinical trials.

Finally, Phase IV research involves the post-marketing study of a new drug. This research is intended to detect problems with safety or efficacy which were not observed during Phases I through III, and to follow up on any inconclusive data which may have raised questions in the previous phases. Phase IV research, unlike the earlier phases, often is performed in the community hospital or in private practice, rather than the academic medical center. This may raise ethical questions about physician reimbursement for the enrollment of patients in these studies, and any potential conflict of interest which may exist.

The structure presently employed in this country has come under criticism by advocates of speedier approval of new drugs, especially for those agents that may have potential utility in the treatment of acquired immunodeficiency syndrome (AIDS). This powerful political pressure has prompted the FDA to open a "fast-track" for drug approval, which attempts to expedite the process for therapy of lethal conditions. This change in the current policy represents an effort to balance the needs of the public for protection from unsafe drugs with the needs of patients for better and quicker access to new therapies.

Institutional review boards (IRBs) are local committees mandated by the federal government to evaluate research proposals on both ethical and scientific grounds. All hospitals and medical centers where human subject research is performed are required to establish IRBs, and no research may be performed without IRB approval. Pharmacists should be actively involved in the IRB process. They can bring to the committee a unique and crucial knowledge base that physicians, ethicists, researchers, and nurses may not possess, and can make an important contribution to the process of research evaluation and approval. Further information about the responsibilities and functions of IRBs is found later in this chapter.

CODES AND STANDARDS FOR DRUG RESEARCH WITH HUMAN SUBJECTS

Pharmacists should be familiar with some of the professional codes and standards dealing with human experimentation that have evolved in Western culture. The FD&CA and IRB regulations are but an extension of these standards that are recognized worldwide to protect humans involved in experimental research protocols. Like the FD&CA, one might say that the standards exist because of tragedies.

The Nuremberg Code (1949)[10]

Uncontrolled and unrestricted limits to human experimentation have led to abuses; witness the Nazi atrocities, which some called "experiments to benefit mankind." Nazi physicians used utilitarian arguments to support their experimentation on condemned individuals "so that some good might come from their deaths." With the conviction of these physicians for "crimes against humanity" came the first international declaration of rights for persons who are the subject of human experimentation—the Nuremberg Code. Among the rights enumerated are:

- The voluntary consent of the human subject is absolutely essential.
- The experiment should be of such use to yield fruitful results for the good of society, unprocurable by other methods or means of study, and not random and unnecessary in nature.
- The experiment should be so conducted as to avoid all unnecessary physical and mental suffering and injury.
- The experiment should be conducted only by scientifically qualified persons. The highest degree of skill and care of those who conduct or engage in the experiment should be required through all stages of the experiment.
- During the course of the experiment the human subject should be at liberty to bring the experiment to an end if he has reached the physical or mental state where continuation of the experiment seems to him to be impossible.
- During the course of the experiment, the scientist in charge must be prepared to terminate the experiment at any stage if he has probable cause to believe, in the exercise of good faith, superior skill, and careful judgment required of him, that a continuation of the experiment is likely to result in injury, disability, or death to the experimental subject.

The World Health Organization (WHO) Declaration of Helsinki (with Recommendations Guiding Medical Doctors in Biomedical Research Involving Human Subjects) (1964; revised 1975, 1983, 1989)

The principles of the Nuremberg Code were extended by the WHO with the Helsinki Declaration emphasizing that "[t]he health of the patient will be the [physician's] first consideration;" and reiterating that "[a]ny act or advice which could weaken physical or mental resistance of a human being may be used only in his interest." The Declaration includes statements of basic principles as well as guidelines for offering medical research combined with professional care (the real thrust of the Beecher's article) and for nontherapeutic biomedical research involving human subjects.

National Commission For the Protection of Human Subjects of Biomedical and Behavioral Research (established 1974) and the Belmont Report (1978)[11]

The *Belmont Report* recommended that IRBs (as discussed below) be established as the local institutional authority to "regulate" human experimentation and research activities; the present research system and structure thus grew from the National Commission recommendations. The *Report* also described in detail the underlying ethical principles that allow research: respect for persons (autonomy), beneficence, and justice.

President's Commission For the Study of Ethical Problems in Medicine and Biomedical and Behavioral Research: Protecting Human Subjects (1981)[12] and Implementing Human Research Regulations (1982)[13]

Even with the Nuremberg Code and the Declaration of Helsinki, problems in human research still exist in the world and in the United States.

The President's Commission noted many of these difficulties in 1982. (These documents are the latest governmental attempt to identify and suggest remedies for the primary concerns that surface in human research.) However, in the United States, the largely-voluntary system of institutional self-regulation through IRBs has worked reasonably well with relatively few governmental measures to ensure oversight and regulatory compliance.[14]

Department of Health and Human Services (HHS)[15] and FDA Regulations Governing Human Experimentation

IRBs are institutional (e.g., university medical center, hospital, clinic, or HMO) committees formally designated by the facility to review and approve biomedical research protocols and applications involving human subjects.[16]

IRBs are to assure that:

- Risks to subjects are minimized (e.g., procedures are consistent with sound research design, subjects are not unnecessarily exposed to risks, and trial procedures are not used over standard procedures without reason).
- Risks are reasonable in relation to anticipated benefits.
- Subject selection is fair.
- The research plan makes adequate provision for monitoring data to ensure safety to subjects.
- Subject privacy is protected.
- Vulnerable populations are safeguarded.

Compliance is voluntary with the institution, but

> no individual may receive department [i.e., U.S. Department of Health and Human Services] support for research covered by these regulations unless the individual is affiliated with or sponsored by an institution which assumes responsibility for the research under the assurance satisfying the requirements of this part [of the Code of Federal Regulations covering IRBs].[15]

If research protocols routinely involve drug (including clinical trials) research, it might be prudent for IRBs to have a pharmacist as member.

INFORMED CONSENT

Informed consent is a relatively new concept in the history of medicine, but may be the most important safeguard against the abuse of human subjects in biomedical research. Pharmacists must understand informed consent to understand the ethical issues in drug research. The obligation of the physician and/or investigator to obtain informed consent reflects the primary commitment to respect for autonomy in both medical care and the conduct of clinical research. However, in practice, informed consent has been criticized as being too easy to undermine, and simple clinical observation suggests that there can be tremendous variability in the quality of informed consent.

For legal purposes, informed consent is represented by a document explaining the risks and benefits of a research study which is signed by the subject. By contrast, morally valid informed consent requires a conversation rather than a signed piece of paper. While the signed consent form may suffice for adequate documentation, real dialogue with the potential subject is the key to ethically important consent. This distinction is described by Faden and Beauchamp as "two distinct senses" of informed consent:[17] the former a *policy* function, and the latter an *autonomous action*. In contrast to the mere fulfillment of institutional requirements, the latter sense of informed consent actually can serve to empower patients and subjects to play a meaningful role in important decisions.

It is important to recognize that the history of informed consent is relatively recent: before this century, the phrase did not exist,[18] and the very existence of the concept was questionable.[19] Only with the shift in emphasis from a medical model based on beneficence to one of autonomy did the concept of informed consent gain prominence. Modern ideas of informed consent are derived from two independent realms of legal thinking: medical malpractice and product liability.[20] The concept was first applied to human research subjects after Nazi doctors performed grotesquely abusive experiments on human subjects during World War II.[21] Unfortunately, the exploitation of research subjects was not limited to Nazi Germany, and some outrageous human subject research was performed in the United States. These include the Tuskegee Study, where hundreds of African-American men were left untreated despite the advent of effective therapy for syphilis,[22] and the Willowbrook Studies, where mentally retarded children were deliberately infected with viral hepatitis.[23] More recent disclosures of post-World War II radiation experiments sponsored by the United States government have stirred further controversy, and led to the creation of a Federal advisory panel to investigate these studies.[24]

Although the most significant ethical function of informed consent has been to safeguard against research abuse, the informed consent doctrine has evolved to become a requirement for the "standard practice of medicine." Where verbal informed consent should suffice, written consent is now obtained for procedures as routine as childhood immunization.

In their standard textbook of medical ethics,[25] Beauchamp and Childress cite four elements required to make consent morally valid. The first is truly a prerequisite: competence. The other three elements cannot be fulfilled without the presence of a competent decision maker. Compared with other definitions of competence, the threshold for medical decision-making capacity is relatively low. That is, individuals who might be considered legally or psychologically incompetent may still be morally competent to participate in medical decisions for themselves. Competence literally means "the ability to perform a task," and the task at hand in this context is to understand the options, and make a free and voluntary choice. Our discussion of vulnerable populations below will focus, in some cases, on individuals who are incompetent. If, however, the requirement for medical decision-making competence is fulfilled, there remain three important elements of informed consent.

The first of these elements is *disclosure*. Initiated by the health care professional, disclosure requires that the patient be given an explanation of a proposed treatment, and an appraisal of the risks and benefits involved. In practice, pharmacists play a major role in this element of informed consent by providing patients with important information on the side effects of medications prescribed by physicians. Because it would be both terrifying and impossible to disclose every possible risk of every medical treatment, balance is very important in a reasonable disclosure. Side effects that are frequent, and those that are very serious, even if not frequent, should be discussed with a patient when obtaining consent. But the question of the extent and limits of disclosure in informed consent can be perplexing.

Faden and Beauchamp address the question of standards for disclosure by elaborating on three distinctive standards found in legal and moral theory of informed consent:[26] 1) The professional practice standard suggests that the nature of disclosure be determined by the general practices of a particular professional group. This standard could apply to pharmacists as well as physicians or other professionals. 2) The reasonable person standard of disclosure dictates that information that is "materially relevant" to an objective reasonable person must be disclosed. The major limitation of this standard is the hypothetical construction of what a reasonable person would find relevant. 3) The subjective standard is both the most demanding and the morally superior disclosure standard. This guideline for disclosure calls for attention to the specific information desired by, and relevant to, the particular subject with whom informed consent is being discussed. Only the subjective standard for disclosure truly fulfills the duty of respect for autonomy which underlies the concept of informed consent.

The second important element of informed consent is *understanding*. Simple disclosure is not sufficient because an individual patient may not comprehend everything he or she is told. The health care professional who is discussing a proposed therapy or procedure must make an effort to ensure that the patient has at least a basic understanding of the relevant issues. This can be accomplished most easily by assessment of the questions a patient may ask if given the opportunity, or by simply asking the patient to repeat the risks and benefits so that one can be sure that he or she understands. In addition to fostering the patient's comprehension, this part of consent encourages dialogue, a key feature of informed consent. Disclosure at the level of the subjective standard discussed above will facilitate understanding on the part of the subject.

The third component of consent is a freedom to act without compulsion. This element serves to prevent coercion. Patients may be vulnerable to pressure from nurses, physicians, spouses, children, or other family members. While persuasion clearly has a role in many health care decisions, a choice to undertake a particular therapy ultimately must be made by the particular individual on a voluntary basis if that individual is competent. Undue manipulation by well-meaning friends, family, or professionals can undermine the autonomy of a patient or subject. Health care workers should try to persuade their patients to make what they feel are good decisions, but they must not go beyond persuasion to coercion.

An important distinction between consent for medical treatment and consent for participation in research must be noted. Specifically, the standard of disclosure is more exhaustive for subjects asked to participate in drug research compared to patients receiving drug therapy. Clearly, for a subject to participate in a research project he or she generally should have received disclosure of the nature of the study, understand the fundamental issues, consent voluntarily, and be competent to do so. This requirement must be even more stringent for research subjects than for patients receiving medical care. In drug research trials, the goal of obtaining further scientific knowledge may conflict with the goal of helping the research subject, and the scientific investigator may not serve as an advocate for the interests of the research subject to the same extent that the physician is committed to the well-being of his or her patient.

PRIVACY AND CONFIDENTIALITY

Medical patients, and by extension research subjects, are entitled to the protection of their privacy and confidentiality. These two concepts are related but not identical. When a patient enters into a therapeutic relationship with a physician, the duty to protect the privacy of the patient becomes the obligation to respect confidentiality in the context of that particular relationship. While privacy is a general right of individuals in our society, confidentiality describes a professional's relationship with a particular patient. For example, a pharmacist may not disclose the medication profile of a patient to an interested newspaper reporter. Doing so would violate the privacy right of the patient and the pharmacist's confidential relationship with that patient. The expectation of privacy and confidentiality is nearly absolute. Only morally compelling arguments that outweigh this obligation can justify the violation of this trust.

The same principle generally should apply to research subjects. Participants in research may wish to remain anonymous, even if results of a study are to be published in the medical literature. Investigators must ensure that this obligation is fulfilled, and if information that may jeopardize the subject's anonymity is to be published, the investigator must obtain full consent from the subject.

In addition to the moral requirement for confidentiality and privacy, some research designs rely on these principles as the scientific basis of a study. These methodologies include blinded studies: single blinded studies, where the subject does not know which arm of a treatment he or she is assigned to, and double blinded studies, where neither subject nor investigator is aware of assignment. These designs may have great methodologic merit in their ability to reduce or eliminate bias in the collection of data. They do, however, have potential practical and ethical problems. Pharmacists sometimes may be the only individuals who are aware of treatment assignment in blinded studies, so they must have a good understanding of both the research design and their role in these studies.

PLACEBO CONTROLLED TRIALS

Controlled clinical trials refer to the study of any diagnostic or therapeutic intervention in which the study design requires that one group be compared with another. The importance of controlled clinical trials in the advancement of medical science cannot be overstated. The ethical conduct of such trials can, however, raise important questions which any overview of research ethics must address. The next sections of this chapter will focus on two particular mechanisms for "controlling" clinical trials: placebos and randomized studies. These designs can be used independent of one another or in conjunction in the same study design, but they should not be confused, because they represent two distinct concepts.

Placebos are agents without pharmacologic effect that nonetheless may have clinical effect arising from a patient's or physician's expectation of therapeutic benefit. While placebos in clinical practice clearly violate a physician's obligation to be honest with his or her patients, in clinical research the issue is more complex. Placebo controlled trials can be an effective way to evaluate the efficacy and toxicity of a new therapy. Problems of honesty, which can make the use of placebos in clinical practice clearly unethical, may be more subtle in the conduct of a placebo controlled clinical trial.

Placebo controlled trials are an especially important issue for pharmacists because of the central role a pharmacist must play in the design and execution of such a study. Pharmacists must be responsible for the actual preparation of both active drug and placebo, making certain that there will be no perceivable difference between the two. In doing so, the pharmacist ensures that nurses, physicians, and subjects remain completely unaware of treatment assignment. Often, the pharmacist will be the only individual who knows or has access to treatment assignment before the code is broken and analysis can proceed. This serious responsibility for pharmacists demands that they have a full understanding of the ethical implications of this study design.

From a moral perspective, the use of placebos might be justified if 1) there is no reasonable standard therapy with which to compare the new therapy, and 2) subjects are completely informed of the trial design so they understand that there is some probability they are receiving placebo rather than the study drug. Even with these requirements, placebo controlled trials deserve careful scrutiny before they are actually employed.[27]

RANDOMIZED CLINICAL TRIALS

Randomized clinical trials (RCTs) have come to be synonymous with controlled clinical trials. It must be pointed out that these are not identical terms. In fact, randomized trials are only one type of controlled trial. RCTs are defined as any research design that randomly assigns interventions to those entered in the study in order to produce cohorts that are comparable.

The need to evaluate clinical data in a scientifically rigorous manner can conflict with important values such as patient autonomy and physician beneficence. This conflict should not be framed as a tension between good science and good ethics, because there is clear moral import to the production of clinical research which ultimately improves health care for patients. Good science is itself of important moral worth. The questions really become: 1) whether alternative study designs will produce data of similar reliability, and 2) if not, is some sacrifice in quality of data acceptable in order to maintain the confidence of the patient/subjects and the clinicians who enroll them on research protocols?

The doctrine presently taught at most medical schools and on the wards of teaching hospitals is that no clinical research provides reliable data unless it is derived from an RCT. This statement is clearly not true. Other methods to control data, including crossover trials, historical controls, and other innovative study designs, can provide reliable data. In crossover study designs, more than one intervention is applied to subjects on each arm of a study at different times, so that subjects are guaranteed access to all possibly beneficial treatments over the time of the study. Historical controls use data published in the literature on a similar patient group to compare the efficacy and toxicity of a new intervention. These and other alternative study designs are well described elsewhere.[28]

Ethical problems with RCTs have been discussed in the medical literature for years. The problems of RCTs are well established by Hellman and Hellman in a paper entitled "Of Mice but not Men."[29] The arguments against RCTs relate to interference with patient autonomy and interference with physician's judgment. Both of these concerns stem from the fear that the requirements of good research will take precedence over medical treatment which is in the patient's best interest, of the patient's own choosing, or both. The latter objection often is dealt with by advocates of RCTs by stating that subjects who consent to enrollment on the trial understand the random allocation of treatment arms, and therefore make a free choice when they agree to participate.

The objection that RCTs may conflict with medical care in the patient's best interest often is handled by pointing out the fallibility of individual clinical judgment and the frequency of bias in treatment decisions. Defenders of RCTs may invoke the somewhat circular logic that dictates that if the right treatment choice were known, there would be no need to do the research in the first place. The suggestion here, stated most forcefully by Chalmers,[30] is that clinicians often act on intuition without scientific basis in their treatment decisions, and enrolling patients in randomized clinical trials at least allows for objective evaluation of therapies over time.

Benjamin Freedman makes a more subtle argument describing the need for equipoise before the initiation of a randomized trial.[31] He defines equipoise as "a state of genuine uncertainty on the part of the clinical investigator regarding the comparative therapeutic merits of each arm in a trial." Freedman broadens the conventional definition of equipoise for an individual investigator by suggesting that a better criteria for an ethically appropriate study would be a standard of "clinical equipoise," reflecting the opinion of the expert medical community.

The debate over RCTs has at times been fierce, and there is a real need for a balanced view. In a previous paper, one of us (Eric Kodish) proposed some ethical guidelines for RCTs.[32] The first recommendation is directed at physicians who enter patients on RCTs, and suggests that they should enroll patients in an RCT only if they cannot judge which arm of a protocol is preferable for a particular patient. This requirement would be more restrictive than Freedman's clinical equipoise concept because the responsibility for the decision would rest entirely with the individual clinician, rather than the community of experts. The second suggestion is for those who design clinical trials. This guideline states that RCTs may need to be modified when patient preferences for one treatment or another can be elicited.

Specifically, this would require that the autonomy of subjects be given more emphasis than in current RCT design, and that investigators include subjects and/or their advocates in the early stages of research planning.

Finally, it is difficult to generalize about RCTs as a whole, because each trial must be evaluated on its individual merits. Although RCTs may have been overused, to the exclusion of other study designs, they offer much as a statistically powerful tool in the evaluation of medical therapies. Pharmacists can bring an important and unique understanding to deliberations on the ethics of drug research studies. Because of their crucial perspective, and their necessary involvement with the conduct of any drug research trial, pharmacists have an obligation to become actively involved in the ethical assessment of drug research programs.

SPECIAL CONSIDERATIONS FOR VULNERABLE POPULATIONS

One of the most difficult areas in the ethics of clinical research is the need for protection of vulnerable subjects. The recognition that certain populations may be at risk for abuse in the research setting is relatively new, and it is worthwhile to consider several different groups who have needed or potentially could need protection. It must be said, however, that despite a vast array of bureaucratic mechanisms designed to protect research subjects, the single most important and powerful protection for subjects is the integrity of the scientific investigator. Further, all research subjects are potentially vulnerable because of the tremendous amount of power and respect generally commanded by physicians in our society.[33] Potential research subjects generally are uneducated in medical matters, and many may not understand the distinction between clinical research and medical practice; thus, subjects may agree to enroll on research trials without a morally adequate education and consent process. In some instances, the combination of trust in the physician/investigator and intimidation resulting from the power imbalance may result in the abuse of research subjects on clinical trials.

Children have been used as subjects in medical research in many settings, but their participation in research continues to be controversial. The extreme positions on this question have been put forth by Ramsey[34] and McCormick.[35] Ramsey suggests that children should never be involved in research because they are never capable of actual valid consent, while McCormick goes so far as to claim that children may have an obligation to participate in research so long as it involves no "discernible risk."

In most cases, parents act as a proxy decision maker for their child, whether consent is for therapy or research. This reflects a commitment to respect for families, with a presumption that the parent speaks for the child. Autonomy in pediatrics is more complex than in adult research or practice, and those who perform research on children undertake special responsibilities of protection for their subjects. Although parents may have the legal right to consent for medical therapy or research on behalf of their children, this does not excuse physicians or investigators from discussing the relevant issues with the child in an age-appropriate manner.[36]

It also must be pointed out that there is a potential to over-protect children from research. Because different diseases occur in children, and many diseases affect children in different ways than adults, it often is not possible to directly apply data obtained in adult research to pediatrics. Further, children with life-threatening diseases can be precluded from access to the most innovative treatments if they are protected too well from research participation.[37] For these reasons, balance is required when attempting to protect children from research abuse.

An even more controversial area in research ethics involves experimentation with embryos and fetuses. This type of research holds great potential for advances in diabetes, neurologic problems, cancer, and other diseases. Here, however, the potential scientific gains must be considered along with respect for the embryo and fetus: the question of how much respect depends on the moral standing of the embryo or fetus, balanced against the rights of women (and men) to control reproduction and fertility. In other words, these questions relate directly to the divisive questions surrounding abortion. Stephen Post has pointed out the moral peril of the scientific establishment becoming dependent on a constant supply of aborted fetuses.[38] This potential supply and demand relationship threatens to make involved scientists morally complicit in the abortion decisions of individuals. Another important question also has been raised: If this research should be permitted, who, if anyone, should provide consent?[39]

A related topic in research ethics, of special relevance to pharmacists, is the controversy surrounding the study and eventual marketing of RU-486, the abortion pill. The discovery of this drug changes the mechanism of pregnancy termination from a surgical procedure to a medical therapy. Because of this change, the introduction of this agent carries dramatic moral, political, and economic implications. Despite the potential for tremendous financial profit by pharmaceutical companies in the United States through the marketing of RU-486, the drug is currently not available in the United States, and is being tested and marketed in Europe. This may be because the potential for economic gain is outweighed by the expected losses that would come with the threatened boycott by anti-abortion groups if this drug is marketed. It also may be that moral, medical, or practical/political considerations have prevented the pharmaceutical industry from introducing RU-486, or it may be related to a combination of these factors. Since embryos and fetuses often are viewed as vulnerable populations, pharmacists should remain well informed about new developments in the medical facts relating to RU-486 and the abortion debate.

Patients with major psychiatric disorders and mentally disabled patients may be vulnerable because they cannot make decisions for themselves. Because of this lack of competence, such potential research subjects may not have the capacity to protect themselves from dangerous experimentation. Retarded individuals were routinely sterilized without their consent up until very recently. A higher level of consent is necessary for participation in research than for medical treatment. While mentally ill or disabled persons should not be denied treatment because of their inability to consent, participation in research is a more complicated matter. Research that has the potential for therapeutic benefit to the subject may be appropriate for mentally incompetent persons, but projects that are strictly designed to produce generally applied knowledge should probably not recruit incompetent subjects. In cases where potential research subjects are mentally incompetent, an independent proxy or family member can make an important contribution by acting as an advocate for the potential subject and providing consent if participation would be in the subject's best interest.

With the dramatic growth of the elderly population in the United States, Alzheimer's disease and other senile dementias are becoming more prevalent. Although morally preferable to proxy consent, obtaining consent from individuals who were once competent, but now may be demented, requires great care. This change usually occurs gradually, and patients may be in various stages on a continuum of decline. If the actual subject rather than a proxy decision maker is approached for consent, honest disclosure of the underlying diagnosis must precede informed consent to participation in a research trial for the treatment of Alzheimer's disease.[40] One example of this problem that pharmacists should be aware of has been the clinical evaluation of tacrine, an agent reported to enhance cognition in some patients with dementia, but which also may be the cause of significant toxicities.[41] When the level of competence of a potential research subject fluctuates because of the underlying disease, questions of appropriate consent and reasonable protection from research abuse become complex and difficult. While progress in the therapy or prevention of dementias can be made only through good clinical research, great caution must be exercised by investigators involved in this type of research.

Fatally ill patients constitute another potentially vulnerable research population. These individuals may be at risk because of desperation on the part of the patient, or the potential for coercion by family members who are not ready to give up hope. Although consent may be given, patients facing terminal illness may feel like there is no alternative to participation in a research project.

Many subjects in Phase I oncology research have no proven therapeutic approach available to treat their disease, and are, therefore, referred for treatment with an investigational agent. Although the scientific purpose of the study is to gain information on the toxicity and pharmacology of the drug being tested, most of these subjects would like to believe that they will get therapeutic benefit. While the potential for psychological benefit from such altruistic behavior cannot be overlooked,[42] investigators who obtain informed consent have a moral obligation to explain the purpose of the study, and the risks and benefits of participation, to all potential subjects.

Human nature is such that most physicians, investigators, patients, and family members prefer not to discuss bad news or dwell on depressing subjects. It is much easier to offer another investigational drug than to talk about the imminent death of a patient. Despite this difficulty, all the relevant alternatives, including no further treatment and a hospice philosophy care plan should be presented as options to terminally ill patients before they consent to enrollment in a research project. Hospice philosophy includes emphasis on the comfort of the patient rather than prolonging life, and attention to the psychological and spiritual as well as physical needs of the dying patient. Pharmacists can play an integral role in the delivery of hospice care by dispensing the appropriate liberal doses of narcotic and anxiolytic medications ordered by the managing physician, and by teaching involved health care workers about the physiologic concept of tolerance and infrequency of addiction in this setting.[43]

Prisoners commonly were used involuntarily for medical research until this century. More recently, prisoners have been paid for participation in research. The potential for coercion or manipulation in either of these circumstances is very problematic. While prisons present a great opportunity for the conduct of clinical research, this practice generally is discouraged or forbidden at this time because of the huge potential for exploitation.

Up until this decade, a great disparity existed in participation in clinical research, with men involved much more frequently than women. This disparity resulted in two problems: 1) Large-scale studies of men were applied to women without clear scientific correlation in females (e.g., coronary artery disease, hypertension). There was an incorrect assumption that data obtained from men would be applicable to women.[44] 2) There was relative neglect of research on common diseases of women such as breast and ovarian cancer. The federal government recently has moved to remedy this problem with a major women's health initiative including greatly increased research funding.[45]

Despite this policy shift, inequities remain and women may be both 1) at more risk for research abuse because of their gender and 2) excluded from participation in research studies by virtue of gender. A recent example is data demonstrating that pregnant women have been excluded from clinical trials in the treatment of AIDS.[46] These data suggest that what may appear as beneficent protection of women and children from research abuse actually can reflect an impingement on the autonomy of women to make their own decisions regarding research participation.

Many of the issues raised above for vulnerable populations apply to various ethnic and religious minority groups. The issues will vary with the circumstances of the particular study and the minority group involved. The Tuskegee Syphilis study, described previously, and the horrendous Nazi experimentation on Jews and other minorities stand as clear examples of the potential for research abuse in minority populations. These historical examples demand that scientific investigators remain vigilant in their sensitivity to the potential for exploitation in clinical research.

CONCLUSION

What does the future hold for research with human subjects? In 1994, the federal Department of Energy established an advisory committee under chair Ruth R. Faden, Ph.D., to report on the history and ethics of the government's radiation experiments on humans during the late 1940s and early 1950s.[24] The particular research itself may have been acceptable in its day; much of it was reported in leading medical and scientific journals. However, bioethicists now suggest more strongly that the "objective" standard of informed consent may not be sufficient *morally* any more. Some patients have special fears or need additional information to make sensible choices, requiring more data than "the reasonable person"; therefore, the required consent standard of the future may be more "subjective" to take into account each patient's knowledge and feelings separately. This individualized standard would place medical practitioners in a very precarious position legally and perhaps impose greater duty on other health care professionals (particularly pharmacists and nurses) involved in human research. However, practitioners must remember that the goal of human research and health care delivery is to help patients, whether individually or collectively, and to improve the quality of their life by putting *their* interests first.

Discussion Questions

1. What are the four phases of drug research, and how does each contribute to the goal of thorough evaluation of new pharmacologic agents?
2. Describe two different senses of informed consent, and discuss the four elements necessary to make consent morally valid.
3. How should drug researchers balance the need to protect vulnerable subjects with fair access to their participation in clinical studies?

REFERENCES

1. Smith M et al. Pharmacy Ethics. New York: Pharmaceutical Products Press; 1991:29–33.

2. Talbert RL. Ethics in clinical pharmacy practice and research: an introduction. Pharmacotherapy. 1993;13:521.

3. Ethical issues related to clinical pharmacy research [American College of Clinical Pharmacy White Paper]. Pharmacotherapy. 1992;13:523–30.

4. First Alzheimer's Drug. FDA Medical Bulletin. 1993;23(3):5.

5. Neergaard L. Something terrible happened. The Knoxville News-Sentinel. 1993;1 Sep:A8.

6. Beauchamp TL, Childress JF. Principles of Biomedical Ethics. 3rd ed. New York: Oxford University Press; 1989:120–255.

7. Apfel RJ, Fisher SM. To Do No Harm: DES and the Dilemmas of Modern Medicine. New Haven: Yale University Press; 1984:107–25.

8. Temin P. Taking Your Medicine: Drug Regulation in the United States. Cambridge: Harvard University Press; 1980:18–46, 58–87, 120–26.

9. Beecher HK. Ethics and clinical research. N Engl J Med. 1966;274:1354–360.

10. Katz J. Experimentation with Humans. New York: Russell Sage Foundation; 1972:283–322.

11. National Commission for the Protection of Human Subjects of Biomedical and Behavioral Research. The Belmont report: ethical principles and guidelines for the protection of human subjects in research. Washington, D.C.: U.S. Government Printing Office, 1978; (stock number 040-000-00452-1).

12. President's Commission for the Study of Ethical Problems in Medicine and Biomedical and Behavioral Research. Protecting human subjects. Washington, D.C.: U.S. Government Printing Office, 1981; (stock number 040-000-00471-8).

13. President's Commission for the Study of Ethical Problems in Medicine and Biomedical and Behavioral Research. Implementing human research regulations. Washington, D.C.: U.S. Government Printing Office, 1983; (Library of Congress card number 83-600504).

14. Sobel S. Ethical issues in study design. P&T. 1992:10:1559, 1560, 1567–569.

15. 45 C.F.R. 46 et seq.
16. Levine RJ. Ethics and Regulation of Clinical Research. 2nd ed. Baltimore: Urban & Schwarzenberg; 1986:19–35.
17. Faden RR, Beauchamp TL. A History and Theory of Informed Consent. New York and Oxford: Oxford University Press; 1986:274.
18. Katz J. The Silent World of Doctors and Patients. New York: The Free Press; 1984.
19. Pernick MS. The patient's role in medical decision making: a social history of informed consent in medical therapy. In: President's Commission for the Study of Ethical Problems in Medicine and Biomedical and Behavioral Research, Making Health Care Decisions. Washington, D.C.: U.S. Government Printing Office, 1982.
20. Charrow RP. Informed consent: from Canterbury Tales to *Canterbury vs. Spence*. Journ NIH Research. 1993;5:75–7.
21. Lifton RJ. The Nazi Doctors: Medical Killing and the Psychology of Genocide. New York: Basic Books; 1986.
22. Brandt AM. Racism and research: the case of the Tuskegee syphilis study. Hastings Cent Rep. 1978;8:21–9.
23. Katz J. Experimentation with Human Beings. New York: The Russell Sage Foundation; 1972.
24. Hilts PJ. Study on tests. New York Times. 1994;30 Jan:15.
25. Beauchamp TL, Childress JF. Principles of Biomedical Ethics. New York: Oxford University Press; 1989.
26. Faden RR, Beauchamp TL. A History and Theory of Informed Consent. New York and Oxford: Oxford University Press; 1986:3–49.
27. Rothman K, Michels K. The continuing unethical use of placebo controls. N Engl J Med. 1994;331:394–98.
28. Kalish LA, Begg CB. Treatment allocation methods in clinical trials: a review. Stat Med. 1985;4:129–44.
29. Hellman D, Hellman S. Of mice but not men: problems of the randomized clinical trial. N Engl J Med. 1991;324:1585–589.
30. Chalmers TC et al. Controlled studies in clinical cancer research. N Engl J Med. 1972;287:75–8.
31. Freedman B. Equipoise and the ethics of clinical research. N Engl J Med. 1987;317:141–45.

32. Kodish E et al. Ethical considerations in randomized clinical trials. Cancer. 1990;65:2400–404.

33. Brody H. The Healer's Power. New Haven and London: Yale University Press; 1992.

34. Ramsey P. "Unconsented touching" and the autonomy absolute. IRB: Rev Human Subjects Res. 1980;2:9–10.

35. McCormick RA. Proxy consent in the experimentation situation. Perspect Biol Med. 1974;18:2–20.

36. Mahowald MB. Children and moral agency. In: Women and Children in Health Care. New York and Oxford: Oxford University Press; 1993:Chapter 11.

37. Levine C. Children in HIV/AIDS clinical trials: still vulnerable after all these years. Law Med Health Care. 1991;19:231–37.

38. Post S. Fetal tissue transplant: the right to question progress. America. 1991;164:14–16.

39. Hurd RE. Ethical issues surrounding the transplantation of human fetal tissues. Clin Res. 1992;661–66.

40. Drickamer MA, Lachs MS. Should patients with Alzheimer's disease be told their diagnosis? N Engl J Med. 1992;326:947–51.

41. Relman AS. Tacrine as a treatment for Alzheimer's dementia. N Engl J Med. 1991;324:349–52.

42. Kodish E. Ethical issues in Phase I oncology research: a study of investigators and IRB chairs. J Clin Oncol. 1992;10(11):1810–16.

43. Jacox A et al. New clinical-practice guidelines for the management of pain in patients with cancer. N Engl J Med. 1994;330:651–55.

44. Healy B. The Yentl syndrome. N Engl J Med. 1991;325:274–76.

45. Merkatz RB et al. Women in clinical trials of new drugs—a change in Food and Drug Administration policy. N Engl J Med. 1993;329:292–96.

46. Caschetta MB et al. FDA policy on women in drug trials. N Engl J Med. 1993;329:1815.

Appendix 1

Code of Ethics For Pharmacists[a]

Preamble

Pharmacists are health professionals who assist individuals in making the best use of medications. This Code, prepared and supported by pharmacists, is intended to state publicly the principles that form the fundamental basis of the roles and responsibilities of pharmacists. These principles, based on moral obligations and virtues, are established to guide pharmacists in relationships with patients, health professionals, and society.

I. A pharmacist respects the covenantal relationship between the patient and pharmacist. Considering the patient-pharmacist relationship as a covenant means that a pharmacist has moral obligations in response to the gift of trust received from society. In return for this gift, a pharmacist promises to help individuals achieve optimum benefit from their medications, to be committed to their welfare, and to maintain their trust.

II. A pharmacist promotes the good of every patient in a caring, compassionate, and confidential manner. A pharmacist places concern for the well-being of the patient at the center of professional practice. In doing so, a pharmacist considers needs stated by the patient as well as those defined by health science. A pharmacist is dedicated to protecting the dignity of the patient. With a caring attitude and a compassionate spirit, a pharmacist focuses on serving the patient in a private and confidential manner.

III. A pharmacist respects the autonomy and dignity of each patient. A pharmacist promotes the right of self-determination and recognizes individual self-worth by encouraging patients to participate in decisions about their health. A pharmacist communicates with patients in

---

[a] *Adopted by the membership of the American Pharmaceutical Association, October 27, 1994.*

terms that are understandable. In all cases, a pharmacist respects personal and cultural differences among patients.

IV. A pharmacist acts with honesty and integrity in professional relationships. A pharmacist has a duty to tell the truth and to act with conviction of conscience. A pharmacist avoids discriminatory practices, behavior or work conditions that impair professional judgment, and actions that compromise dedication to the best interests of patients.

V. A pharmacist maintains professional competence. A pharmacist has a duty to maintain knowledge and abilities as new medications, devices, and technologies become available and as health information advances.

VI. A pharmacist respects the values and abilities of colleagues and other health professionals. When appropriate, a pharmacist asks for the consultation of colleagues or other health professionals or refers the patient. A pharmacist acknowledges that colleagues and other health professionals may differ in the beliefs and values they apply to the care of the patient.

VII. A pharmacist serves individual, community, and societal needs. The primary obligation of a pharmacist is to individual patients. However, the obligations of a pharmacist may at times extend beyond the individual to the community and society. In these situations, the pharmacist recognizes the responsibilities that accompany these obligations and acts accordingly.

VIII. A pharmacist seeks justice in the distribution of health resources. When health resources are allocated, a pharmacist is fair and equitable, balancing the needs of patients and society.

Appendix 2
Resources in Pharmacy Ethics

The following bibliography is a compilation of suggested readings from Chapters 3, 4, and 10, and from Haddad AM et al. Curricular guidelines for pharmacy education: ethics course content committee council of faculties. Am J Pharm Educ. 1993;57:34S–43S.

Journals

Anon. Home test kits offer patients active role in health care. Calif Pharm. 1987;May:32–5.
> Review and guide to home test kits for pharmacists. Good opportunity for patient care.

Anon. Pharmacists and Physicians: Professional Allies or Professional Adversaries? Schering Report XI. Kenilworth, NJ: Schering/Key Laboratories; 1989.
> Report deals with the relationship between the physician and pharmacist. Empirically based answers regarding pharmacist's functions.

Anon. Pharmacy ethics. Am J Hosp Pharm. 1989;46:75, 116–19.
> Handy resource of reprinted articles on a variety of issues in pharmacy practice.

Appelbaum PS, Grissot. Assessing patients' capacity to consent to treatment. N Engl J Med. 1988;319(25).
> The legal standards for competence are reviewed and include four related patient skills. The role of the clinical examiner is discussed.

Arnold RM et al. Ethical issues in a drug information center. DICP. 1987;21:1008–11.
> Abstract: The frequency and nature of ethical issues faced by pharmacists have not been well documented. To address these issues a retro-

spective study of the potential ethical problems encountered by pharmacists in a drug information center was conducted. Of the 744 calls received over a 13-month period, 50 raised ethical issues. Consumer calls were more likely to raise ethical issues than were health provider calls. The calls mainly fell into five categories: Drug identification, assessment of a physician's recommendations for consumers, conflict between callers' needs and legal or public-health considerations, therapeutic issues in the pharmacist-patient relationship, and paternalistic treatment of 'difficult' callers. These questions raised ethical issues related to confidentiality, truth telling, and pharmacists' societal obligations. Pharmacists may confront an increased number of ethical issues as more drug information centers provide consumer services. Although there is no empirical evidence regarding pharmacists' ability to deal with ethical issues, there are reasons to believe that training in medical ethics will better equip pharmacists to recognize, analyze, and resolve ethical dilemmas.

Bagley JL. New products spur sales of home tests. Am Druggist. 1987;Apr:118–25.
Review of common home test kits.

Bell JA et al. Clinical research in the elderly: ethical and methodology considerations. Drug Intell Clin Pharm. 1987;21:1002–7.
Abstract: Clinically oriented research in the elderly is of growing interest because of increasing numbers of older persons, the relative lack of research data with this population, and recent Food and Drug Administration mandates to study drugs in the elderly. Studies of young, healthy persons cannot necessarily be extrapolated to the elderly due to changes associated with aging and the increased number of concomitant disease states and medications. Subject recruitment may be more time consuming in finding subjects with the appropriate inclusion criteria and lack of exclusion criteria who are willing to participate. Additional concern must be placed on protecting the subject's rights while allowing autonomous decision making. Likewise, protocols may need to be flexible enough to include persons with concomitant disease and medications.

Bok. The ethics of giving placebos. Sci Am. 1974;231:17.

Boyce EG et al. Cross-sectional study of the ethics of pharmacy students. DICP. The Annals of Pharmacotherapy. 1989;23(7-8):590–92.

Brody H. The lie that heals: the ethics of giving placebos. Ann Intern Med. 1982;97(1):112–18.

Brown LJ, DiFranza JR. Pharmacy promotion of tobacco use among children in Massachusetts. Am Pharm. 1992;32:45–8.

As with the articles relating to suicide, these papers provide good background reading prior to a discussion of the ethics of selling tobacco products in pharmacies.

Brushwood DB, Weinstein BD. Ethical and legal issues in pharmacy: deception. US Pharmacist. 1990;Sept:88–91.
> While there is much debate among ethicists concerning which principle is of paramount importance, this debate may be reconciled if we interpret the principle of beneficence to mean that pharmacists should do for patients the good those patients would choose for themselves. One would then be led to conclude that pharmacists ought never to dispense placebos to which patients or research subjects have not consented. Catherine Baker thus should not substitute a lactose placebo. She might instead urge Dr. Scirocco to discuss honestly his concerns with his patient.

Buerki RA, Vottero LD. The changing face of pharmaceutical education: ethics and professional prerogatives. Am J Pharm Educ. 1991;55:71–4.
> Discussion regarding the differences between ethical mandates and professional prerogatives. Practical discussion regarding the implementation of pharmaceutical care in practice and education.

Callahan D. Ethics and health care: the next twenty years. Am J Hosp Pharm. 1985;42:1053–57.
> Discusses shifts in moral values in health care both past and future. Future decisions will be made on the 'common good.'

Chi J. Drug giveaways for the needy: altruism or marketing ploy? Hosp Pharm Rep. 1991;Feb:26–7.

Cohen EP. Direct-to-the-public advertisement of prescription drugs. N Engl J Med. 1988;318:373–76.

Coons SJ, Fink JL. The pharmacist, the law and self-testing products. Am Pharm. 1989;29(11):35–8.
> Discusses the pharmacist's role in providing self testing products and concludes that this is an opportunity with some liability issues.

Cowen DL. Pharmacists and physicians: an uneasy relationship. Pharm in History. 1992;34:3–16.
> Good companion piece to *Schering Report XI*. Historical account of relationship between medicine and pharmacy.

Dyck AJ. Ethical aspects of care for the dying incompetent. J Am Geriatr Soc. 1984;32(9):661–64.
> Discusses active versus passive euthanasia and the need for strong consensus in decisions affecting care of the dying incompetent patient.

Engelhardt HT. Morality for the medical-industrial complex. N Engl J Med. 1988;319(16):1086–89.

Erwin WG et al. Ethics course work at colleges of pharmacy: differentiation by practice degrees awarded. Am J Pharm Educ. 1987;51:24–7.
Comparative study regarding status of ethics education in Pharm.D. and B.S. pharmacy programs.

Feinberg J, ed. Pharmacy professionalism challenged by Washington Post. PAS-Washington Line. 1987;2(10).

Finley RR. Withholding treatment. Drug Ther Elder. 1986;1(11).
Pharmacy case discussion of passive euthanasia.

Gebhart F. Is there a problem of sexual harassment in pharmacy? Hosp Pharm Rep. 1991;Nov:9–10.
This paper is useful in discussion about sexual harassment in pharmacy, particularly when combined with a one-page case (written by Bruce Weinstein, West Virginia University) of a potential sexual harassment in which the class is asked to identify at what point in the case harassment may have occurred.

Goodman LE, Goodman MJ. Prevention—how misuse of a concept undercuts its worth. Hastings Cent Rep. 1988;Apr:26–38.
Discussion of the 'overselling' of certain aspects of medicine as prevention. Mass prevention programs may become 'fads' without solid scientific support.

Gossel TA. Home testing products for self-monitoring. Am J Hosp Pharm. 1988;45:1119–126.
Review of current and future home test kits and considerations for pharmacists.

Graubert JI. Pharmacy managers use planning, education to accommodate high cost drugs. Am J Hosp Pharm. 1988;45:1007–12.

Gunby P. Gifts to physicians from industry. JAMA. 1991;265(4):501.

Haddad AM. Ethical problems in pharmacy practice: a survey of difficulty and incidence. Am J Pharm Educ. 1991;55:1–6.
National random survey of pharmacists regarding incidence and difficulty of ethical problems in practice.

Haddad AM et al. Confidentiality and pharmacy practice: urban versus rural perspectives. Am J Pharm Educ. 1992;56:16–20.
Report of a quantitative descriptive study which explores the beliefs of urban and rural pharmacists regarding confidentiality.

Hastings Center Report, Journal of Clinical Ethics, Bioethics and New England Journal of Medicine regularly feature essays on ethical issues in health care, though generally they do not pertain to pharmacy directly.

Heacock MV, McGee GW. Whistleblowing: an ethical issue in organization and human behavior. Business and Professional Ethics J. 1986;6(4):35–46.
> Criteria for determining when to report suspected misconduct and a survey of categories of "whistleblowing."

Hepler CD, Strand LM. Opportunities and responsibilities in pharmaceutical care. Am J Hosp Pharm. 1990;47:533–43.
> Seminal work in pharmaceutical care. Lays groundwork for ethics in new practice paradigm.

Hepler CD. Unresolved issues in the practice of pharmacy. Am J Hosp Pharm. 1988;45:1070–81.
> The author discusses the issues of technology, economics, and social values as they affect the future of pharmacy.

Hulstrand EP. Pharmaceutical companies should offer reliable information, not freebies. Am J Hosp Pharm. 1989;46:702.

Koffer KF, Gerbino PP. Home laboratory test (part 2). Am Druggist. 1986;Apr:103–8.
> Review of home test kits using case situations.

Koop CE. The challenge of definition. Hastings Cent Rep. 1989;19(1):2–3.
> Philosophical essay in opposition to 'mercy killing.'

Lachman BG. Legal and ethical issues: their effect on home health care. Calif Pharm. 1988;July:18–20.
> These are some of the ethical issues facing health care in general and home health care in particular. Pharmacists can set an ethical example in the community by providing services, charging true costs for them and working with other professionals to provide home care that will improve and maintain the patient's quality of life. In the final analysis, that's the best bottom line.

Lachman BG et al. Offering referral fees to physicians for home health care patients. Am J Hosp Pharm. 1989;46:738–41.

LeBlang TR. The pharmacist's duty to warn of hazards to non-patients. Am Druggist. 1990;Nov:72–4.

Lo B, Steinbrook RL. Deciding whether to resuscitate terminally ill patients. Arch Intern Med. 1983;143:1561–563.
> A discussion of the use of DNR orders based on a case.

Lo B, Doinbrand L. Guiding the hand that feeds: caring for the demented elderly. N Engl J Med. 1984;811:402–4.
> The role of nutrition and feeding tubes in the case of a severely demented patient.

Lowenthal W. Ethical dilemmas in pharmacy practice. J Med Humanit Bioeth. 1988;9(1):44–9.
> Survey study of pharmacists regarding ethical problems in practice.

Manasse HR. Medical use in a imperfect world: drug misadventuring as an issue of public policy, part 1 and part 2. Am J Hosp Pharm. 1989;46:929–44, 1141–152.
> Outlines crisis that mandates pharmacist's role in expansion into pharmaceutical care.

Mangione RA. Getting involved in child abuse prevention and detection. Pharm Times. 1989;Dec:29–32.
> This article provides an introduction to students about their potential ethical responsibility in an area not generally considered part of pharmacy practice.

Manolakis ML. Why APhA should reject its code of ethics. Am Pharm. 1991;31:46–8.

Marsh FH. Informed consent and the elderly patient. Clin Geriatr Med. 1986;2(3):501–10.
> A case study is used to review the ethical issues related to informed consent and clinical research.

Marvell MJ, Anderson RJ. Concerns with postmarking surveillance. Am J Hosp Pharm. 1984;41:54, 56.

McCann J. Pharmacists play an important role in suicide prevention. Drug Topics. 1993;Oct:14–5.

McCart GM et al. Maintaining patient confidentiality in a case of potential drug abuse. Am J Hosp Pharm. 1989;46:116–19.

McLaughlin SS. Novel promotional activities, direct-to-consumer advertising subjects of FDA scrutiny. JASHP. 1989;46:870–75.

Meyer LE et al. Impact on perception of side effects. DICP. 1985;19:213.
> Ninety employees of a large company were studied to see if those who were counseled on meds experienced more side effects than those who where not counseled. No difference was noted.

> Care must be taken to present understandable written material so patient confusion or disregard does not interfere with the administration of medicine. However, this present study supports previous findings

that no practical clinical difference in the incidence of reported side effects occurs when specific verbal and written information on drug side effects is given to the patient. We believe the inability to detect a difference in side effects as perceived by patients weighs against any practical adverse clinical significance for side effects forewarning.

Middelton WS. Speaking out against freebies. Am J Hosp Pharm. 1989;46:2001.

Millstein LL. The regulation of prescription drug advertising. Am Pharm. 1983;23(9):54–7.

Morreim EH. Am I my brother's warden? Responding to the unethical or incompetent colleague. Hastings Cent Rep. 1993;23(3):19–27.
Distinguishing levels of adverse consequences of and types of professional misconduct helps to guide colleagues in fulfilling their policing responsibilities; focused specifically on physicians but directly applicable to other health care professionals.

Mossinghoff GJ. Reasons for high cost of high tech drugs. Am J Hosp Pharm. 1988;45:1865–866.

Nelson LJ et al. Taking the train to a world of strangers: health care marketing and ethics. Hastings Cent Rep. 1989;Sept/Oct:36–43.

Nielsen JR. The doctor, the pharmacist, the patient and the placebo; or, you're not my mother, Doctor. Food Drug Cosmetic Law Journal. 1989;44(6):639–57.

Oddis JA. Direct-to-consumer advertising. Resid Staff Physician. 1989;35(8):110.

Parrish RH. Stop big government. Drug Topics. 1990;Nov:9.

Perri M. Patient-directed prescription drugs ads. Merck Minutes. 1988;5(3).

Poikonen JC et al. Distributing soon-to-expire medications to the Commonwealth of Independent States. Am J Hosp Pharm. 1992;49(11):2772–777.
One in a series of articles in the American Journal of Hospital Pharmacy that consists of a brief case and commentary by two pharmacists/ethicists and final analysis by Robert Veacth, Ph.D.

Popovich NG. Home diagnostic agents and testing devices. Wellcome Trends in Hospital Pharmacy. 1990;July:2, 3, 13, 15.
Brief review on home test kits and the role of the pharmacist.

Prime R. What is pharmacy's biggest ethical problem today? Drug Topics. 1987;Aug:14–5.
>Interviews with four practicing pharmacists.

Prince R. What is pharmacy's biggest ethical problem today? Drug Topics. 1987;Aug:14–5.

Randall T. Does advertising influence physicians? JAMA. 1991;265(4):443.

Randall T. Ethics of receiving gifts considered. JAMA. 1991;265(4):442–43.

Randall T. Kennedy hearings say no more free lunch—or much else—from drug firms. JAMA. 1991;265(4):440–41.

Reidenberg MM. The state of drug development in the United States in 1990: a view from the academic community. Clin Pharm Ther. 1990;48(1):1–9.

Rosendahl I. Decisions decisions—ethical dilemmas facing pharmacists. Drug Topics. 1989;Feb:44–50.
>Review of ethical dilemmas facing pharmacists and a survey asking for response to eight cases.

Ross JW et al. Treatment decision making. Handbook for Hospital Ethics Committees. American Hospital Association. 1986:87–92.
>Brief review of competence and consent, advanced directives, living wills, and uniform Anatomical Gift Act.

Schafer A. The ethics of the randomized clinical trial. N Engl J Med. 1982;307:719–24.
>The physician who enlists his patient in a randomized trial faces at least the possibility of a conflict of obligations. In many cases the tension between the physician's traditional role as healer and his modern role as scientific investigator can be resolved without serious cost either to the patient or to science. In other cases, however, the tension may reach the level of outright commitment to patient welfare, with its corollary of totally individualized treatment, may sometimes properly be modified so as to permit randomized clinical trials to proceed with a statistically significant sample of subjects. The circumstances in which it is ethically permissible to abrogate the Hippocratic principle are in need of careful definition.

Simonsmeier LM. Motorist sues pharmacist for failure to warn patient. Pharm Times. 1988;Feb:117–19.
>The plaintiff in this month's case was seriously injured when her automobile was struck by a car driven by John Smith. Mr. Smith was under

the treatment of a psychiatrist and had received a prescription for an antidepressant which was dispensed by the defendant pharmacy. After having breakfast one morning, Mr. Smith drove his automobile through a red light and hit the plaintiff's car.

The court concluded that Michigan should adopt the rule that a pharmacist has no duty to warn a patient of possible side effects of a prescription drug when neither their physician nor the manufacturer has required that any warning be given to the patient by the pharmacist. It did hint that a warning might be appropriate when the pharmacist knows of a particular patient's unique problems or when a pharmacist fills two incompatible prescriptions. However, until the court is presented with such a fact pattern, the rule will remain, in the Michigan jurisdiction, that a pharmacist has no duty to warn a patient.

Smith MC, Smith MD. Instruction in ethics in schools of pharmacy. Am J Pharm Educ. 1981;45:14–7.

Smith WE. Ethical, economic and professional issues in home health care. Am J Hosp Pharm. 1986;43:695–98.
Patient services issues in HHC involve the ethics of providing high-technology feeding therapies to terminally ill patients and the controversies surrounding drug products, such as the appropriate amount of drug to be dispensed, the appropriate individual to compound home-care drug products, acceptable types of product packaging, and the impact of a switch in vendors on the drug products supplied to patients. Economic issues include reasonable profit for HHC services, methods used to charge for products and services, payments to physicians for patient referrals, and pharmacies owned and operated by the HHC industry. Pharmacy relations issues center on the influence of nonpharmacists on pharmacy-based HHC services on intraprofessional relations.

Sox HC. Probability theory in the use of diagnostic tests. Ann Intern Med. 1986;104:60–6.
Analytical evaluation of sensitivity and specificity as it relates to diagnostic testing. The value of Bayes theorum is also presented.

Starr C. Pharmacists' ethical dilemmas: an abused child. Drug Topics. 1989;Aug:21.
The response from pharmacists regarding their opinion of case of child abuse.

Steinbrook R, Lo B. Decision making for incompetent patients by designated proxy. N Engl J Med. 1984;310:1598–1601.
Discusses the California durable power of attorney for Health Care Law of 1984 and other related advanced directives.

Taylor HG. Pharmacists who choose not to sell tobacco. Am Pharm. 1992;32:49–52.

Ukens C. Sexual harassment a fact of pharmacy life, some find. Drug Topics. 1991;Nov:16–8.
> This paper is useful in discussion about sexual harassment in pharmacy, particularly when combined with a one-page case (written by Bruce Weinstein, West Virginia University) of a potential sexual harassment in which the class is asked to identify at what point in the case harassment may have occurred.

Veatch RM. Drug research in humans: the ethics of nonrandomized access. Clin Pharm. 1989;8:366–70.
> Seriously ill patients without other alternatives may reject randomized access to the only hope of therapy. The author evaluates the ethics of this research dilemma.

Veatch RM. Ethics of drugs for un-approved uses. US Pharmacist. 1983;8:69–72.

Veatch RM. Hospital pharmacy: what is ethical? Am J Hosp Pharm. 1989;46:109–15.
> Excellent article to use as an overall introduction to the application of normative ethics to pharmacy practice.

Veatch RM. Professional prerogatives: perspectives of an ethicist. Am J Pharm Educ. 1991;55:74–8.

Vogel AV et al. The therapeutics of placebo. Am Fam Physician. 1980;22(1):108–9.
> The use of placebo is not old-fashioned, ineffective, or unethical. It requires an ongoing, trusting relationship between the physician and the patient. Deception of the patient and self-deception must be avoided. Under these conditions, there are specific situations in which placebo is the treatment of choice.
>
> A placebo might make him feel better, but it won't really help him. This is not true. Some well-demonstrated physiologic effects of placebo action include antitussive effects, antiemetic effects, changes in gastric acid production, and release of endorphins.
>
> Relief of pain via endorphin release [placebo action can be blocked with naloxone (Narcan)]. Increased or decreased gastric acid secretion and gastric motility, depending on what the patient is told. Decreased exercise-induced bronchospasm in asthmatics (40% of patients). Fifty percent decrease in the rapid-eye-movement (REM) phase of sleep.

Vottero LD et al. Ethics in pharmacy practice: a code of professionalism. Tomorrow's Pharmacist. 1985:Nov/Dec.

Walters KD. Your employees' right to blow the whistle. Harv Bus Rev. 1975;53:26–34, 161–62.

>Suggestions of institutional mechanisms to obviate the need for external "whistleblowing."

Weinstein BD, Brushwood DB. Confidentiality: an ethical issue. US Pharmacy. 1990;May:53–5.

Welty TE. Ethical considerations for pharmacists. Am J Hosp Pharm. 1985;42:273.
>Letter asking pharmacist to get more involved in medical ethics.

Wertheimer AI, Serradell J. Informed consent and prescription drugs. Leg Aspects Pharm Pract. 1986;9(1).
>In the current climate, in which patients commonly sign consent forms without either reading them or receiving any reasonable explanations as to what their consent involves, [and] physicians and other health professionals frequently proceed in their work as if no explanation are necessary and as if it would be presumptuous for patients to question their judgment, the application of informed consent to pharmaceuticals probably will evolve slowly—initially for drug therapy for cancer and transplant surgery, followed by more common uses. We can expect to see the development of specific data systems or instructions and informed consent materials for each drug or therapeutic category for physicians and pharmacists. Pharmaceutical companies may distribute materials with their drugs like patient package inserts.

Williams RL. Sale of tobacco products in pharmacies. Am J Hosp Pharm. 1988;45:1279.

Woods JS. Nursing home care. Clin Geriatr Med. 1986;2(7):601–15.
>Overview of ethical issues in long-term care for physicians.

Zellmer WA. Reiterations. Am J Hosp Pharm. 1988;45:1295.
>Birth defects caused by isotretinoin; nicotine addiction caused by smoking—two serious but quite different public health problems that have their pharmacy connections. If we ignore these problems, we sharpen further the profession's stereotype. If we do our unique part to address these problems, we set the stage for the profession to contribute to the needs of the nation on a broader scale.

Zoloth AM. The need for ethical guidelines for relationships between pharmacists and the pharmaceutical industry. Am J Hosp Pharm. 1991;48:551–52.

Textbooks

Almond B. The Philosophical Quest. London: Penguin Books; 1988:Ch.2.

Beauchamp TL. Philosophical Ethics: An Introduction to Moral Philosophy. New York: McGraw Hill; 1982.
> This is an excellent introduction to the nature and methods of ethics as an intellectual discipline.

Beauchamp TL, Childress JF. Principles of Biomedical Ethics. 3rd ed. New York: Oxford University Press; 1989.
> A classic text in biomedical ethics; provides an indispensable analysis of the nature and relationship of ethical rules and principles in the context of health care.

Bok S. Whistleblowing and professional responsibilities. In: Callahan D, Bok S, eds. Ethics Teaching in Higher Education. New York: Plenum Press; 1980.

Clark B. Whose Life Is It Anyway? Woodstock: The Dramatic Publishing Company; 1974.

Dubler NN, Nimmons, D. Ethics on Call: Taking Charge of Life-and-Death Choices in Today's Health Care System. New York: Vintage Books; 1993.

Engelhardt HT Jr. The Foundations of Bioethics. New York: Oxford University Press; 1986.
> This difficult but immensely rewarding book presents a libertarian account of ethical issues in health care and is one of the few works in bioethics that can genuinely be called a classic.

Frankena WK. Ethics. 2nd ed. Englewood Cliffs: Prentice-Hall; 1973.

Garrett TM et al. Health Care Ethics, Principles and Problems. 2nd ed. New York: Prentice Hall; 1993:307.
> A new text that divides the subject matter into two parts: the principles of health care ethics, and the problems. Discusses at some length current relevant problems. Written clearly with many pertinent cases.

Hollis M. Invitation to Philosophy. New York: Basil Blackwell; 1985:Chs. 7 and 8.

Munson R. Intervention and Reflection, Basic Issues in Medical Ethics. 4th ed. Belmont: Wadsworth Press; 669.
> Text which deals briefly with the ethical principles then moves directly into salient issues. There is heavy emphasis on readings by current thought leaders and many case presentations and scenarios.

Nagel T. What Does It All Mean? New York: Oxford University Press; 1987:Chs. 7 and 8.

Petersen JC, Farrell D. Whistleblowing: Ethical and Legal Issues in Expressing Dissent. Dubuque: Kendall Hunt Publishing; 1986.
> Focused primarily on engineering, but relevant to all professions and a variety of employment settings.

Raphael DD. Moral Philosophy. New York: Oxford University Press; 1981.

Seedhouse D. Ethics: The Heart of Health Care. New York: Wiley Publications; 1991:157.

Smith M et al. Pharmacy Ethics. Binghamton: Haworth Press; 1991:555.
> Weak on ethical theory. The cases and in-depth analyses, presented in part two of the book, are excellent. Useful as a secondary text.
>
> Essentially a compilation of essays, some of which are from the 1970s. Only minimal reference to standard ethical principle theory. Would have more use as a reference than as a text.

Wertheimer AI, Smith MC. Pharmacy Practice: Social and Behavioral Aspects. 3rd ed. Baltimore: Williams and Wilkins; 1989.
> Some of the topics discussed therein are relevant; however, the primary utility of this text is as a source of excerpts that can be used for particular applied topics in the course.

Encyclopedias

Reich WT, ed. Encyclopedia of Bioethics. New York: Free Press; 1978.
> While slightly outdated, this work is a standard reference source and is available in most libraries. The second edition currently is being prepared.

Newspaper, Magazine, and Other Articles

Knox RA. Poll: Americans favor mercy killing. The Boston Globe. 1991 Nov 3.

Lazzareschi C. Drug ads: prescription for controversy. Los Angeles Times. 1988 May 1.

Mahar M. The genentech mystique. Barron's. 1988 Jan 11.

Pollack A. High cost of high-tech drugs is protested. New York Times. 1988 Feb 9.

Robin E. To administer B12, or not to administer B12? San Francisco Examiner. 1988 Sept 8.
> Many physicians have looked down at the practice of administering Vitamin B12 as a nonspecific tonic. Physicians advising this form of therapy have regarded the practice as, at worst, giving a harmless potion and, at best, improving the patient's sense of well being.

Sullivan J. Drug store owner bans Camels. The Boston Globe. 1991 Dec 19.
> As with the articles relating to suicide, this paper provides good background reading prior to a discussion of the ethics of selling tobacco products in pharmacies.

Searches of the Literature

The National Reference Center for Bioethics Literature at Georgetown University will run computer searches of the literature on any topic and mail them to you at no charge. Phone toll-free 1-800-MED-ETHX.

Codes and Law

Buerki RA, ed. The Challenges of Ethics in Pharmacy Practice. Madison: American Pharmaceutical Association. American Institute of the History of Pharmacy; 1985:60–4.
> The Code of Ethics of the Association (1852, 1922, 1952, 1969, 1981) have been collected in the appendix.

Harris P. An Introduction to Law. 4th ed. London: Butterworths; 1993.

Inappropriate business practices. Policy Statement: American Society of Consultant Pharmacists; 1988 July 19.
> Inappropriate Business Practices
>
> The American Society of Consultant Pharmacists believes some activities to be inappropriate and possibly illegal business practices and strongly encourages its members to avoid such arrangements in their dealings with health facilities, facility representatives, and other health professionals.
>
> Examples of inappropriate business practices include, but are not limited to:
>
> ♦ Paying a physician to sign a certification or a prescription.
>
> ♦ Offering or providing cash or goods to a health facility or its representative in exchange for favorable consideration in obtaining or maintaining the business of the facility.

- Offering or providing supplies and/or equipment to a health facility at no charge or below market value when these items are not integral elements of the medication distribution system.

- Paying rent to a health facility for space that is not used or is unusable or paying a rental rate for space that is significantly greater than the usual and customary rental rate for similar space.

- Paying a health facility or its representative a percentage of patient prescription charges or a flat fee when the facility provides no common or useful business service.

- Offering or providing a discount or direct payment to a health facility or its representative for billing, collection, and/or bad debt coverage services when such discounts or payments are significantly greater than the cost of similar services and/or historical bad debt experience.

- Offering or providing computers, FAX machines, and/or other electronic devices to a health facility when that equipment is not an integral element in providing pharmacy and/or consultant services.

- Offering or providing a health facility consultant pharmacist services at no charge, Below market value, or below cost in exchange for obtaining or maintaining the business of the facility.

Mission statement for the pharmacy profession. Washington, DC: American Pharmaceutical Association; 1990 Nov 1.

Twining W, Miers D. How To Do Things With Rules. 3rd ed. London: Weidenfield and Nicholson; 1991.

Zander M. The Law Making Process. 4th ed. London: Butterworths; 1994.

INDEX

Abortifacient drugs
  ethical dilemma 175–191
Abortion law 179–181
Advertising pharmaceuticals 249–280
Antidiscrimination law 181–183
Autonomy
  application to dispensing 185–189
  conflict with beneficence 30, 44
  principle of respect for 29, 45–53
Belmont report 289
Beneficence
  commitment to patient 34, 38
  conflict with autonomy 30, 44
  conflict with decisions 30
  principle, normative 29, 34, 38, 42–45
Benzodiazepines 259–264
Bioethics 222
Cases
  abuse potential 231
  antihypertensive cost 58
  antihypertensive choice 80
  antihypertensive noncompliance 47
  contraceptive consultation 44
  drug interaction 87
  drug ordering 55
  drug research 282
  education sponsorship 146
  epoetin nonapproved use 42
  resource allocation 140
  therapeutic interchange 2
  hypnotic overdose 32
  impaired colleague 199, 212
  impaired physician 202
  P & T decisions 91
  patient confidentiality 70
  religious conflict 73
  rights to medication 158
  refusal to dispense 176
  stockpiling/suicide decision 49
  two pharmacists' dialogue 112–135

Chemically impaired colleagues 193–220
Code of ethics
  APhA 31, 33, 39, 45, 198–208, 307–308
  role of 183–184
Colleagues, impaired 193–220
Confidentiality
  patient data 70–72, 294–295
Consent, informed 253, 291–294
Counterside conversation 97–110
Decision making
  ethical 29–66, 79–95
  moral 35
  process 79–95
Discussion questions
  counterside conversation 110
  drug research 303
  ethical decision making 90
  ethics and law 76
  impaired colleagues 217
  medicating by media 277
  normative principles 64
  pharmaceutical industry 154–155
  pharmacy as a profession 25
  power and responsibility 244
  refusal to dispense 190
  rights to health care 172
  relationship to physicians 133
Distributive justice
  principle, normative 29, 57–61
Drug research 281–306
Educational sponsorship 146–156
Employment law 178–179
Ethical decision making 29–66, 79–95
  application of process 91–95
  codes of ethics 31, 33, 39, 45, 183–184, 198–208
  conflicting principles 29–36, 61–63
  conflicting with law 70–72, 175–191

narrative approach 97–110
principle-based 106–110
principles of justification 34–38
refusal to dispense 175–191

Ethical dilemmas
abortifacient drugs 175–191
drug research 281–306
conflict with law 70–72, 175–191
conflict with religion 73–75, 175–191
conflicting principles 29–36, 61–63
education sponsorship 146–156
impaired colleague 193–220
impaired physician 201–205
patient interactions 104–106
principles vs rights 162–163

Ethics
APhA code of 31, 33, 39, 45, 183–185
business 1, 12–19
counterside application 97–110
definition 82
professional 1, 12–19, 82–95
principles, normative 29–66
relationship to
    law 67–77, 160–162
    morals 69
    rights 157–173

FDA, human research 290

Fidelity
definition 34
pharmacist to patient 29, 30, 34, 38, 53–57

Halcion 260–264

Health care
rationing 167–169
rights 157–173

Helsinki declaration 289

Human research 281–306

Impaired colleagues 193–220

Law
abortion law 179–181
antidiscrimination law 181–182
conflict with ethics 67–77, 160–162
conflict with religion 73–75
employment law 178–179
pharmacy law 177–178
relationship to morality 69–75
refusal to dispense 175–191
rights 160–162

Loyalty
principle, normative 29, 34, 38, 53–57
pharmacist to patient 30

Media 249–280

Minoxidil 267–269

Moral
conflicts 29, 36
dilemmas 29, 36, 68
justification 34–36
principles, status of 61–63
relationship to ethical 69
relationship to legal 69, 160–162, 175–182
weakness 29

Narrative ethics 97–110

Nuremberg Code 288

Nonmaleficence
application to dispensing 185–189
definition 29
principle, normative 29, 38–42

Norplant 264–267

Paternalistic ideology 45

Patient rights
autonomy 29, 45–53
health care 157–173
medications 157–173
pharmacist confidentiality 70–72
pharmacist as professional 1–28
privacy 72

Pharmaceutical industry 137–156, 249–280

Pharmacist
Also see Pharmacy
confidential patient privileges 70–72
duty to provide 170–172
education support 146–153

Index

empowerment 221–247
ethical decision making 29–66, 79–95
impaired colleagues 193–220
mediations 222–226
obligations 1–28
professional integrity 148–154
professional virtues 19–24
refusal of prescription 73–75, 175–191
relationships to
    colleagues 193–220
    media 249–280
    patients 1–28, 29–32, 34, 38, 52–57, 70–72, 112–135, 182–185, 222–247
    pharmaceutical industry 137–156
    physicians 30, 32–33, 112–135, 235–240
    research subjects 281–306
    society 221–247
responsibilities 97–110, 221–247
roles
    professional 1–28, 30–31, 67, 182–185, 221–247
    technician 31
self-regulation 194–199

Pharmacy
    Also see Pharmacists
    education 235–237
    ethical practice 82–83
    ethical principles, norms 29–66
        beneficence 29, 34, 38, 42–45
        distributive justice 29, 57–61
        loyalty 29, 34, 38, 53–57
        nonmaleficence 29, 38–42
        respect for persons 29, 45–53
    laws 177–178
    media influence 249–280
    profession 1–28, 30–31, 67, 182–185
    relationship to industry 137–156
    self-regulation 194–220
    social context 221–247

Physicians
    relationship with pharmacists 30, 32–33, 112–135, 235–240
    impaired 201–205

Privileges
    compared to rights 157–173
    self-regulation 193–199, 205–208

Professions 1–28, 30–31, 67, 182–185

Relationships
    colleagues 193–220
    health care personnel 112–135
    media 249–280
    patients 29, 30, 32, 34, 38, 52–57, 70–72, 112–135, 182–185
    pharmaceutical industry 137–156
    physicians 30, 32–33, 112–135, 235–240
    research subjects 281–306
    society 221–247

Religious conflicts
    with duties 73–75

Research, drug 281–306

Respect for autonomy
    application to dispensing 185–189
    conflict with beneficence 30, 44
    principle of respect for 29, 45–53

Rights
    definitions
        compared to privileges 160
        ethical rights 160
        legal rights 160
        natural rights 159
        negative rights 160
        positive rights 160
    to
        confidentiality 70–72
        health care 157–173
        know 251
        medications 157–173

Societal relationships 221–247

Triazolam 260–264

WHO research 289